Mindfulness-Based Cognitive Therapy for Cancer

Praise for *Mindfulness-Based Cognitive Therapy for Cancer*

A profoundly compassionate offering of affirmation and possibility in the face of the difficult and the unwanted. Trish Bartley and her colleagues are to be congratulated on a magnificent contribution to the field of mindfulness and cancer care. May it touch the millions who could benefit from it.
Jon Kabat-Zinn, Professor of Medicine Emeritus, Author of 'Coming to Our Senses: Healing Ourselves and the World Through Mindfulness'

Trish Bartley has succeeded in writing a book that speaks to the deepest fears of cancer sufferers with such compassion that no-one can fail to draw hope and healing from her words. Drawing on her own experience of cancer, and on her skill as a mindfulness teacher, she has pioneered a combination of mindfulness and cognitive therapy. The implications of what she says goes far wider than any clinic – to the heart of what it means to be fully human and fully alive in the presence of our own death.
Mark Williams, Director of the Oxford Mindfulness Centre, Co-author of 'The Mindful Way Through Depression and Mindfulness: A Practical Guide to Finding Peace in a Frantic World'

What a gift of a book. Alongside her own experience of living with cancer, Trish Bartley also has many years' experience of teaching and developing the MBCT-Ca programme – this combination of the personal and professional makes for a beautiful combination of personal story; a clear and practical manual for the eight-week programme; and poems and insights from the many people Trish has taught. This book will be invaluable to patients and health professionals alike. Read this book carefully. It is a precious jewel.
Vidyamala Burch, Author of 'Living Well with Pain and Illness: The Mindful Way to Free Yourself From Suffering'

As mindfulness becomes more main stream, what we need are mindfulness developments guided by clear intentions, adapted to new populations with creativity while maintaining the essence and integrity of MBCT and MBSR. *Mindfulness-Based Cognitive Therapy for Cancer* offers such an adaptation. It has a clear rationale, pragmatic and clinically tested innovations, clear guidance for MBCT teachers and poignant clinical illustrations. The book is imbued with compassion, courage and a sense of common humanity. It will be highly valued both by people with life threatening diseases and health care professionals offering mindfulness classes to people with cancer. Trish Bartley is an MBCT therapist who teaches mindfulness with enormous heart, drawing from a well of experience and knowledge. She writes with a clear, authoritative, compelling and inspiring voice.
Willem Kuyken, Professor of Clinical Psychology and Co-Founder of Mood Disorders Centre, University of Exeter, UK

Mindfulness-Based Cognitive Therapy for Cancer

Gently Turning Towards

Trish Bartley

⟨W⟩WILEY-BLACKWELL

A John Wiley & Sons, Ltd., Publication

Wiley-Blackwell is an imprint of John Wiley & Sons, formed by the merger of Wiley's global Scientific, Technical and Medical business with Blackwell Publishing.

Registered Office
John Wiley & Sons Ltd, The Atrium, Southern Gate, Chichester, West Sussex, PO19 8SQ, UK

Editorial Offices
350 Main Street, Malden, MA 02148-5020, USA
9600 Garsington Road, Oxford, OX4 2DQ, UK
The Atrium, Southern Gate, Chichester, West Sussex, PO19 8SQ, UK

For details of our global editorial offices, for customer services, and for information about how to apply for permission to reuse the copyright material in this book please see our website at www.wiley.com/wiley-blackwell.

Library of Congress Cataloging-in-Publication Data
Bartley, Trish.
  Mindfulness-based cognitive therapy for cancer : gently turning towards / Trish Bartley.
       p. ; cm.
  Includes bibliographical references and index.
  ISBN 978-1-119-95405-7 (cloth) – ISBN 978-0-470-68383-5 (pbk.)
  I. Title.
  [DNLM: 1. Neoplasms–psychology.   2. Neoplasms–therapy.   3. Cognitive Therapy–methods.
QZ 266]
  LC classification not assigned
  616.99'40651–dc23

                                        2011024246

A catalogue record for this book is available from the British Library.

This book is published in the following electronic formats: ePDFs 9781119960058;
Wiley Online Library 9781119960041; ePub 9781119954958; eMobi 9781119954965
Set in 13 on 16 pt Times by Toppan Best-set Premedia Limited

1   2012

To

Jules, Christos, Eleni and Aris,
Christopher and Natasha,

and

all those who journey with uncertainty,
especially the Alaw mindfulness course participants,
my teachers all.

Contents

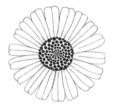

Contributors

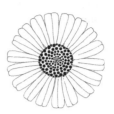

Author

Trish Bartley
Mindfulness Teacher at Alaw Unit
Ysbyty Gwynedd Hospital
Bangor, Gwynedd
Wales, UK

Mindfulness Teacher Trainer
The Centre for Mindfulness, Research and Practice (CMRP)
School of Psychology
Bangor University
Wales, UK

www.trishbartley.co.uk / trish@trishbartley.co.uk

Contributors

Ursula Bates
Director of Psychosocial and Bereavement Services
Principal Clinical Psychologist
Blackrock Hospice
Our Lady's Hospice and Care Services
Blackrock
Co. Dublin, Ireland
00-353-1206-4000
ubates@olh.ie

Stirling Moorey
Consultant Medical Psychotherapist
South London and Maudsley NHS Foundation Trust and Honorary Senior Lecturer
Institute of Psychiatry
London, UK

Nicholas SA Stuart
Consultant Medical Oncologist
Alaw Unit,
Ysbyty Gwynedd Hospital
Bangor
Gwynedd, UK
n.stuart@bangor.ac.uk

Foreword

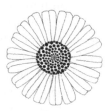

Mindfulness-based cognitive therapy (MBCT) is already well-established as a treatment for the prevention of recurrent depression. Now, in this important book, Trish Bartley describes how, over a ten-year period, she has extended and developed the original MBCT framework to meet the needs of cancer patients. The impetus for this mindfulness-based cognitive therapy for cancer (MBCT-Ca) programme came from Trish's own first personal encounter with cancer (she has had a further encounter while actually writing this book). This experience, together with her involvement with teaching and training in MBCT from the early days of its development, make Trish uniquely suited to the task she has undertaken.

In common with all mindfulness-based approaches to the relief of distress, MBCT-Ca is grounded in the view that our suffering actually arises more from the way in which we *relate* to experiences of pain, discomfort and difficulty than to the experiences themselves. This view suggests the possibility that we can substantially reduce distress by learning a different relationship to unpleasant and unwanted experiences, even if we can do little to change the experiences themselves. Anyone who works with cancer, who has cancer themselves, or who cares about someone close to them who has cancer, will know only too well that cancer and its treatment can offer one opportunity after another to experience pain, discomfort, anger, fear, and despair. It can seem wholly natural and understandable that we might be very distressed by these experiences, to the point where any suggestion that 'there may be another way to relate to these experiences' has to be approached with great sensitivity. It is here that Trish's direct personal experience of being both a cancer patient and a teacher of, literally, hundreds of cancer patients passing through the MBCT-Ca programme are so helpful.

This fertile interface, coupled with Trish's personal background in meditative disciplines, has led very naturally to a focus on the heart quality of compassion as a central feature of MBCT-Ca. The emphasis on opening to and caring for others' suffering, as well as one's own, on connecting with the common humanity shared with all who are touched by cancer, and on reaching beyond the isolation that pain and distress can so often reinforce, is one of the most lovely and powerful features of this approach. The fundamental importance of kindness and compassion within mindfulness-based applications has not always been explicitly acknowledged. This is changing – we now, for example, have empirical evidence that increases in *self*-compassion are one of the main routes through which MBCT for depression has its beneficial effects (Kuyken et al., 2010). I hope that the sensitive and heartfelt focus on compassion within this book may further alert those working with mindfulness-based applications more generally to the healing qualities of this universal capacity we all share.

The book also describes many further creative adaptations of the basic MBCT framework to the particular needs of patients with cancer – the development of a range of new brief practices, of ways to become more sensitive to the messages of the body, and of ways to 'deconstruct' experiences of suffering into their elements, to name but a few. Throughout, the description of the details of practice is held in a wider container of warmth, compassion, and a great sensitivity to the dynamics of group process.

Trish invites us to think widely: 'Maybe we can play with the possibility that what we do as teachers and as participants in mindfulness classes affects far more than we imagine. The ripples that spread out may continue spreading a long way, for a long time, maybe forever'. I hope that many who are touched by cancer will feel the benefits from this timely book and of the care that has led to it.

John Teasdale, PhD.,
Cambridge, England, April 2011

Preface

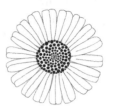

Our experience is the only experience there is. This is the ultimate teacher.

(Pema Chödrön, 1997)

I have written this book for all those who are interested in the potential of mindfulness for people with cancer. You may be a health professional wanting to learn about the relevance of mindfulness to your work. You may be a mindfulness-based teacher currently working with people with cancer – or you may be teaching in a different context, and considering translating your experience into oncology, or work with people who have life threatening or life limiting illness. You may be someone who has had cancer and want to read about mindfulness and what it might offer people like you.

Central to this book is the voice of those who are bringing mindfulness into their lives as they journey with cancer. There is an intention in writing this that their experience will inform and inspire those of us working in the fields of mindfulness and oncology – influencing our professional practice in the care of those we work for. There is also an aspiration that this book will support further research into the psychological impact of mindfulness-based interventions for people with cancer.

This is the first published outline of Mindfulness-Based Cognitive Therapy for Cancer (MBCT-Ca), which has been specifically adapted for cancer patients. The eight week programme described in detail here was developed directly out of Mindfulness-Based Cognitive Therapy (MBCT) for Depression (Segal et al., 2002) and Mindfulness-Based Stress Reduction (MBSR) (Kabat-Zinn, 1990). This book shares the learning from teaching MBCT-Ca to over thirty groups of cancer patients. It is drawn from over ten years' experience of evaluating, developing and refining the programme. If there is any heart in these pages, it comes directly from the course participants and their courage in turning towards their experience. If there is any lack of clarity or confusion, it is entirely mine as author.

Who am I as teacher?

This book is also a little unusual. Most of it is written by me, a mindfulness-based teacher, who was myself a cancer patient before I trained as a teacher. This programme draws from my experience both as patient and as teacher on the same oncology unit. Whilst writing this book, I was diagnosed with another cancer and had to pause as teacher, to become a patient again.

There is a profound process within mindfulness-based teacher training programmes, where we ask ourselves, 'Who am I as teacher?' In reflecting on that now, I have to honour my experience of not knowing, in a new way. The boundaries between patient, teacher, practitioner and participant have become less clear for me after the experience of becoming a cancer patient again. As practitioner, I have had an opportunity to test what I teach in a real live 'laboratory' – namely my own mind and body. I am still teacher when leading a session – holding the process of the group and the curriculum of the programme, but with a knowing that I could be 'patient' again – as they could – and as we all can. We practice holding that uncertainty from moment to moment.

What this book is and is not

This book is *not* a definitive version of Mindfulness-Based Cognitive Therapy for Cancer (MBCT-Ca). Every time an eight week mindfulness-based course is led, there are changes and adaptations, tweaks and inspirations – in response to the group, the context, the moment, the process and the experience of the teacher. It is vital to have a map to guide us, and know the important staging posts that are needed to mark the way, but we also need awareness of the present moment to allow an organic flow to what unfolds, session by session, group by group.

If you are a mindfulness teacher – as you read this, you are bound to come across ideas or sections that are unclear, or that you may want to question or challenge. This may be all to the good. My purpose is not to lay down a prescriptive form, but to offer you an opportunity to reflect on your own approach and on the shape of this particular adaptation. See what it offers you and your participants. Use what is interesting and helpful and ignore the rest. It is up to all of us to continue to develop and deepen this work, with whoever we connect with. I hope that this book will be of some service to that process and in some way support what you do.

If you are not involved in teaching mindfulness, I hope that there will be enough signposts along the way, to enable you to get an experience of mindfulness and a taste of the course process and what it offers people with cancer. If it engages you in wanting to explore further, you may choose to participate in a mindfulness-based course yourself and perhaps look at training as a teacher in due course. In which case, there are some links at the back of the book that might help you find teachers or training resources.

Some practical writing issues

I have used the feminine form 'she' and 'her' for all references to teachers and participants. Obviously, there are many teachers who are men. There are fewer men than women participants in my experience. However, to save endlessly typing 'she or he', I chose to keep to 'she'.

Participants' names have all been changed, except those in the personal stories and original poems – when only first names are used. The examples that are dotted through the chapters have all genuinely taken place in sessions. Participants were informed of my writing and were willing for me to use their experiences, if it might benefit others. I decided to refer to people within the text as patients before they joined a course and participants once they had.

After this preface, the text almost always uses 'we' throughout. 'We' are the teachers, the process, the author/s and often, the participants. The voice of people with cancer, who were participants on the course, is the most significant and vibrant. Their experience and learning is essentially what this book offers.

'Practice' and 'practising' are terms that are dotted through this book. Some mindfulness teachers happily refer to 'meditation' in connection with mindfulness. We prefer to use the more neutral term of 'practice'. Some cancer patients, especially in rural areas such as North Wales, may have some tricky cultural associations and be put off by the term 'mediation'.

A process focus

Working with people on cancer journeys, and as a former development worker, the process of the course is as important to me as the task of teaching the programme. A number of areas therefore receive particular attention in this intervention. This includes an emphasis on the group process – on *how* the learning is facilitated, not just *what* learning is there – and on the connection between teacher and participants. Compassion and kindness also feature strongly. People who are journeying with cancer have great need of both.

Ten years of adapting the course, reflecting on the process, and bringing this together as a book, has offered much learning. Awareness of the many ways that I fall short as teacher and practitioner helps me realize that I am barely 'five minutes' ahead of my participants. If fate had been different, it might well have been one of them as teacher and me as a participant. It always seems important to me to emphasize the common venture that we are engaged in, the human capacities that we share and the practice and learning that connects us.

Therefore, it is not me and them – teacher and participants with cancer – but we, who go together on these 8 week marathons. After the course, we often stay in touch in the months and years that follow. So, when recurrences occur for people, we may still be in contact and I may be able to offer some moments support. As teachers and fellow travellers, we sometimes journey together along the same path – all the way to the end, with some. When recently I became 'patient' again, many of the course participants who I have taught, brought me into their mindfulness practice, as at times I have brought them into mine.

Mentors and colleagues

You may question what a development worker is doing working clinically with people with cancer. Fortune brought me to this work, and colleagues and mentors have supported my learning within it. Mark Williams generously offered his guidance and encouragement at the beginning. Jon Kabat-Zinn has been an important teacher and inspiration to me. John Teasdale, most significant of all, has been friend, mentor and supervisor for many years. He has had an important influence on my teaching and on this intervention. I have indeed been fortunate.

Ursula Bates has collaborated closely with me over this book. She has generously contributed her clarity, skill and theoretical flare. We have been lucky to find friendship and creativity in our connection. The three-circle model that captures the formulation of the MBCT-Ca is one that she and I have developed together.

Finally, my colleagues at the Centre for Mindfulness Research and Practice (CMRP) in Bangor have been very significant. I have learnt much from them over many years. When I was diagnosed, they were the ones I turned to – who sat with me, taught courses in my absence, came to clinic appointments and offered their encouragement through it all. They are my mindfulness teaching community.

A personal intention

When starting to draw out what underpins MBCT-Ca, Ursula Bates and I were excited to find Kristen Neff's research on self compassion (Neff, 2003) and her use of the term of 'common humanity'. This speaks of the interconnection between people, forged through a shared experience of suffering, of being human. It is meaningful. It comforts us.

In Africa, Ubuntu has this same quality.

> Ubuntu (is) the essence of being human. Ubuntu speaks particularly about the fact that you can't exist as a human being in isolation. It speaks about our interconnectedness. You can't be human all by yourself, and when you have this quality – Ubuntu – you are known for your generosity. We think of ourselves far too frequently as just individuals, separated from one another, whereas we are connected and what we do affects the whole world – what we do ... spreads out ... it is for the whole of humanity (Tutu, 2000).

I have met many families embodying Ubuntu who have been impacted by HIV and Aids in rural South Africa. Grandmothers are raising grandchildren and great grandchildren on their own, often with their adult children's graves in the yard. One such woman, I remember, changed into her white church uniform to have her photo taken – a wonderfully strong face, which had experienced so much, full of resolution and dignity.

Maybe we can play with the possibility that what we do as teachers and as participants in mindfulness classes affects far more than we imagine. The ripples that spread out may continue spreading a long way, for a long time, maybe forever. We can join with the intention of practitioners and teachers long before us, influencing what we are and what we do. I find this comforting and inspiring, especially when I doubt myself as teacher. It is not just me. What we are practising in this work is more than any individual, or any specific class or any group that is taught. Staying in touch with this, whilst not ever giving up on our commitment to teach and practise with integrity, heart and presence, we can find rest in the wisdom and inspiration of the teachings and the heart essence of our interconnectedness. Within this, we can be whole and in touch with love for our fellow beings – and a wish to offer them support.

The Other

There are nights that are so still
that I can hear the small owl calling far off
and a fox barking miles away.

It is then that I lie in the lean hours awake
listening to the swell born somewhere in the Atlantic
rising and falling, rising and falling,
wave on wave
on the long shore by the village,
that is without light and companionless.

And the thought comes to me
of that other being
who is awake too,
letting our prayers break on him,
not like this for a few hours,
but for days, years, for eternity.

R. S. Thomas (1993)

Acknowledgements

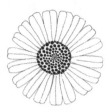

I am very grateful to all those who have helped in the writing, reading and producing of this book. Particular thanks go to Ursula Bates, Stirling Moorey and Nick Stuart for their very fine chapters. To Jill Teague for her kind and patient encouragement and skilful advice. To Josephine Seccombe, Cindy Cooper and Christina Shennan for their invaluable feedback. I am especially grateful to John Teasdale for his foreword and wise guidance, generously given.

There are a further group of people who have been important in supporting reflections, sharing ideas and contributing to how this book has developed. These include Andrew Patching, Katie Morrow, Jill Teague, Tina Usherwood, Linda Gwillim, and David Rynick. I greatly appreciate Andy Peart, Karen Shield, Kathy Syplywczak, Kevin Fung and all at Wiley, who have been consistently kind and encouraging, and have offered me much support during the creation and production of this book. I am very grateful to Katie Green (www.katiegreen.co.uk) for her considerable skill in creating the three circle diagrams and other models – to Evan Herbert for his daisy logo, produced in an instant – and to Jas Lehal (www.jaslehalphotography.co.uk) for her photograph of me, generously given. I also want to acknowledge my teaching colleagues and all the staff at the Centre for Mindfulness, Research and Practice at Bangor University, for all that they have given me, the students and teachers who I have taught, trained and supervised. I have learnt an immense amount from you all.

I am very grateful to my friends and family for their love, kindness and support especially during my recent treatment – particularly Janne Foster, Joan Burgen, Mariel Jones, Diana and Jim Allanson, Josephine Seccombe, Evan and Delphine Herbert – and to friends in South Africa, especially Loretta van Schalkwyk, Davine Thaw and all at Woza Moya. Much appreciation also goes to Jill Bishop, Laura Edge and her team, Rachel

Williams, Chas Muskett, Jilly Wilcox Jones, Nick Stuart, Derek Crawford, Beryl Roberts and the radiotherapists at Ysbyty Glan Clwyd, for their care and kindness.

I want to acknowledge the very significant learning I have gained from all participants of the Alaw mindfulness courses. The programme described in this book rests entirely on their experience. Special thanks goes to those who were willing to be interviewed, and whose personal stories and poems are in this book. My gratitude also to all those Alaw mindfulness folk, who stayed in touch and travelled with me during my recent treatment. Particular thanks goes to Gwenlys Williams and Heli Gittens for their skilful and generous support of the follow up sessions.

I greatly appreciate and want to thank all my teachers for their wisdom, inspiration and generosity – especially Rigdzin Shikpo, Jon Kabat-Zinn, John Teasdale, Ferris Buck Urbanowski, Mark Williams, Melissa Blacker, Andrew Patching, Christina Feldman, and the late Francis Batten.

This book would not have happened without Ursula Bates. Her inspiration, energy and ideas are rooted in these pages.

Finally I wish to acknowledge my love and appreciation for my children Jules and Christopher, their partners Christos and Natasha, and my grandchildren Eleni and Aris. I dedicate this book to them.

Introduction

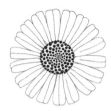

Contents Overview

Part One – Mindfulness and The Cancer Journey

There are three parts to this book. The first serves as an orientation to the rest. We start by describing mindfulness in very general terms. Then we meet three people with cancer, who all participated on mindfulness-based courses. Through their experience, we build a picture of what mindfulness can offer people like them. After this, we learn about the psychological and medical implications of the experience of cancer and treatment. The last chapter in this section maps out a model of the psychological patterns of cancer distress.

This first section of the book involves a number of authors, who draw from their own rich experience to describe different aspects of the cancer journey. Ursula Bates, Stirling Moorey and Nicholas Stuart lend much needed weight and wisdom to the overall text and I am very grateful to them.

Part Two – The MBCT for Cancer Programme

The second part of the book moves up close to the eight week MBCT-Ca programme, from before the course begins to after it ends. The first chapter

Mindfulness-Based Cognitive Therapy for Cancer: Gently Turning Towards,
First Edition. Trish Bartley.
© 2012 Trish Bartley. Published 2012 by John Wiley & Sons, Ltd.

outlines the ways we recruit people with cancer and describes how we prepare them for the course. The following chapters explore the eight week programme, in detail, week by week with many anecdotes from participants. The second of the circle diagrams comes next, drawing out the central underpinnings of the programme and the development of mindful awareness. After that, we look at the mindfulness practices in the programme – both in terms of adapting them for people with cancer and outlining the short practices we use. We describe ways of supporting participants after the course and of the one to one work with people who are unwell. There is a welcome chapter outlining a mindfulness-based intervention for people receiving palliative care. This is written by Ursula Bates. Finally, we draw the last circle diagram, which takes us beyond the course, to the practitioner who is using mindfulness to live her life and be with cancer.

Part Three – The Practitioner Teacher and a Three Circle Model

We then move on to explore the role of the mindfulness-based teacher, who is working with people with cancer. We discuss some of the challenges she will meet in this work and the qualities she might need. We look at issues of practice and intention in teaching mindfulness and draw out the significance of the group process within MBCT-Ca. We suggest that the teacher is facilitator of the participants' learning and explore some ways in which she can develop this. In the last chapter, which is co-written with Ursula Bates, we bring all three circle diagrams together as a proposed formulation for the MBCT-Ca intervention.

Personal stories and participants' poems

Interconnecting these sections are some personal stories drawn from interviews with people who have been touched by cancer – either personally or through those they care for. They have all attended MBCT-Ca courses and use mindfulness to support them in their lives. Some participants have also contributed poems to the book. These were written at the end of their mindfulness course, inspired by their own experience of the practice and those they had practised alongside. Other poems are written by me or are included by kind permission of the poets.

Daisies

The cover of this book is decorated with daisies, which grew in my garden. They are known as moon daisies and grow wild beside roads, on verges, in gardens and fields. They have a circle of hundreds of white petals with a centre of bright yellow that becomes seeds later in the year. I chose these daisies for their beauty and good cheer. They crop up all over the place, often unplanned, but lovely for all that, turning towards the sun for warmth and light. They speak to me of the mindfulness community of people with cancer, who find courage to turn towards their suffering with the light of their awareness practice and the warmth of their heart intentions.

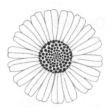

Personal Story

Trish

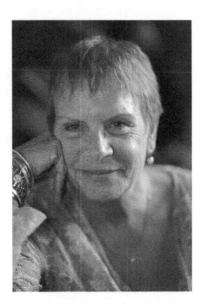

Trish was 50 when first diagnosed with breast cancer. Ten years later a new cancer was found. She has a much loved family and lives on a mountain in North Wales. She is the author of this book.

Mindfulness-Based Cognitive Therapy for Cancer: Gently Turning Towards,
First Edition. Trish Bartley.
© 2012 Trish Bartley. Published 2012 by John Wiley & Sons, Ltd.

Diagnosis

'I was first diagnosed on a cold, snowy afternoon in February 1999.

I had moved to North Wales the previous summer, after working in a remote area in South Africa. Sitting, waiting in the Llandudno clinic, it crossed my mind that some of the women waiting with me would be diagnosed before the end of the day. (I later heard there were seven of us). I remember wishing them well whoever they were. I didn't feel concerned about my small lump. I was there to fulfil a promise made to my daughter that I'd get checked out once back in the UK.

I had a mammogram and a laugh with the female radiographer. On my return to the waiting area, I was called into another room. A consultant radiographer Dr. G said he was concerned about my mammogram. Surprised, I asked him how concerned and he said about 3 out of 5. My insides lurched. A biopsy followed and Dr. G said that the pathologist next door would test the cells straight away. 'Time for him to put down his copy of the Beano and do some work', he joked, but my mind was racing. The nurse seemed to be crying quietly.

I had 30 minutes to wait, so I drove into town, intent on finding a church. I wanted to light a candle. If I could do this, all would be well. It was dark and snowing. There was no-one to ask. Eventually I found a large gloomy church but it had no candles, so I sat shivering in the dark cold, trying to steady myself.

On my return, Mr. C the consultant surgeon told me I had breast cancer. There was no doubt. A lot of information followed. I wept. I felt shocked. I couldn't take in what was being said. I was immediately and intensely thirsty. After a while, I drove myself home.

Impact

Ten months of treatment followed – including surgery, chemotherapy and radiotherapy. With luck, it had been caught in time. Lots of feelings surfaced. Treatment removed any opportunity to work with people, and I missed this. Waiting in the oncology unit, I found myself sitting with people who were clearly suffering. We rarely spoke, but I found I could meditate as I sat there. This felt comforting.

Letting go

Work commitments had to be shelved. A kind friend brought me a new diary. It seemed best just to start again with blank pages. I felt sick and easily got tired. It was a tough time. Happily, losing my hair was not a problem. I wore African headscarves and felt connected to my village friends in South Africa.

I was a keen meditator but once I started treatment, my practice felt dull and lifeless, except when I went for chemotherapy. I found I could drop into the process, which was strangely uplifting.

Kindness and connections

Friends and family, shocked by my news, offered me much kindness. On going down to surgery, I felt an almost tangible sense of being held by them.

My daughter was nearing the end of medical training. I had been reluctant to tell her my news. The medics were insistent. I can see her now, standing in the kitchen of my little Welsh cottage, visibly drawing herself up. She was upset, but almost immediately said that she now knew why she was doing medicine. My son was often the first to phone after treatment. At a family picnic, soon after losing my hair, he gave me a baseball cap. It was the softest he could find, he said. It still hangs behind my kitchen door.

Kindness became my hallmark of best medical care. A few years later, I recounted my experiences as a patient to an audience of nurses at a cancer training day. I told them how I had dreaded seeing my scar after surgery but the gentleness of the nurse who removed the bandages, meant that what could have been traumatic was reassuring and nurturing. As I walked away from the podium after the talk, coming towards me was the very same nurse who had been so kind. I had not seen her since that time. She had tears in her eyes. 'I never knew,' she said.

I was lucky to receive chemotherapy in a small oncology unit where patients are treated with much kindness. My first treatment was given to me by the sister on the unit who was half way through a mindfulness course at the University. It seemed an amazingly good omen. We practised together as the chemo dripped in. We often talked about the potential of mindfulness for cancer patients.

Looking back on that year of treatment, with the gift of hindsight, I can now appreciate that almost every aspect of the experience has been useful. No longer taking life for granted; living each day with a sense it might be the beginning of the last; and doing work that connects me with people and offers us the capacity to be more compassionate and alive.

Mindfulness

Back in August 1999, about half way through treatment, I attended a mindfulness retreat. Mark Williams, John Teasdale and Zindel Segal had just completed their MBCT for Depression study and wanted to develop mindfulness teaching. It was a wonderful week, with Ferris Urbanowski from the Centre for Mindfulness, skilfully guiding us.

Staying on Bardsey was a great leveller. The island has no electricity or modern plumbing. There were some advantages in being mid-treatment, when let off the toilet emptying rota! Mark and I spoke of developing mindfulness within oncology. In the event, Becca Crane taught a course to staff and one to patients less than a year later. In January 2001, I started teaching cancer patients on the same unit where I had received my treatment. Courses have run three times a year since.

The above was written in 2009, when half way through this book. What follows are some adapted extracts from my journal.

Thursday 10th December – Last follow up clinic appointment.

My last regular mammogram: A new surgeon prods me – and discharges me from the clinic. I am cured. What a great day! I text my family and celebrate with P over lunch. Ten years!

Tuesday 15th December – Recall.

Driving into town I pick up my post. I open a hospital envelope and read that I am recalled by the radiology department.

An empty sharp lump lands in my belly. Disbelief. It must be a mistake. I check my name several times.

Later I called my meditation instructor.

> *Asked A. to help me connect with my practice. He reminds me there are others experiencing something similar. Could I connect with those who are afraid? he asks – yes I could do that. We discuss who to tell. My plan is to keep this to myself. My family would be worried. Why put them through it? A. asked me to imagine I am supporting someone else in this situation. What would be best for them? I see straight away that I must tell them. I phone my kids and email my sisters.*
>
> **15th – 22nd December – The Yo-Yo.**
>
> *I try to convince myself that it is a smudge on the plate. The radiologist will say, 'We just need to check. It often happens'. And from here, I quickly move into: 'You are making such a meal of this. You have worried people unnecessarily'.*
>
> *There is no comfort here. The only solace is that I know what I am doing. I feel it deep in my belly.*
>
> *At the other end are some awful possibilities. The prognosis may be bleak. Images of lingering death – my funeral – intense fear and loss. But as soon as this appears, in comes, 'Stop making a fuss. It will turn out to be nothing'.*
>
> *I intensify my practice. 'Quickly dispel the pain of sickness and misery for all beings'.*
>
> **Tuesday 22nd December – Diagnosis**
>
> *Dr. G was standing in the doorway. As soon as I saw him, I knew I had not made a fuss. I felt a moment of shock, but also noticed calm. An ultrasound followed. He eventually found it and said it was definitely cancer – a new primary, nothing to do with the first. It was small and quite early. I heard that clearly. It was strangely peaceful in the dark womb like space.*

Coming out, I called E into the changing room and told her. Crying a little, my head spinning with thoughts: treatment, telling my family, my book, ongoing work, would I need chemo? Could I face it again? E asked me if I could drive. She was gentle and clear. I didn't need to look after her. She had been a perfect choice.

We went to Centre for Mindfulness, Research and Practice (CMRP). Some of us practised together. My head was still busy, but it was held in the stillness. I was cold and wore B's shawl. It was comforting. Talking later over tea – connecting around suffering, I felt very close to people, very open. I phoned my family. J was in Greece. I heard LB, my two year old granddaughter, ask, 'Mummy why are you crying?' This was the worst part – asking them to go through it again with me.

Surgery follows in the New Year. Ten days after, Mr. C tells me that my prognosis is good. A week or so later, Dr. B my oncologist, tells me she definitely recommends chemotherapy. I cannot go to South Africa as planned.

I wrote this soon after:

The tender softness of your face,
the way you hold mine in your hands
and kiss me, looking straight into my eyes.
The sweetness, not anticipated, of this new love.

At the clinic, the doctor told me
that I could not follow my heart south,
to be with those special Woza Moya people,
to support their courage, their intention,
their dogged hard work with the sick and the dying.

Well, I cried. …
I cried over the doctor,
who until then had seen me as this respected psychologist
helping her patients capture some calm
(wrong there on several counts).
And I cried into the phone to poor Jo,
who is always there at the other end.
'How can I do this again?'

And then my new love called me
and we sang our songs, and she invited me to tea.
'Danny (her two year old version of Granny)
would you like to come to my house in a minute?'

I knew later as she drove away,
With her mother and brother in the car
That of course I must do this,
to have more time with this glorious being.

10 February, 2010

It is now August and my treatment is finished and I am feeling strong and well.

My practice has accompanied me closely on this second journey – as has kindness from many sources. Both have been deeply nurturing and inspiring. There have been dips and troughs, twists and turns – and many times when the sun came out.

Part One
Mindfulness and The Cancer Journey

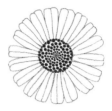

Chapter One
Mindfulness and Cancer

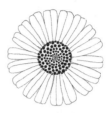

Mindfulness practice is really a love affair with what we might call truth, which includes beauty, the unknown and ... how things actually are, all embedded here in this very moment.

(Kabat-Zinn, 1990)

Mindfulness practice is central to my own experience of being with cancer. In the previous section, I write about this and the ways that cancer and mindfulness have impacted on me personally.

Now, in this first chapter, we ponder questions, such as:

What is mindfulness?
What does a mindfulness-based course involve?
What might a mindfulness practice offer someone with cancer?

After suggesting some basic descriptions of mindfulness, we look through the eyes of three different people with cancer, all of whom made their way to a Mindfulness-Based Cognitive Therapy for Cancer (MBCT-Ca) course in North Wales. Their stories will help to orient us towards what mindfulness offers those who are living with cancer.

Mindfulness-Based Cognitive Therapy for Cancer: Gently Turning Towards,
First Edition. Trish Bartley.
© 2012 Trish Bartley. Published 2012 by John Wiley & Sons, Ltd.

Introduction

Being mindful is to be fully present with your direct experience, whatever you are doing, thinking or feeling – here and now.

Mostly, we are *not* aware. We are rarely fully *with* the experience we are having *now*. We tend to wander back, dwelling in the past – or run forward, anticipating the future. We can be driving a car, but functioning on automatic and only partly aware, whilst worrying about something about to happen, or thinking about something someone said earlier.

When we practise being mindful, we do something and know that we are doing it – like eating and actually tasting the food – or going for a walk and noticing the full scope of the view – or turning on the radio and actually hearing the programme. Becoming more mindful offers us many possibilities. It helps us to become more aware, centred and balanced. We may find more to appreciate in the ordinary experiences of our day.

Mindfulness also helps us learn to respond differently to difficult situations. Instead of reacting, in a knee jerk way, immediately imagining the worst – we learn to stop, and come back to the direct experience we are having now. This changes things and gives us an opportunity to find other ways of managing what is challenging us.

We now turn to the experience of three people. Their stories will help us begin to understand what mindfulness might offer people with cancer.

Will Mindfulness Help Me?

> Jane was only 32 when she was told that she would probably not survive breast cancer. A single parent with three young children, she tolerated nearly twelve months of an aggressive treatment regime and seemed to manage pretty well. After it was all finished, her doctor told her that she might be fine after all.

Almost immediately, Jane started feeling awful. 'My head is all over the place', she told me. 'I'm angry – not sleeping well – and horrible with the kids'.

Family and friends had withdrawn, assuming she was alright now that treatment had finished and her prognosis was so much better. In reality, Jane was only just beginning to get in touch with her feelings and finding them hard to manage. She could not understand what was happening and thought she was being 'really stupid'.

After a clinic appointment with her oncologist, she was referred to a mindfulness course.

When Jane heard that what she was experiencing was entirely normal, and that others also get in touch with strong emotion after the end of treatment, she immediately felt a bit better.

On hearing about mindfulness and the course, she could see that it might help her to be more 'present', although just talking about it did not give her much of a clue as to how she could do that. However, she was well aware that she was spending a lot of the time anxiously brooding on what might happen – worrying about the children, and fretting over every twinge of pain thinking it might be the beginning of the cancer returning.

In describing persistently critical thoughts, 'that do my head in', Jane can connect with the possibility that learning to stop and be more aware of the habits of her mind, might be a first step in helping her to develop ways of being kinder to herself. She knows that she blames herself for everything – getting cancer, losing patience with the children, and even for feeling so awful. She would love not to do that and feel more herself again. It is a long time since she has felt happy.

'Count me in', she tells me 'I can't wait to start'.

What Does Mindfulness Offer? Is It Safe?

David is a retired professional man in his sixties with incurable cancer. He finished a recent round of treatment last year and is currently in remission. He is a fairly cautious person, who does not easily engage with new people or situations. His doctor referred him for a mindfulness course, because he is not sleeping well, and is feeling low and lethargic.

David meets me to hear about the course. He is not sure it will help him, but he says he thinks he ought to give it a go. 'I haven't much to lose', he says 'I wonder if it will work for me'.

What might mindfulness offer someone like David? And how could he be helped to commit to the vital home practice involved. On the face of it, he is very different to Jane. He is a lot older, more set in his ways, and clearly sceptical about the approach.

David was not much interested in hearing about learning to be more present. It did not sound like his sort of thing, and anyway he did not understand. He became a bit more engaged when he was told about some research, which demonstrated evidence of the benefits of mindfulness. This was more his line.

The first mindfulness-based course was developed by Jon Kabat-Zinn in Massachusetts over thirty years ago, for groups of people with a wide range of different health conditions. Since then, Mindfulness-Based Stress Reduction, (MBSR for short) has spread to many parts of the world (Kabat-Zinn, 1990). Part of that development includes some research undertaken by a leading psycho-oncology team with cancer patients in Calgary, Canada over the last ten years. They are getting some good outcomes from MBSR. Evidence is building that mindfulness holds much promise for cancer patients (Shennan et al., 2010).

David was relieved to hear this. He had already decided to take the course, because his doctor advized it, but if mindfulness was not the flaky, touchy feely approach that he first assumed, it might have something genuine to offer him. The news got better the more he heard. A form of mindfulness for people with depression, known as Mindfulness Based Cognitive Therapy

(MBCT) has been found to significantly reduce the risk of relapse in people with a history of depression (Segal et al., 2002). NICE (the National Institute for Clinical Excellence), the UK health standards body, explicitly recommends MBCT for people who have had three or more depressions.

David was currently on medication for depression. He heard that the mindfulness course he would be going on had been adapted directly from MBCT for Depression, and targeted to the needs of people with cancer. It had been running for over ten years. Regular evaluations of course outcomes suggest that participants experience improved levels of sleep and wellbeing after attending. 'I could do with that', said David wistfully 'I wonder if it will work for me'.

What is Involved on the Course?

The last person we meet is Sheila. A married woman in her early 40s, with two children, she was traumatized by a diagnosis of ovarian cancer, eighteen months earlier. She has never forgotten the look on her mother's face when the doctor told them.

After treatment, her prognosis was said to be fairly good, but she did not believe it. Sheila is convinced that she is going to die, but can't bear to think about it. She dreads going to bed at night. As soon as she closes her eyes, everything crowds in – especially that expression on her mother's face.

She broke down when she last saw her specialist nurse. Sheila admitted to be feeling terribly tense. 'It is as if there is a dark cloud blocking out the light', she said 'I know I can't go on like this. It is making me ill. Even my husband, who is very laid back, is really worried'.

When Sheila met me, we discussed how she was feeling and touched on what she had been through. It was hard for her to talk about it, but she said that she was desperate to feel better. She had been referred to counselling but had not chosen to continue. 'Talking about it doesn't help', she told me.

Like David, she would have to develop some confidence in mindfulness before she could commit to the course. Unlike David, hearing about research findings would not be much help to her. Sheila needed to make a personal connection with me, her teacher, and feel that she could trust the course. It helped her to hear about practical details, such as what to expect, and how the sessions were structured.

I told her that the course ran for eight weeks, with a session every week lasting for two and a half hours, with about ten people in the group. Sheila admitted that she was quite nervous with people she did not know. I explained that it was not a self help support group. We practise a mindfulness-based exercise, guided by me, the teacher, and then we explore our experience of it. Then we experience another practice or exercise and discuss that. 'There is no need for you to say anything unless you want to', I told her. At times the group breaks into pairs or small groups to discuss the mindfulness exercise, and sometimes we stay in the larger group.

Sheila quickly appreciated that she would have to commit herself to the home practice. I was clear that whatever she got out of the course was mainly up to her – and the home practice was an important ingredient in it all. She said that she was so desperate to feel better that she would do whatever was needed. I explained that she would follow one of the thirty minute practices every day at home using a CD.

There are also a number of short practices which she would learn to weave into her day. Some of these could be helpful to turn to when things felt tough. It seemed very important to explain to Sheila that mindfulness involves having the courage to turn towards what is difficult little by little, with sense of friendliness and kindness for herself. She said that 'turning towards' sounded scary, and she was not sure she could do that, but something inside told her that learning to be kinder to herself was probably exactly what she needed.

As she left the room after our exchange, she looked a little brighter.

Developing Course Themes

Jane, David and Sheila all decided to join an MBCT-Ca course. They were not told about the themes that would build through the course. It was too soon for that and would not have made sense to them. Mindfulness is best learned through direct experience.

However, over the weeks that follow the start of the course, they all became more familiar with awareness of sensations in the body. Jane found this naturally much easier than David and Sheila, but they all engaged in the practice of scanning the body. They were learning to be curious about their physical sensations.

Sheila got on well with practices involving the breath. She found she was able to bring her focused attention to sensations of breathing quite easily. This helped her feel less tense and gave her something to concentrate on at night. Jane liked to focus on the sensations of the contact of her feet on the floor. This helped her to feel more settled and steady. David said he particularly enjoyed the practice of mindful movement. He was rather surprised by this, as he was not a particularly active person, but he found he felt better after doing the gentle stretching postures. In different ways, they were all learning to bring their attention back to the 'anchor' of their present moment experience, in the body and the breath.

The movement practices helped Sheila come closer to awareness of her body and helped her to practise gentleness. She found the body scan hard and struggled with the stillness of it, but she noticed that it was possible to open into the intensity of a stretch, by breathing into it. She could be aware of strong sensations in her body, without feeling so frightened. David also found it was easier for him to be mindful when moving and stretching. His mind seemed to wander much less and he felt more alive and alert after the practice.

These and other practices helped them to develop:

• The intention to step out of automatic reacting and come back to the anchor of present moment in the body and the breath.
• The practice of turning towards what is difficult little by little.
• The possibility of bringing kindly, curious and gentle attention to their experience.

As time passed, and their practice developed, it became easier for them to become aware of the way their minds wandered. They began to notice when judging, worrying or despairing thoughts crept in and were less likely to be swept away by them. Through the building momentum of their mindfulness practice, it was sometimes possible to respond to these troubling moments with one of the short practices they were learning. They were becoming more mindful in their everyday lives. This offered them choices that enabled them to live more fully, and manage difficulties with more kindness and compassion.

A Cognitive Model of Cancer Distress

About half way through the course, we share a cognitive model of cancer distress with participants. It is known as a vicious circle of anxious preoccupation (Moorey & Greer, 2002). Jane and Sheila immediately recognized it from their own experience. David's patterns were a bit different, but he knew that he too could be swept up like this.

The vicious circle starts with some general anxiety, which is often present in the background experience of people with cancer. This inevitably triggers tension in the body, which is felt as an ache or a pain. Attention is drawn to these feelings and because they are unpleasant and not wanted, negative interpretations soon start forming. 'It is getting worse'. 'It might be a recurrence'. 'Maybe it will kill me'. These thoughts are added to the feelings of anxiety and 'not wanting', fuelling the tension and physical pain. This simply increases the negative interpretations making them more and more apparently convincing. A vicious circle of anxious preoccupation quickly builds.

Individuals have different patterns in their adjustment to cancer. Unlike a mental health condition such as depression, there is no one cognitive model that comprehensively explains the mechanisms that fuel distress in everyone with cancer. However, the vicious circle of anxious preoccupation comes closest to offering a cognitive model of cancer distress that applies to the people who find their way onto a mindfulness-based course for people with cancer. This is discussed in much more detail in the next chapter. Other relevant cognitive models that contribute to cancer distress are also explained.

Through practising mindfulness, participants learn to notice and interrupt the cycle of anxious preoccupation. Thoughts may still arise, anxiety may still be felt, interpretations may even start to build – but it may be possible to recognize the thoughts, feelings and body sensations for what they are – not necessarily true facts. Once noticed, it is always possible to come back to the 'anchor' of the breath in the body. This offers connection to present moment awareness and an opportunity to choose what to do next, rather than be at the mercy of overwhelming thoughts and feelings.

Jane, David and Sheila

We conclude this first chapter by returning to our three participants.

By the end of the course, Jane had relaxed a fair bit. She continued to feel anxious, especially around clinic times, but she used her own versions of some of the short practices most days, came to mindfulness follow up sessions now and again, and used a longer practice when she felt she needed to. She said she felt a lot happier, and was definitely steadier at home with her children. When I last heard from her, she was well and hoping to start work again soon.

David was surprised at how much he gained from the course. Of the three, he probably benefitted the most. He continued to do the movement practice and also followed a short sitting practice regularly. He joined a choir, which he loved, and reported that he was sleeping better and feeling pretty good much of the time. Last heard, he was still in remission, no longer depressed and continuing to practise.

Sheila was less troubled by flash backs by the end of the course. She used some short breathing practices, when thoughts and feelings were troubling her. She said that she could see more chinks of light at the end of the tunnel. Her specialist nurse was impressed with these changes, and subsequently regularly referred other patients to courses. Sheila wrote a poem, which she posted to me some time after the end of the course, praising mindfulness for giving her back her life.

Not everyone who participates on MBCT-Ca courses is necessarily as motivated or gains as much as these three. However, they are by no means unusual.

What Comes Next

In the next chapter, Stirling Moorey and Ursula Bates draw out the psychological implications of having a cancer diagnosis and of receiving treatment. They present a clear picture of the mechanisms that perpetuate the distress experienced by cancer patients. Then in the following chapter, Nicholas Stuart describes the medical implications of cancer and treatment. This might be especially relevant to those of you who are unfamiliar with the world of oncology and treatment for cancer. We conclude this first section with a circle diagram that summarizes the patterns of suffering for people with cancer. In later chapters, other circles will be added that draw out the development of mindful awareness, from the picture of suffering with cancer, to learning to practice mindfulness through the eight week course, and finally to living mindfully and being with cancer.

From Blossoms

From blossoms come
this brown paper bag of peaches
we bought from the boy
at the bend in the road where we turned toward
signs painted *Peaches*.

From the laden boughs, from hands,
from sweet fellowship in the bins,
comes nectar at the roadside, succulent
peaches we devour, dusty skin and all,
comes the familiar dust of summer, dust we eat.

O, to take what we love inside,
to carry within us an orchard, to eat
not only the skin, but the shade,
not only the sugar, but the days, to hold
the fruit in our hands, adore it, then bite into
the round jubilance of peach.

There are days we live
as if death were nowhere
in the background; from joy
to joy, to joy, from wing to wing,
from blossom to blossom to
impossible blossom, to sweet impossible blossom.

Lee Li-Young (1986)

Chapter Two

Cancer – The Psychological Implications

Stirling Moorey and Ursula Bates

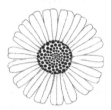

Our sorrows and wounds are healed only when we touch them with compassion.

(Jack Kornfield, 1994)

Introduction

Cancer is the second leading cause of death in developed countries and accounts for nearly 13% of deaths worldwide (World Health Organization, 2006). In the United States, the lifetime risk of being diagnosed with cancer is 46% for men and 38% for women (Ries et al., 2004). Although the overall 5-year survival rate is 64% and continues to improve, a diagnosis of cancer is still perceived by many as a death sentence. Knowing that the cells of your own body are out of control and can proliferate to the point that they might kill you, has a symbolic significance shared by no other disease. The sense of uncertainty in the face of a condition that could progress or recur at any time; and loss of control of your body and life, are common themes in the experience of people with cancer. Mindfulness offers a radical approach to living with these feelings.

This chapter will consider the traumatic effects of the diagnosis and treatment of cancer on the psychological equilibrium and distress experienced through the course of the illness. It will also review two coping styles which have been consistently found to be associated with poorer psychological adjustment – avoidance and rumination. As will be seen later in this book, mindfulness presents a middle way between attempting to escape from painful feelings and getting caught in unhelpful loops of thinking about them. It allows us to face the fear and respond more effectively. This chapter will give a brief overview of the evidence available for the effectiveness of mindfulness and other therapeutic approaches in the treatment of psychological distress in people with cancer.

The Trauma of Cancer

Many aspects of cancer can be shocking: the discovery that you have a life threatening illness, the side effects and consequences of treatments, learning that you have a recurrence, or being given the news that your disease is incurable. Distress tends to be more prevalent at these times. A study which followed 222 women with breast cancer over 5 years found rates of anxiety and depression of 33% at diagnosis, 15% at 1 year, when most women had been successfully treated and were disease free, and 45% when there was a recurrence (Burgess et al., 2005). Feelings of numbness and disbelief, overwhelming emotions, intrusive catastrophic thoughts, and confusion are common at these times. These may be signs of emotional processing, as the person struggles to incorporate new information about their mortality into their previous view of themselves and the world (Moorey, 2010).

Greer (1985) suggested that the initial diagnosis is often viewed in a catastrophic manner as a death threat. Gradually as time progresses the patient is able to revaluate the threat in the light of his or her growing understanding of the medical condition. He or she also begins to consider how much coping and control they themselves can bring to bear on the illness and treatment. Greer and colleagues identified five common adjustment styles that patients develop following the initial shock (Moorey & Greer, 2002):

- fighting spirit
- avoidance or denial
- fatalism
- helplessness
- anxious preoccupation

Studies of stress related processes in cancer patients have focused on intrusions and avoidance of thoughts about the illness. These show that they have high levels of preoccupation and distress with general illness related events (Kaasa et al., 1992; Kelly et al., 1995). Intrusive memories are associated with poor coping, specifically anxious preoccupation, helplessness and hopelessness (Watson et al., 1994).

It is not uncommon for patients to experience intrusive images and memories of the time they were told of their diagnosis, or of the time when they received treatment. In some cases this may become so severe that it warrants a diagnosis of post traumatic stress disorder (PTSD). The National Cancer Institute (2009) reported that the incidence of PTSD ranges from 3% in early stage patients to 35% following treatment (see Andrykowski & Kangas, 2010 for a discussion of the difficulties in diagnosing PTSD in people with cancer).

Distress

After the initial adjustment phase, most cancer patients settle into a more stable psychological state. If they see the disease as a challenge which they can meet, they have what Greer has termed a 'fighting spirit'. If they focus on their inability to manage the illness or its consequences, they have a 'helpless-hopeless' adjustment style, while if they focus on the uncertainty of the situation, they may have an 'anxious preoccupation'. These adjustment styles tend to be associated with greater or lesser degrees of psychological distress with helplessness/hopelessness correlating with depression and anxious preoccupation with anxiety (Moorey & Greer, 2002).

The distinction between 'normal' anxiety and low mood in response to cancer, and 'clinical' anxiety and depression is to some extent an arbitrary one, since these symptoms are distributed across a spectrum of severity. Therapeutic approaches, including mindfulness, can be helpful across this spectrum, even if a patient does not meet criteria for a clinical diagnosis. A helpful way to consider anxious and depressive reactions is through the functional impairment experienced by the patient. A common pattern associated with low mood is a tendency to think in a helpless/hopeless way which leads to further low mood, fatigue and lack of motivation. Negative thoughts then lead to behavioural and social withdrawal. 'What's the point in doing anything? If I can't do what I used to do, it's not worth it', which further lowers the mood.

A vicious circle can also be seen in anxiety. Here for instance, worries about recurrence can lead to hypervigilance for symptoms, with constant checking and reassurance seeking. Reassurance has a temporary effect but quickly wears off, while checking may make the patient more aware of everyday aches and pains, which become signs of disease progression. Understanding these cycles of helplessness/hopelessness and anxious preoccupation can help the cancer patient identify ways out of their repetitive patterns of reactivity.

Unhelpful reactions tend to include more severe emotional distress and more functional and social impairment. Signs of a more clinical level of depression include:

• Pervasive and distorted negative thoughts about the self (e.g. self criticism, guilt and low self-esteem).
• The future (e.g. unrealistic pessimism in the light of an objectively good prognosis).
• More physiological symptoms of depression (fatigue, loss of pleasure and interest, weight loss, insomnia).

It can obviously be difficult to separate physical symptoms of depression, from those of cancer or its treatment – and this may require close co-operation with the patient's oncologist to disentangle the symptomatology. More severe anxiety is also characterized by extreme and distorted thinking, which goes beyond the reality of the situation. This may include overly catastrophic thoughts about the future, and an underestimation of the patient's ability to cope, or to find help and support.

Among one large sample of cancer patients, researchers found an overall prevalence rate for psychological distress of 35% (Zabora et al., 2001). A recent study by Stark (2002) found that 44% reported some anxiety and 23% had significant anxiety. The most common presentation is adjustment disorder with anxious mood, directly related to the illness. Other anxiety disorders, such as phobia or panic disorder, generally predate the illness. Depression affects between 15–25% of cancer patients (National Cancer Institute 2009). Long after treatment is over, difficulties involving body image, fear of recurrence, and sexual problems are reported by a large proportion of survivors (Kornblith & Ligibel, 2003).

Psychological distress has been shown to increase the experience of pain (Massie & Holland, 1992), decrease overall functioning (Noyes, Holt, & Massie, 1998) and is a major risk factor for suicidal ideation and suicide attempts (Rosenfeld, Breitbart, Krivo, & Chochinov, 2000).

Distress across the three stages of cancer

The distress experienced by patients varies across the three stages of cancer (curative, chronic/incurable and palliative – see chapter 3). In early stage cancer, the treatment rather than the disease itself may be the cause of significant symptoms. A woman with breast cancer, for instance, might discover a lump, but otherwise feel well. Treatment may involve surgical removal of the lump or a mastectomy, followed by chemotherapy which may cause fatigue, nausea and hair loss. These treatments can all have an effect on mood, but also have major effects on a woman's body image, and self-esteem (Moorey, 2007). The psychological problems faced by patients whose disease is curable often tend to be focused on fears of recurrence, or the psychosocial consequences of treatment.

In more advanced or chronic disease, patients may face the challenges of living with a long term medical condition. As the disease advances further, the illness itself may increasingly limit the person's life. About half of people at the end of life do not consider themselves to be suffering, 25% report only minimal or mild suffering and 26% moderate to extreme levels of suffering (Wilson et al., 2007). In Wilson et al's study, 21% of patients met diagnostic criteria for depression, and 14% for anxiety. Physical problems, for example: pain, functional loss, weakness etc., were mentioned most frequently as a source of suffering. Other respondents referred to concerns that were psychological (for example, mental stress), existential (for example, lack of control and worry about death) and social-relational (for example, dependence, isolation and worries about others).

Coping with Cancer

Each individual's experience of cancer is unique, and there is no right way to cope. People tend to draw on past strengths and coping strategies when they face a crisis. If we have had experiences of facing and overcoming difficulties, we will have a sense that we can solve new problems as they are presented to us. However, if we have not encountered difficulties, or have been overwhelmed by them, we may doubt our capacity to cope. Cancer may evoke core beliefs that we are vulnerable, and that others are unable or unwilling to support us.

In other situations we may try to employ coping strategies too rigidly. For instance, if someone has developed a belief like 'if I can control my life I will be safe', she or he may react by trying harder than ever to exert control over their situation. While their perfectionism and overcontrol may be adaptive in other circumstances, the uncertainty of the cancer experience makes it impossible to achieve the levels of control they yearn for. Consequently their distress and sense of vulnerability may be worsened (Moorey, 2010). Factors associated with better adjustment include adopting an optimistic attitude, problem solving, and social support. The coping strategies that tend to correlate with poorer adjustment are avoidance and rumination.

Avoidance

Avoidance is an almost universal response to painful experience. It is part of the behavioural repertoire available in the face of danger, where the body is physiologically primed to go into fight, flight or freeze mode. Avoidance may be conscious or more automatic, and can operate at the level of cognition (deliberately not thinking about aspects of the diagnosis), behaviour (avoiding situations that remind you of cancer) or affect (distracting oneself from negative emotions). At its extreme end, avoidance can become denial: of the seriousness of the illness, or even of the diagnosis of cancer itself.

At the behavioural level, people with cancer sometimes try to avoid anything that might be associated with the illness, such as television programmes about medical matters; newspaper articles; or even using the word 'cancer'. Because it is difficult to insulate yourself in this way, they are often caught off guard, and experience overwhelming rushes of anxiety. The feeling of shame in being labelled a 'cancer patient', may lead people to avoid contact with other patients, and so deprive themselves of sources of support. They avoid previous sources of social activity, because the constant well meant inquiries about their health are too upsetting or intrusive. They often feel extremely alone while surrounded by loved ones, as they avoid any real intimacy in an effort to protect their family members.

Some patients may become so anxious about scans or hospitals, that they are unable to attend appointments. Often, it is only when a mindfulness practice is established, that patients will recall how disturbed and fearful they were during scans and treatment. They become fearful of specific body movements related to illness sites, and restrict their activity levels in an attempt to protect their fragile bodies. The cycle of anxious preoccupation leads them to catastrophize, with thoughts like 'if I get pain, it might make the cancer worse', and then avoid doing things, which contribute further to anxiety and depression.

At the cognitive level, there may be a conscious avoidance of thoughts about the disease, or a more subtle tendency to change the conversation, or move away from uncomfortable topics.

In one sense, behavioural and cognitive avoidance can be seen as driven by avoidance of unpleasant emotions. A cue may cause a momentary pang, which becomes a trigger for moving away from the experience through action or thoughts. Mindfulness helps people to identify these cues, and their rapid emotional reactions, and to develop the courage to allow the emotions to arise without immediately distracting themselves. Sometimes, emotional avoidance may take the form of dissociation, which is a more automatic cutting off of emotion, akin to the freeze response. This can sometimes be problematic for people learning to practice mindfulness, as they may cut off or 'zone out' when facing painful emotions – and these dissociative reactions require sensitive handling by the mindfulness teacher.

Rumination

In contrast to the strategy of avoidance, rumination is characterized by an inability to let go of thoughts about painful experiences, either from the past or the future. Rumination is a recognized factor in the maintenance of generalized anxiety disorder (Roemer & Orsillo, 2002) and in recurrent major depression (Teasdale et al., 2000). Both these mental states have been shown to respond to mindfulness interventions, which support a letting go of repetitive patterns of thought.

Rumination is the opposite of mindfulness, since it is never focused on the present moment. In cancer, the focus is often on what might happen in the future – 'Will the disease come back?' 'Will I be able to cope?' 'Will I be in pain?' 'How will my children manage without me?' Worry usually leads to ineffective attempts at problem solving. Rather than being able to identify a plan for dealing with a possible future threat, the worrier engages in repetitive loops of thought. A possible solution is imagined, but then doubts set in about its effectiveness, and so the process has to be repeated, or another problem suddenly comes to mind.

It has been suggested that worry may actually be an attempt to avoid the more emotive aspects of a problem, since it tends to be a verbal process, which avoids the more imagery based catastrophic thoughts about the future. Rumination about the past can also occur in people with cancer, with regrets about what one should or should not have done, dominating the person's life. This may be particularly troublesome in people whose behaviour may have contributed to their illness (e.g. through heavy smoking or drinking). There may be a persistent attachment to the story of one's life, combined with an inability to reconcile that story with the current reality of loss and illness. The person is then left with a continuous gap between the desired identity and the present identity which is causing deep suffering.

Treatment for Distress

The strong evidence for the effectiveness of cognitive behaviour therapy (CBT) in a wide range of psychological difficulties such as depression, anxiety disorders suggests it will be effective for the distress experienced by people with cancer. Sage and colleagues (2008) indicated that there is a strong overlap between issues which occur in a mental health context, and those that happen in relation to life-changing illness/terminal illness.

Overall, CBT has been shown to be effective in enhancing the quality of life for people experiencing cancer. For instance, past studies (Greer et al., 1992; Moorey et al., 1994; and Moorey et al., 1998) have found that six sessions of adjuvant psychological therapy (APT – adaptation of CBT for cancer patients) was more effective with newly diagnosed and recurring cancer patients, than no treatment at all. Furthermore, the research evidence suggests that CBT is more effective when applied later rather than earlier after a cancer diagnosis has been made (Edgar et al., 1992). This could be due to the fact that initial distressing emotions after a diagnosis, may interfere with an individual's ability to utilize CBT effectively (Edgar et al., 1992).

Savard et al., 2006 demonstrated that cognitive therapy was an effective treatment for depression in women with advanced breast cancer. Several psychosocial interventions that effectively ameliorate the distress, or improve the quality of life of cancer patients have been developed. These interventions have been reviewed several times over the past decade (e.g. Schneiderman et al., 2001; Newell et al., 2002). Though the methodology of many trials has been less than optimal (see Lepore & Coyne 2006; Coyne et al., 2006 for a critique of the literature), most reviewers have concluded that psychosocial interventions can effectively decrease distress and improve the quality of life of cancer patients. It appears the effectiveness of the mode of treatment depends on the time period of the illness trajectory, that is; diagnosis/pre-treatment, post-treatment or during extended treatment.

Scientific investigation of mindfulness-based interventions for people with cancer has been prolific in the past decade as cited in chapter one. Though MBSR promotes an orientation of non-doing, highlighting awareness of being rather than goal-orientated behaviour, patients do often learn experientially how to moderate their level of arousal. This knowledge can assist them in managing symptoms of cancer and side effects of treatment such as pain or nausea that are exacerbated by anxiety (Mundy et al., 2003). This allows them to assume an active and effective role in the healing process.

However, the bulk of the research is in the area of supportive and cognitive behavioural interventions. Trials directly comparing MBSR with other treatment modalities for cancer patients have not been reported; thus, an evidence base for drawing distinctions concerning the differential effectiveness of MBSR is not available. Comparing MBSR with other validated psychosocial treatments for cancer patients would be a useful avenue for future research.

Summary

Cancer poses threats on many levels: to our survival, our physical integrity, our relationships, and our sense of our self. An initial adjustment phase is characterized by fluctuating emotions, and intrusive thoughts and images, alternating with feelings of numbness. After this, most people settle into a more stable mode of coping with their illness. For some, this initial traumatic reaction persists, while new cancer stressors, such as recurrence or side effects of treatment, can tip patients back into trauma. A significant percentage of people with cancer experience ongoing distress, with symptoms of anxiety and depression. Everyone copes with cancer in their own way, but strategies of avoidance and rumination tend to be associated with poorer adjustment.

Mindfulness offers new ways to relate to trauma and distress, together with an alternative to avoidance or rumination – through learning to be present for our emotional experience, as it is, from moment to moment. There is good evidence for the effectiveness of cognitive behavioural techniques with this group of patients and encouraging evidence for the effectiveness of mindfulness.

The Raku Bowl

Like a raku bowl
that goes into the dark
without mould or cast,
a true warrior lives
and dies with uncertainty,
knows how to reconcile
two halves of the whole,
knows that to be vulnerable
is like the fragile beauty
of a vessel holding life
on the edge of breaking.

So from a lost crow's nest,
the iridescence
of a bird of paradise
is found.

Jill Teague (2010)
Maentwrog, North Wales

Chapter Three
Cancer – The Medical Implications

Nicholas S. A. Stuart

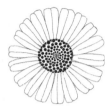

The greatest mistake in the treatment of diseases is that there are physicians for the body and physicians for the soul, although the two cannot be separated.

(Rudolph Friedrich, 1961)

Introduction

Cancer – one of the most terrifying words in the English language. The word no one wants to hear.

A diagnosis of cancer is often associated with fear – of pain, surgical mutilation, toxic treatment and imminent death. Whilst this is no longer true, thanks to modern medicine, there is no doubt that a cancer diagnosis will be life-changing. What previously seemed certain is suddenly uncertain. What previously seemed important is now unimportant. An ordinary life that seemed stable, organized, planned, and in control is suddenly turned upside down. It is in this context that we need to understand the cancer journey and

Mindfulness-Based Cognitive Therapy for Cancer: Gently Turning Towards, First Edition. Trish Bartley.
© 2012 Trish Bartley. Published 2012 by John Wiley & Sons, Ltd.

the role of MBCT-Ca in helping patients cope with the psychological challenges that arise from a cancer diagnosis.

Diagnosis

Every cancer patient will have their own experience and their particular journey. This reflects the varied behaviour of different cancers and the diverse reactions of different people. Nevertheless, some common patterns do exist.

A few cancers will reveal themselves dramatically, leading to emergency medical care and a rapid route to diagnosis. This may be very distressing but it allows little opportunity for delay, prolonged anxiety or rumination over possible test results. For most patients, the cancer journey will begin in a mundane way. A troublesome cough, a hoarse voice, a nagging pain, something odd when using the lavatory, a lump felt in the shower – a first symptom – an awareness that all is not right. Indeed, there is no symptom that could not be a first sign of cancer.

Having realized that something might be wrong, the patient is faced with a decision to seek medical advice or not ('Oh, I'm sure it's nothing'). This often comes after a period of reflection, thought and consideration. It is well recognized that many patients delay seeking medical advice for a considerable time after their first symptom. In some, this may become a fertile area for future guilt, recrimination, or rumination – 'If only I'd been to see the doctor sooner', 'Why did she tell me it was nothing to worry about?'

For most patients, the first step is to visit their general practitioner. This may lead to initial reassurance (which may subsequently prove to be false). This is followed by investigations such as blood tests, a scan, or referral to a specialist. While a diagnosis may be suggested at any stage, for most patients, it is only confirmed after a biopsy (removal of a piece of tissue for examination under the microscope). This is inevitably followed by a wait for the results – as processing and examining the biopsy takes several days. Each test is a further opportunity for anxious waiting, worry about results and speculation as to the nature of the problem. This step-by-step process towards diagnosis provides so many opportunities for anxiety and endless rumination.

The final and crucial assessment involves staging the cancer. Staging is a process that determines the size of the tumour and how far, if it all, it has spread. This will usually require one or more body scans (ultrasound, CT or MRI). The stage of the tumour is the critical fact that will determine the sort of treatment the patient will require, and their prognosis, and prospect of survival. In general, the further advanced the cancer is, the lower the chance of cure.

Treatment

Cancer treatment options continue to evolve, develop and improve. The prospect of survival for most common cancers has increased year-on-year, for at least the past decade. This may be partly due to earlier diagnosis, but is mainly the result of improvements in treatment. It could be said that there has never been a better time to get cancer.

The broad categories of treatment nonetheless remain unchanged:

- Surgery – when the cancer is localized and can be removed in its entirety.
- Radiotherapy – when the cancer is localized but can't be removed surgically or in order to reduce the chance of the cancer re-growing after it has been removed
- Drug treatment – often known as chemotherapy but nowadays this involves an increasingly wide range of treatments, some of which are given as tablets. This treatment option may be used for cancers that are too widespread for surgery or radiotherapy, or that have re-grown despite previous treatment. Drug treatments are also widely used after surgery to reduce the chance of the cancer relapsing. While there have been improvements in all areas of treatment, it is in this area of drug treatment that most improvements have been made.

All of these treatment options offer their own benefits. However, they also make their own demands on patients. Some of these involve simple practical matters such as the frequency with which the person has to attend the hospital for treatment - or whether they have to travel to a different hospital. Clearly, the type and severity of side-effects and each individual's attitude to possible complications are also critical to the experience of treatment.

Surgery

With surgery, there is a single event to focus on. A date is set in advance for admission to hospital. The person with cancer may be understandably anxious, but she or he knows what will happen and when. Following the operation, a period of time in hospital is needed, followed by further time to recover at home. The duration in hospital and the time taken to recover will depend on the nature of the surgery but in most cases, clear guidance can be offered as to what to expect. The patient will also be informed of the possibility of complications from surgery. These may detain him or her in hospital, may delay their full recovery, or could even be life-threatening. Complications from surgery are generally rare however, and clear advice can be given on how often they occur.

Radiotherapy

Radiotherapy uses powerful X-rays to treat cancer. Complex equipment is needed that is not available in most hospitals. Therefore, the first practical problem facing patients is the need to travel to a radiotherapy centre. In some cases, this may be 100 miles away or more. Radiotherapy is usually given as repeated, daily treatments. Although each treatment may only take a few minutes, the treatments may continue for up to 6 weeks, though 3–4 weeks is more typical. In addition, visits may be required, before the treatment starts, in order to plan the treatment. Post treatment visits may also be needed to assess the results. Radiotherapy may therefore be very disrupting to the patient's life. Those who live some distance from the radiotherapy centre may need to stay at the hospital for several weeks, returning home each weekend. Accommodation is usually in a hostel rather than in a hospital ward. This will inevitably impact on employment, and require more sickness leave. It will also reduce the patient's contact with their family and friends, and distance him or her from normal mechanisms of social and psychological support.

The side effects of radiotherapy depend largely on the area of the body being treated. In many cases there will be a tendency to tiredness, weakness and loss of appetite, maximally for a week or two after treatment. However, radiotherapy will cause some damage and inflammation to the tissues in the area treated – like 'internal sunburn'. This will be more likely to cause symptoms in those parts of the body sensitive to inflammation. For example if the mouth, throat or gullet are treated, the inflamed tissues may make eating difficult or even impossible for a time. Skin inflammation over the area of treatment is also common. Radiotherapy that involves the abdomen, directly or indirectly, will commonly cause nausea or even vomiting, as well as loss of appetite. Fortunately, radiotherapy side effects generally subside over a few weeks and many can be ameliorated with appropriate treatments.

Chemotherapy

Chemotherapy is the use of drugs to treat cancer. Traditionally these drugs are given as an intravenous drip with treatment once or twice every three or four weeks. However, treatment may be given as frequently as weekly or as infrequently as monthly. There are also a number of new chemotherapies that are given orally. In each case, the treatment will be repeated in order to achieve maximum benefit. Patients may therefore have four, six, twelve or even more treatments over a period of several months.

All types of chemotherapy can cause distressing side-effects, although some types are less likely to than others. Medical knowledge around preventing or controlling side-effects has greatly improved. In most cases, patients find the experience of chemotherapy 'not as bad as I thought it would be'. Nonetheless, all patients experience some degree of adverse effects. Tiredness, reduced energy, loss of appetite, nausea, hair loss, and bowel disturbance are all common. A few people experience severe side-effects that lead to hospitalisation, and can be life threatening or prevent further treatment being given. It is impossible to predict which patients will suffer severe side-effects and which will have none. Chemotherapy is therefore always a bit of a gamble.

Side-effects from treatment tend to be worst within the first few days of treatment and have usually resolved by the time of the next treatment is due. This means that the patient, has to both cope with the side-effects, and also be faced with the knowledge that the next treatment is approaching. They will have to face this experience again and again – perhaps many more times. Although most chemotherapy side-effects do not build up during treatment, lack of energy, and physical and mental weariness certainly do. The psychological challenges of a patient's first treatment (anxiety, uncertainty, fear, etc.,) will be quite different from their last (mental and physical fatigue, and depression).

New drug treatments

In recent years a range of new drug treatments have been introduced that are quite different to standard chemotherapy, in relation to how they work. These may be called antibody-therapies, biological therapies, or small molecule drugs. As evidence of their benefits grows, more and more patients are being given them. Many can be given as tablets and most do not have the standard side–effects associated with chemotherapy. Nonetheless, they do have their own patterns of effect. Interestingly, several still cause fatigue as a major problem. Many can cause a marked skin rash that, whilst not life threatening, can be distressing, and inhibit social interaction and impair quality of life. Unlike chemotherapy, these drugs are not given for a few weeks or months, but often for a year – or sometimes indefinitely, while the patient continues to respond. In this situation, even minor side-effects that persist for months can acquire a major significance in someone's life.

Treatment combinations

An increasingly common feature of modern cancer treatment is the use of multiple treatments. Nowadays, many patients will have a combination of two of three types of treatment. For instance:

- Surgery may be followed by a period of radiotherapy or chemotherapy treatment.
- Radiotherapy may be combined with chemotherapy and given at the same time.
- Chemotherapy may be followed by surgery and then further chemotherapy.
- Surgery can be followed by chemotherapy, and then radiotherapy.

While these complex treatment plans lead to a greater chance of cure, they are increasingly challenging for the patient. Rather than simply having an operation with the aim of getting over it in a few weeks, many patients are now faced with a program of treatment extending over many months. Treatment lasting six, twelve, or even more months is not uncommon. This inevitably increases the possibility of psychological problems, particularly depression. The challenge of coping with the side effects of multiple treatments, and the length of time involved means that the prospect of full recovery can seem a long way off.

Treatment Choices

Deciding which course of treatment to offer individual patients is the essence of oncological medical practice. These decisions are not straightforward. In many cases, a balance needs to be struck between trying to achieve maximum benefit from treatment, whilst seeking to minimize the disruptive effects on the patient's quality of life. In many cases, the patient's own views and attitudes – should she or he wish to express them – will influence the oncologist's decision.

For most patients the dominant consideration revolves around the best chance of cure. This generally outweighs concerns about the effects of treatment. For some patients though, the acceptability of treatment is greatly influenced by the possibility of experiencing certain adverse effects. This is particularly the case for those patients where palliation of symptoms or prolongation of life is the aim of treatment. For some patients, hair loss is devastating and may sufficiently impair their quality of life to make the treatment unacceptable to them. Even the practical considerations, such as the frequency with which the patient has to attend the hospital, may be a genuine concern for some people. In working out how best to help patients cope with their cancer, it is important to understand from the beginning, what is important to each person. Only then can they be offered the treatment with the best chance of benefit and the least chance of detrimental effects.

Physical Effects of Treatment

Weakness or fatigue from treatment may prevent normal family or social activities such as cooking, shopping, or entertaining. All these exacerbate feelings of failure, low self-worth and guilt. Other physical effects such as hair loss, bowel disturbance or loss of libido may also inhibit social interaction and contribute to depression.

When treatment is complete most of the immediate physical effects of treatment resolve within weeks. Patients experiencing fatigue and mental changes tend to be slower to recover. Some people experience temporary muscle and joint aches in the weeks following treatment. Few patients feel fully recovered within six months and some may take considerably longer. Indeed some patients feel they never fully recover their energy and fitness, even when cured of cancer. Psychological problems also tend to resolve and usually do so in parallel with the resolving physical effects.

After Treatment

The end of treatment is a period of transition and has its own specific challenges. Most patients report an increase in anxiety as frequent hospital visits, support, and opportunities to discuss their concerns are replaced by infrequent out-patient clinic visits. Some say they feel 'abandoned'. Many say they feel 'at a loss', not knowing what to do with their time or how to return to normal activities. Some patients remain depressed, withdrawn or anxious despite resolving physical effects.

The period of recovery, when the effects of treatment are largely resolved and when normal life is returning, is one where new psychological techniques to enhance wellbeing; to prevent recurrent depression; and to enable people to cope with future problems can be particularly helpful. Mindfulness-based courses certainly have a role.

Three Groups of Patients

For all patients, the shadow of the cancer remains. The future is uncertain and patients know it and feel it. It might be helpful at this point to broadly categorize patients into three groups with different prognosis and with different psychological needs.

The first group of people are those who have been treated in the expectation of cure. Such patients can live in the hope that they have beaten their cancer. Generally their need is to recover from the physical and psychological effects of treatment and return to full, normal life. However, even when the statistical chance of cure is high, there is always the possibility of relapse. For some patients this fact is difficult to deal with, leading to continued ongoing anxiety or depression that needs management. Some patients may also have to cope with permanent physical consequences from their treatment, for example; mastectomy, amputation, the presence of a stoma or the long-term effects of radiotherapy. These patients have a permanent reminder of their illness and the possibility of relapse as well as possibly greater psychological challenges.

A second group of patients are those who sadly have a type of cancer for which current treatment is ineffective. Such patients are likely to experience a continued physical deterioration usually leading to a short life-expectancy. For these people, their need is to cope with awareness of their short prognosis and live with the implications of this. They may also need to manage persistent symptoms, even when expert palliative care is offered.

The third group is especially important because it is increasing in size, as a result of improvements in cancer treatment. These are patients who have a cancer that can not be cured but which can respond well to treatment – at least for a time. Such patients often undergo a roller-coaster ride of treatment experiences with periods of remission, with possible elation at encouraging hospital visits, followed by inevitable relapse with associated anxiety and depression. As a consequence of improved cancer treatments patients may now have several periods of remission and relapse before treatment becomes ineffective and is abandoned. For this group, the challenge is to maintain stable mood and avoid anxiety and rumination. As with other groups the permanent physical consequences of treatment may add to the patient's burden and give greater psychological challenges.

While each person has to find their own way through their cancer journey, as oncology clinicians we need to offer guidance and help on coping with that journey. While the benefits of mindfulness-based cognitive therapy for cancer (MBCT-Ca) are far from fully understood, and certainly require more research, the experience in our department over the past ten years suggests that many cancer patients can benefit from this approach. Most of those who have attended our MBCT-Ca courses report an improvement in their levels of wellbeing. They also experience reduced levels of anxiety and depression.

This third group of patients (those with treatable but incurable cancer) seem to be the group likely to benefit the most, given that they have both the time to learn and apply the approach whilst in remission – and the opportunity to have the support of mindfulness when they relapse. This group is increasing in number and deserves specific research. If the benefits we have shown are confirmed in more detailed studies then MBCT-Ca could logically be offered to all patients diagnosed with such cancers. The curative and palliative groups may also benefit from MBCT-Ca, but courses may need to be adapted to the special needs and prognoses of different groups of cancer patients. (There is a description of the way that Ursula Bates has adapted MBCT-Ca for palliative patients in Dublin, towards the end of this book.)

Of the patients who have attended MBCT-Ca courses, I bring three especially to mind.

The first is a young woman who was diagnosed with cancer soon after the birth of her child. There was a good chance of her treatment being successful and she seemed to get through surgery and chemotherapy well. However when I saw her on follow up, she appeared tired, tearful and depressed. She attended a mindfulness group soon after this and reported some months later, that her sleep was improved and she felt more herself. 'I've got the old me back', was what she told me.

The next patient is a young man who very sadly had an aggressive disease and a poor prognosis. We gave him what medical and psychological treatment was available. He was clearly depressed and very anxious and was referred for counselling, which seemed to help a little. He was not well enough to attend a mindfulness group, nor would it have been entirely appropriate – but he benefitted from working one to one with the teacher and learned some basic approaches, which he practiced at home. He died on the unit.

The last patient is a middle aged woman who had incurable cancer. A strong woman, she took on her diagnosis and treatment very bravely, wanting to do whatever she could to live her life as fully as possible. She was very disappointed when her first recurrence was diagnosed and after treatment, she attended a mindfulness course. She seemed to get some benefit from it. Her words to me were along these lines: 'It somehow helps me be a bit more 'selfish' and take better care of myself. It taught me that it isn't weak to ask for help. I admit defeat more easily. I am strong in a different way'.

I Just Want to Live

'I just want to live …', I said
when told I had cancer.
'I'll do anything …'
I poisoned my body with chemo.
I disfigured it with two operations.
I burnt my body with radiotherapy
All because
I just wanted to live.

'I just want to live …'
'Yes, yes', she said, 'but why not try a different way?
Why not try living with
Awareness
Love
Kindness
Peace?'

Because *now* I don't just want to live,
I want to live with meaning and with feeling.
So thank you for starting this journey with me,
And whatever happens in future,
May we all go in peace
Because at the end of the day,
We *all* want to live.

Helen (July, 2009)

Chapter Four

The First Circle – Cancer and the Circle of Suffering

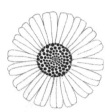

When this book was in planning, Ursula Bates and I started experimenting with diagrams. A three-circle model developed. These circles are introduced in this book one at a time. We lay out the integrated model in the final chapter, when we bring all three circles into a formulation for MBCT for Cancer. If you prefer to see this overview first, turn to chapter 15.

This first circle draws out the patterns of suffering that accompany a cancer diagnosis and the experience of treatment. The Figure 4.1 captures the essence, albeit in simplified form – of what is described by Stirling Moorey and Ursula Bates in Chapter Two – The Psychological Implications of Cancer. It has three concentric rings within it. The inner ring, **Cancer**, is the focus of the whole system. It radiates out through the middle ring of reactivity, to the outer ring, which describes a cognitive model of cancer distress.

The *Circle of Suffering* is represented with the use of thick dark markings, suggesting heaviness, claustrophobia and obstruction. This links with the nature of cancer and also with the inevitable tightening, closing and resistance that is experienced at diagnosis and probably during treatment. In general, the greater the resistance and tightening, the more suffering will result.

Mindfulness-Based Cognitive Therapy for Cancer: Gently Turning Towards,
First Edition. Trish Bartley.
© 2012 Trish Bartley. Published 2012 by John Wiley & Sons, Ltd.

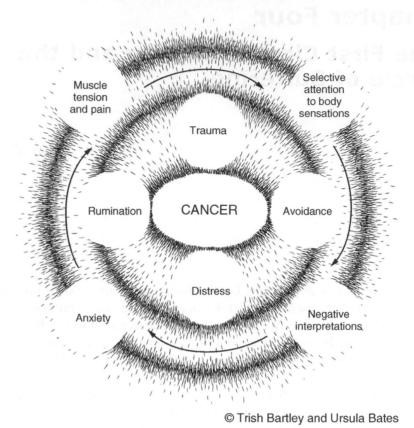

© Trish Bartley and Ursula Bates

Figure 4.1 Circle of Suffering – The Psychological Implications of Cancer.

Inner Ring – Cancer

Once a diagnosis has been made, cancer seems to influence all experience. The centre of the circle is represented here as an elipse, suggesting a lens or an eye. This lens of cancer can easily appear to distort and pervade an entire view of the world. It is as if the disease is everywhere. Newspaper stories, television programmes, societal beliefs and anecdotal tales all reinforce a profound sense of uncertainty and fear of imminent death. Invasive treatments add greatly to physical suffering, increasing dependence, vulnerability and often, a sense of isolation. Cancer is sometimes described as the 'plague' of the 21st century.

Middle Ring – Four Reactions

1. TRAUMA
2. RUMINATION
3. AVOIDANCE
4. DISTRESS

A cancer diagnosis invariably triggers reactivity in various forms. The four reactions or mechanisms that are described here are the ones that people with cancer experience. One or two may be experienced at the same time. For example, avoidance accompanies trauma. However, it is helpful to identify them individually and appreciate that rumination and avoidance (pictured opposite each other on the circle), are the key mechanisms that perpetuate cycles of distress.

TRAUMA has a frozen quality closely connected to intense fear, helplessness, or horror. Intrusive images and memories usually of diagnosis and/or treatment can be re-stimulated at different points on the cancer journey. An initial diagnosis of cancer may be viewed as a death threat. Disbelief, confusion, numbness and catastrophic thoughts are also experienced. Shcila, who we met in chapter one, was traumatized by her diagnosis of canccr. She kept seeing the look on her mother's face at the time of her diagnosis. This experience triggered catastrophic thoughts that she would die of cancer.

Some level of DISTRESS is widely experienced – especially around diagnosis; recurrence; at treatment decisions and at the start and end of treatment. For some, this leads to low mood, feelings of hopelessnes and helplessness, fatigue and increasingly pessimistic thoughts. In some, cycles of anxiety build (see outside ring) resulting in patterns of worrying, hyper vigilant checking of symptoms, tension and agitation, and thoughts that the disease is progressing.

RUMINATION is characterized by an inability to let go of repetitive verbal thoughts and worry, which often involves self blame and focuses on painful experiences and/or catastrophic events. Rumination is never focused on present experience but moves back into the past or forward worrying about the future. This invariably triggers a downward spiralling of mood. David, who we also met in chapter one, tended to ruminate about his illness. He was often consumed with thoughts about what he should have done to have stayed well and avoided getting cancer. This moved him into regretting aspects of his life, and dwelling on things he wished had been different. As a result, he felt increasingly depressed and hopeless, and spent long periods sitting motionless in his chair.

Experiential AVOIDANCE is a widespread reaction to painful experience, which inevitably increases levels of distress. A strong form of avoidance is denial – of the seriousness of the illness or even of the diagnosis itself. This may lead to doing things such as avoiding people, not sharing diagnosis news, withdrawing from social activities, avoiding television, or even not using the word 'cancer'. The extreme end of avoidance is disassociation. Experiential avoidance can be cognitive or behavoural or both, and inevitably is accompanied by increased anxiety. Jane found that she had to keep busy or a 'cloud of doom' would descend on her. When this happened (and sometimes the cloud appeared whatever she was doing), she felt out of control, angry, anxious and distressed, which triggered strong self blaming thoughts. Her only recourse was to push the distress away, increase her busyness, and try not to think about it. This merely adds to further cycles of avoidance, distress, agitation and self blaming.

Outer Ring – A Cognitive Model of Cancer Distress

As explained in chapter one, as cancer is not a mental health condition, there is no one cognitive model that applies to everyone. However, the vicious circle of anxious preoccupation (Moorey & Greer, 2002) is readily recognizable and applies to most people with cancer. It can be triggered in a number of ways. Anxiety can produce symptoms such as shakiness or sweating or palpitations in the chest. Or anxiety may result in automatic bracing against what is most feared, producing tension in the body that causes pain or aching. Soon, most of the attention is focused on these physical symptoms – in an avoidant way, often increasing the resistance around them. This magnifies the experience, and inevitably results in fueling the tension and intensifying the anxiety.

It becomes evident from this pattern that the mind adds extra layers (of secondary suffering) to the primary suffering (of cancer). As tension is felt and areas of pain, or generalized aching are experienced, inevitable thoughts arise about their possible cause. Negative interpretations soon follow and become more and more convincing as anxiety builds further, tension increases, and hypervigilance of selective sensations follows.

Summary

People with cancer find that the impact of their negative thoughts and emotions is more distressing and uncomfortable, than all the considerable physical challenges involved in having cancer and managing treatment.

This is the picture of suffering for people with cancer, who may find their way to a mindfulness-based course. Individual patterns may vary – as we can see with Jane, David and Sheila – but the tendency of the mind is to add 'extra' to the primary cause of suffering.

As we move into the next section of the book, we encounter the eight week MBCT-Ca course and hear how mindfulness impacts on participants. Their stories and experiences illustrate the way that the *The Circle of Suffering* is brought to the practice of mindfulness. The second of the three-circle diagram, *The Circle of Practice*, follows in chapter seven, representing the development of mindful awareness through the learning and practice of the eight week course. First we meet Beryl, who had cancer in 2004 and uses mindfulness to support her in her life.

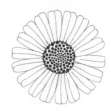

Personal Story

Beryl

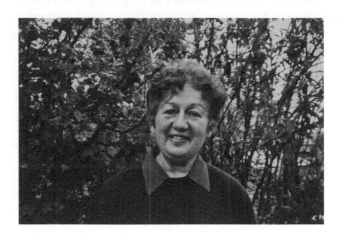

Beryl is retired with two daughters and two grandchildren. She lives in sight of Snowdon with her dog Tolly. She was diagnosed with breast cancer in 2004 and participated on an Alaw[1] mindfulness course the following year. She is well and much enjoying life

[1] ALAW Oncology Department, Gwynedd Hospital, Bangor, Gwynedd

Mindfulness-Based Cognitive Therapy for Cancer: Gently Turning Towards,
First Edition. Trish Bartley.
© 2012 Trish Bartley. Published 2012 by John Wiley & Sons, Ltd.

Diagnosis

I was upstairs spraying deodorant under my arms and just noticed that my breast had changed shape. There was only a line, but I instantly knew what it was. It was the last thing I expected to see. I thought 'How come I'd never noticed it before?' I felt shocked, but I didn't cry.

This was around the end of May 2004. I went to the GP and was sent an appointment for August 24th even though I was meant to be fast tracked. But in that time, I had got my head round it. I knew what it was. I decided not to tell anyone until I was diagnosed. I didn't want to put that on my daughters. 'Has she got it?' 'Has she not?' – all that worry. I told a friend in work and showed her. She said it just looked like stretch marks to her. 'Well, it's not stretch marks' I said, and then put it to the back of my mind until the appointment. I never once thought 'I'm going to die. I've got cancer'. But maybe I was burying my head in the sand, because I never dreamt I'd have to have chemotherapy or radiotherapy. I thought it would be: In. Breast off. Bob's your uncle. Done.

The only thing that really worried me was how I was going to tell people.

I went to the one stop clinic on my own. I had a mammogram and then was called in for an ultrasound. In the waiting room, I looked round and saw these other women with long faces. For me, I knew it was cancer, but what must they be feeling? They were the colour of these walls. No-one spoke and we avoided each others' eyes.

Eventually the surgeon told me I had breast cancer. He said he could fit me in on the 13th September. 'Are you superstitious?' he asked. 'No', I said, 'Let's get it done'. When I got home my friend phoned from work. 'Are you ok?' she asked. 'I'm fine', I said, 'I'll see you tomorrow at work'.

My friend fell apart when I told him. That was the last thing I needed. I gave him the number of the Cancer Back Up people. I didn't tell my daughter who was going on holiday. I told them when they got back. I think they understood in the end. Surgery was ok and I was looked after brilliantly

Treatment

Overall, I felt I didn't have enough information about the chemotherapy. I went on the internet and found a good book I could refer to. With one of the chemotherapies, I was bouncing off the walls for the first day or so, but I wasn't sick. I usually went for chemo on my own. The waiting was difficult. I took a book everywhere with me. It wasn't a particularly anxious time for me, apart from all that waiting. I tried to carry on as normal, whatever that is.

Then I had radiotherapy. Actually I enjoyed the three weeks staying up at the hospital. It was a nice rest, but I burnt to bits. I was fed up that no-one ever told me. I thought it was a thing in the past, burning with radiotherapy. It was dreadful and I had to have it dressed every day. I've still got the scarring.

Post Treatment

After my chemotherapy, I was getting quite awful mood swings. I'd been diagnosed with depression some years before, so I knew the signs and I was going down that slippery slope. I also felt such rage. I'd wake up just as I was going off to sleep and want to smash the bedroom up. I remember sitting up in bed one night and actually beating the mattress. Then I cried because I didn't want to be like that. There was no trigger – and when I woke up the next day there was nothing left – but I was quite irritable with my daughters and grandkids. I'd come home and ask myself, why had I been like that, when they've done nothing to me. But I couldn't stop myself. I was on this rollercoaster and I couldn't get off. It was an awful feeling. It was more painful than the treatment. I actually said to a friend 'I'm never going to me again'. Not physically, but mentally. 'The person I was, is gone. I'd lost her. I'm someone else now and I don't like this person at all'. I'd go off and cry and rage and rant. It was a dreadful feeling. I wasn't so bad at work. I could shove it all to the back of my mind and *work*. But I got tired out. I wasn't doing myself any favours. In fact I was making things worse.

Mindfulness

I heard about mindfulness from my breast care nurse about a week before I started the course. It was the first time I'd heard anything about it. I thought I'd go along and see what it is. I've nothing to lose. I had a meeting before the course and heard more about it, but I'd already decided to do it. I knew I could get drugs off my doctor, but I felt full of drugs with the chemotherapy and Tamoxifen and I really didn't want any more.

The word mindfulness was interesting. I needed something to soothe this mind of mine and gather up the reins of my life again. I wanted to try something different and complementary. I'd had enough medical treatment. To be told it was going to be hard work didn't bother me. It was about getting the old me back again – and it wasn't physical work anyway or even mental work really.

I walked into the room on the first session and although it was all strange, and I didn't know anyone, it was calming just to walk in. I'm not on my own, I felt. Here we are together, all in the same boat. No-one had bits falling off them, everyone seemed quite normal. The door shut, and then it was just me, taking a chunk of that life back – stopping, slowing down and making time for me. I started to get benefit early on.

The group were quite important to me, although I don't see them any more now. I felt quite privileged really. Those people shared their experience with me and were open and honest. We didn't talk much about our lives but we shared the emotions and our experiences without going into detail about what had happened to us with cancer and everything. In some strange way, it allowed me to come to terms with some of my demons. I hadn't expressed them before, but when someone said things in the sessions, I realized 'I do that'. 'I feel that'. I can't begin to tell people how much benefit I got. I just went in at the beginning open minded, thinking I'll suck it and see, and in the end I got myself back – maybe even better.

I've got more time for myself now. I still run around and do too much. I lose my way, but I can come back again. I practice in work now – even if it just for 10 or 15 minutes. I was feeling absolutely wretched one day last week – and stood in the yard where no-one can see me. They knew I was having a bad day, so they all left me alone. I stood in 'mountain' and did some stretches and then I did some very slow mindful walking. I walked back into the office and someone said 'Look at you. You are all smiling. What's happened to you?!' I said nothing. She wouldn't let it go. I felt so much better just taking that time to bring myself back to the present. It only took 10 or 15 minutes.

I dreaded that first All Day on the course. I couldn't visualize myself keeping my mouth shut all day! It was even worse when we were told that we shouldn't have any eye contact with each other. But it was a wonderful experience. I remember on another occasion, doing a hearing practice and finding I hadn't judged anything at all or labelled the sound once. That was amazing.

When I'd tried to meditate before, I'd got lost. I couldn't get my mind blank. I thought that was what you were meant to do. I love being more mindful. Instead of waiting for the flowers to come out, I go out and see the things that are happening now. I am happier. Things still get difficult at times and when they do, I practice. I do mountain and some stretching, and sometimes walking or maybe some sitting practice. I am conscious of that barometer in my body. I really feel it and ask myself 'Let's see what is bothering you'. It doesn't take up masses of the day, but what does it matter if it does. It is a way of life really. Everyone should go on the course. I think we've all got something to give to each other.

My Journey

I've run, jumped, staggered,
Leapt and lunged
Pushed and pulled
Picked it up and not put any of it down
I've tottered and teetered.

I don't believe in co-incidences
But then again …

Now I'll walk the rest of the journey
And will be present
With love.

Beryl (December, 2005)

Part Two
The Mindfulness-Based Cognitive Therapy for Cancer Programme

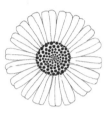

You begin a cascade of goodwill by infusing your intentions and actions with a sincere concern for the well-being of not only yourself, but everyone else as well.

(Carlson & Speca, 2010)

Introduction

Having looked at the context and impact of cancer, we now move up close to the eight week MBCT-Ca programme.

In the following pages, we explore the detail of all eight weeks of the course. Many participants share their experience of their mindfulness journeys. The second of the three-circle diagrams follows, capturing diagrammatically the development of mindfulness on the MBCT-Ca programme. After this, we focus on the practices, used on the programme. We look at how we adapt the core practices for people with cancer, and consider the short practices and their significant role within the intervention.

A description of Mindfulness and Palliative Care, written by Ursula Bates, comes after this. The chapter beautifully captures the approach she takes in a hospice setting to adapting the programme for people, who are terminally ill.

We then look at how to support participants after the course has finished. Finally, the last of the three-circle diagrams draws out the development of mindful awareness in being with cancer in everyday life.

Chapter Five
Starting Out

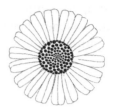

If we really practice curiosity, we will be inspired teachers and creative learners and we will be genuinely interested in understanding the colours and differences in our midst .... in knowing the stranger.

(Sara Lawrence-Lightfoot, 2000)

Introduction

What is involved in setting up and offering MBCT courses for people with cancer?

These tasks – many of them essentially practical – often take longer and need more energy than we might anticipate. However, like skilful gardeners, we prepare the ground as best we can.

Recruiting patients

In order to reach the people who might benefit most from the course, we probably need to understand the context we are working in and the medical and psychological stages that cancer patients go through.

Mindfulness-Based Cognitive Therapy for Cancer: Gently Turning Towards,
First Edition. Trish Bartley.
© 2012 Trish Bartley. Published 2012 by John Wiley & Sons, Ltd.

The MBCT-Ca courses, described in this book, take place in a small, but busy oncology unit, in a regional North Wales hospital. Ideally, we want to reach patients as they finish their treatment – via referrals from medical staff, and through direct contact. Working in different contexts such as in cancer support centres, hospices, or community based settings may need different approaches. Even though our courses have been running for a long time, recruiting always seems to take more time than we expect.

Informing staff

In the first instance, we started by offering a course to staff on the unit. Championed enthusiastically by two members of the team, a sizeable group attended. It proved invaluable in laying down the foundations of support for mindfulness within the department.

Since then, we use various ways to keep staff informed:

- lunch time talks
- presentations at specialist nurse meetings
- mindfulness steering group meetings
- conversations with new staff members take place.

Whenever possible, we guide a short practice:

> At a small gathering, one of the nurses shared the news that a patient had had a serious recurrence. She mentioned this shortly after finishing a short breath practice, and as she talked, she became quite sad. The moment passed, but she commented that normally she would have just rushed on to the next thing. Stopping and breathing had let her get in touch with what was there. She said that she was glad that she had.

We also send regular emails to staff inviting referrals. Sometimes we include research headlines or brief feedback from course outcome measures (averaged across the group), encouraging a sense that MBCT-Ca courses are part of the oncology service – not just something extra at the edges. Some colleagues respond readily, especially after one of their patients has significantly benefited from mindfulness recently.

We find natural allies amongst psychologists and counsellors. Breast cancer specialist nurses and oncologists welcome opportunities to refer their patients, due to the numbers of women affected and the impact of the disease. Staff are welcome to come to courses themselves, (only one per course). This is helpful to them and also serves to boosts referrals and increase understanding about the course.

We obviously cannot rely solely on busy clinicians or oncology nurses to signpost patients to courses. They have too much else to do. Additionally, research suggests that the psychological challenges of cancer tend to be under diagnosed by oncologists, (Passik et al., 1998; Söllner, et al., 2001), although medical colleagues may dispute this. There is also a risk that some patients get screened out by medical staff, due to assumptions about who is suitable and who might be able to manage the home practice, which they themselves found difficult.

Informing patients

We therefore need to find additional ways of reaching participants directly. Information packs are given out to patients at the start of their oncology treatment. Mindfulness leaflets can be included, although they may be overlooked in the numbers of leaflets in the packs. Catchy posters displayed in unusual places can get some good results – such as opposite the chair where bloods are taken, or on radiology notice boards, where breast cancer patients wait for mammograms.

It is worth casting the net wide. We send out occasional press releases or write articles in local papers. A recent national magazine article found its way into several participants' hands. We sometimes get fliers into health food shops, chemists, surgeries and libraries. We might mail-out to GPs and practice nurses, and give talks at cancer support groups. Reflecting on local sources of support guides us to where we target publicity.

Probably the most effective recruiting is by word of mouth. Giving out leaflets to participants as they finish the course gives them something to pass on to friends and colleagues should they too be diagnosed. Participants who arrive via word of mouth are generally well prepared. We also tell past 'graduates' when new courses are due to start. Some may want to attend for a second time.

When is the Best Time to Take a Course?

At an MBCT-Ca research presentation, a consultant oncologist jokingly suggested that a few months *before* diagnosis might be the perfect time to take a mindfulness course!

Some patients ask to join a course soon after their diagnosis. We always encourage them to make contact again after their treatment is over, but might teach a short practice over the phone to help support them with what they are experiencing. Cancer brings with it an 'existential plight' that adds to the shock and distress of diagnosis. (Weisman & Worden, 1976). This usually fades in time – but it is not wise to attend mindfulness classes when feelings are very turbulent.

Others are keen to start a mindfulness course, even whilst they receive their treatment. This is usually counterproductive, except perhaps at the very end. Cancer treatments are physically and psychologically arduous. People tend to get very tired and often feel unwell. This can build over the cycles. Treatment invariably involves patients in many hospital visits and sometimes in-patient treatment. None of this is conducive to steady home practice and regular weekly attendance on the course. There are always exceptions and special circumstances – but we tend to be quite cautious with those who want to combine attending a mindfulness course with receiving treatment. It often proves to be too much.

Mindfulness is best developed when life is reasonably steady. In simplistic terms, we offer the course to people who are experiencing chronic rather than acute difficulties. Ideally, we encourage patients to attend as soon as possible after the end of their treatment. This has specific benefits. Widespread reports suggest that there are three periods when cancer patients are most likely to need support:

- at initial diagnosis
- when a recurrence is diagnosed
- at the end of treatment.

Friends and families may assume that the worst is over, once treatment has ended. In some ways, it may be only just beginning.

A Cancer Patient's Recollection

I remember having my last treatment. It should have been a great day. The nurses kept greeting me with 'Isn't this your last one? Well done!' I'd been looking forward to it for months. I should feel pleased, I told myself – and in a way I was.

But I kept thinking that I'd miss everyone. I felt safe coming back to hospital. I didn't have to worry about it (*cancer*) coming back. I got very weepy on that last day. I held it together during chemo, but when I was getting my prescription made up, I could feel the tears very close. Sister B noticed and took me into a side room and gave me a hug. She told me that many patients felt like that on their last day. I was so relieved. I thought it was just me being stupid.

Almost any time is a good time

Attending a mindfulness course immediately after treatment might be ideal for many people, but any time after that is also fine. Some people find their way to mindfulness many years after diagnosis. Others come after stressful times, such as returning to work, some other major life event, or a recurrence of the cancer. Each participant has his or her own pattern of suffering that draws them to the course.

Preparing for the Course

Developing course resources

As teachers, we need to develop course materials to support home practice, summarize learning, and inspire and refer back to, after the course has finished.

When we first taught this programme, we used weekly handouts that we could tailor to each group. Thanks to the generosity of the original MBCT teachers, weekly summaries and outlines are available free of copyright (Segal et al., 2002) We type them up developing our own course 'style' and carefully acknowledge the original source. The debt to our teachers remain. Their summaries are very clear and form the basis of all those within MBCT-Ca.

Nowadays, we produce workbooks, which look better and are more efficient and effective. Given out on the first week, we encourage our participants to notice the inclination to read from cover to cover at the first opportunity.

We also use practice CDs to give out to participants for them to use at home. At first, we used other, more experienced teachers' practices. Then we recorded our own. It seems that it works better for participants to be guided by the voice of their own teacher. Like the workbook, practice CDs develop over time. Creating, refining and developing course materials probably needs to be an ongoing task.

Support and venue

The venue needs to be big enough for 10–12 people to be able to lie down for the Body Scan and manage mindful movement. We use a seminar room on the oncology unit corridor. It can be challenging for patients to return to the unit after treatment – but it is also an opportunity to 'turn towards' what is difficult, which is what they will be learning to practise on the course.

It is invaluable to have a mindfulness 'champion', who holds some authority within the department. We have been fortunate in having the support of a senior oncology consultant, Professor N. S. A. Stuart (contributing author in this title), who has signed off invoices, chaired meetings, hosted research seminars, reminded medical colleagues about referring patients, and generally taken a lead, by sustaining interest and encouraging contact with the mindfulness 'project.'

The Orientation and Assessment Process

Learning from experience

In the early days, when we met potential participants before the start of the course, we tended to focus on promoting mindfulness. As our experience consolidated, we changed our approach. This was precipitated by one particular group, whose members experienced so many crises that by week 5, over 40% of them had withdrawn. Something was clearly wrong.

After personal reflection and discussion in supervision, we decided to shift from a focus on recruiting participants, to one of preparing them for the course. Now, when someone is cautious about joining the course, we agree that it is not right for everyone. Instead of jollying them along, we talk about the intensity of the course and the challenges of committing to the practice – alongside the potential benefits.

As a result, some people wisely choose not to take part in the course. Others, instead of being put off, jump in with both feet. By promoting individual choice, they are able to decide for themselves; take responsibility for committing to the practice; and own the outcomes that result. Due to the complexity of treatments, and the culture of medical systems, many of us can become dependent on the knowledge and skills of our doctors to keep us healthy. Connecting as one adult to another in the orientation process is helpful in balancing this in an oncology setting. By empowering our participants to make their own decisions, we are supporting them to invest in their own health and wellbeing.

As a result of this approach, attrition within the groups dropped dramatically and outcome benefits have increased. This has been maintained over many years. It is now very unusual for participants to withdraw during the course, unless one of them becomes ill.

Preparing people for the course

Helping to prepare participants for the course starts as soon as we first make contact, or when a referral is received from one of the oncology team. We follow this with a phone call and then send written information by post or email. The benefits and challenges of the course are emphasized equally. Practical details are included such as dates, times and venue.

Eventually, we arrange a one to one meeting between the teacher and each participant, shortly before the course starts. These meetings take place on the same day of the week that the course will run. If participants are unable to show, they are unlikely to make it to the classes.

It is tempting to undertake this orientation process in a group. This would obviously save time and expense. However, we chose to stay with one-to-one meetings. They seem to offer the best opportunity to fully assess and carefully prepare people for the course. The process seems to help teacher and participant make an initial connection. This in turn supports the stability of the group.

An excerpt from the letter sent to potential participants

Dear Joan,

I am writing to give you some information about the Mindfulness Based Course you have expressed an interest in …

I will need to meet you in the unit probably a week or two before the start of the course … This meeting will last for about an hour and it gives you an opportunity to ask about the course, meet me, your mindfulness teacher, and look at what has drawn you to take the course. Most people find it is helpful to know more about what to expect. It allows us to make sure that the course is right for you at this time.

The course, in some ways, is quite hard work. You will need to practice at home every day between classes. This is a very important part of the course and although it is not strenuous as such, it does involve you listening to CDs and practising exercises that we have done during the classes. These practices involve lying down, or sitting, or doing gentle stretches. They last for 30 minutes each. There are also a number of short practices. Participants who are most conscientious about their home practice seem to get the most out of the course. I suppose it is like most things – you get out what you put in – so starting now to develop a commitment to do the practices is very helpful – even if you sometimes find them boring or might feel you have more pressing things to do.

Looking at the roles we take

The orientation meetings with participants cover a lot of ground. As teachers, we can facilitate this by looking at the different roles we take.

The list seems long and is probably not comprehensive. We do not cover everything in one session. Much of it has been included in the written information and perhaps through phone contact.

Table 5.1 Roles that we as teachers take.

Role (not in order)	Questions / Information (examples)
Listener	*What would you like me to know about your illness?* *Do you experience pain or have any challenges in moving or stretching?* *Is there anything else you want me to know?* *What do you hope for from the course?*
Assessor	*Is this the right time for you to take the course?* (implicit question) *How do you find being in groups?* *Have you experienced any significant life events recently (apart from cancer)?* *How do you feel about learning (over time) to be with difficult thoughts?* *Are you on any medication?*
Informer	Venue (show room if possible). Group size. What to expect in the class: Body Scan practice – lying down – in the first class. Length – All Day (very brief). Video permissions. Visitors to classes. Basic mindfulness information – including practical things – e.g., clothing.
Cautioner	*It can be stressful to take the course...* *Sometimes things get more intense...* *Most people find it challenging to keep up with the home practice...* *The course is not a self-help group – minimal sharing about personal stories...*
Connector	Starting to build trust. Hearing personal stories of the cancer journey. Starting to offer appropriate holding connection that can support the participant to have courage to turn towards and be with the process.
Orientor	Emphasizing importance of the practice. *How will you manage this?*
Supporter	*Encouragement just to engage as best you can – and trust you will get out of it what you need.* *Who will support you at home/amongst your friends? When/if you feel like giving up.*
Promoter (not over developed)	Some outcomes others have experienced – including research evidence for mindfulness and cancer. Mindfulness out there in the world. NICE guidelines – recommending mindfulness for people with recurrent depression. Support from the oncology team for the course.

©T. Bartley, (2012). Mindfulness-Bases Cognitive Therapy for Cancer.

Honouring the process

The conversation with each participant is unique and each will have its own emphasis. There is something vital and significant about the process of hearing and being fully present to each person and his or her story. Often, tears are shed as the experience of diagnosis and treatment is shared. It is the beginning of an important connection between participant and teacher.

We allow plenty of time. We used to squeeze these meetings into 30 minutes and always ran late. We now allow an hour per person and run the sessions over 2 days. They can be intense experiences. Looking after ourselves, as teachers, in the process is important. If we see ten people one after another, it will not be possible to be open to each one. Breaks between people are helpful – to pause, breathe and come back.

Special circumstances and different groups of people

We sometimes invite cancer patients to bring a carer with them. It can be invaluable to have support if mobility is a challenge, or if someone is shy and nervous, or if the cancer is advanced. This can be a friend, family member or partner. Sometimes a couple come together, which can help them both, especially in terms of supporting home practice. Anyone who attends the course, whether carer or patient, needs to be willing to participate in their own right – with a strong commitment to practise and stay with the process. This is emphasized in orientation meetings and everyone is seen individually at some point on their own, even if they come as a couple.

Sometimes, ongoing support from a professional psychologist or counsellor enables more vulnerable people to attend the course. This is especially relevant with patients who have had very challenging cancer journeys and difficult adjustment challenges.

Counselling people off the course

In unusual circumstances, it might not a good time to participate on the course. A prospective participant might find it difficult to relate to the give-and-take of group discussion. Occasionally someone might have strong views about conventional oncology treatment, or some other strongly held opinion, which might prove difficult for others in the group. Even more rarely, serious mental health difficulties might result in negotiating a return when things are steadier.

Sometimes people move into denial or strong avoidance in relation to their illness. They may talk about feeling as if they are in 'a bubble', with everything and everyone else appearing rather unreal on the outside. Some cancer patients may have developed strongly defended ways of coping that would mean that it was highly challenging for them to turn towards what was difficult. In this event, we would offer our support to help them understand that it may not be the right time to take the course. One to one talking therapy may be a better option. Others on hearing about the demands of the course may feel that they are coping fine in their own way.

Launching the boat

By the time the first session arrives, ideally everyone taking the course is well prepared to start. We sometimes use a metaphor to illustrate this process.

> *'It is as if we are getting ready to go on a boat journey. We need to make sure we have everything we need. This meeting is part of that. We are going on quite a long journey that will take us eight weeks. This boat, 'Mindfulness', regularly sets out with a group of people three times a year, but each time it does, the experience is always a little different.*
>
> *It may feel a bit rocky when we first meet as a group – just as when you get into a boat – but eventually when everyone has found their place, we will set off. It is my job, as your teacher, to launch the boat – then I hop in with you – and we'll be off, on our way!'*

Sometimes

Sometimes things don't go, after all,
from bad to worse. Some years, muscadel
faces down frost; green thrives; the crops don't fail,
sometimes a man aims high, and all goes well.

A people sometimes will step back from war;
Elect an honest man; decide they care
Enough, that they can't leave some stranger poor.
Some men become what they were born for.

Sometimes our best efforts do not go
amiss; sometimes we do as we meant to.
The sun will sometimes melt a field of sorrow
that seemed hard frozen: may it happen for you.

Sheenagh Pugh (1990)

We now meet Sally, who had cancer in 2005 and came to an MBCT-Ca course very soon after the end of her treatment.

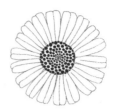

Personal Story

Sally

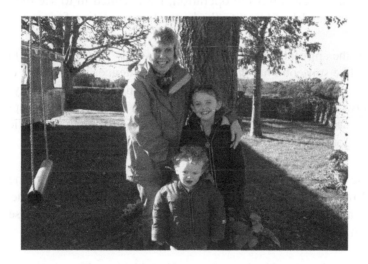

Sally is a farmer's wife in her early forties. She has four children, the youngest born after her illness. She was diagnosed with non-Hodgkin lymphoma in 2005 and attended a mindfulness course just a few weeks after the end of her treatment. She is well and enjoying life.

Mindfulness-Based Cognitive Therapy for Cancer: Gently Turning Towards,
First Edition. Trish Bartley.
© 2012 Trish Bartley. Published 2012 by John Wiley & Sons, Ltd.

Diagnosis

I found a lump in my neck in January 2005 and went to the doctor. I thought it was an infection. The doctor did too. He said to come back if it was still there in a week. It didn't go away, so I went back a couple of times and eventually saw a different doctor, who said that I must see someone straight away. I got an appointment within a fortnight and saw Dr. B., an ear, nose and throat surgeon. I had surgery the following week and everyone seemed to think it was ok and that was the end of it. But they sent away for tests to Cardiff just to make sure.

As the weeks went by, I wondered if I would ever be the same again. I looked awful. I was having a lot of night sweats and I felt really tired. I was sure things were not right.

Nine and a half weeks after the operation, I was called in to see the surgeon again. He said that I had to go to the haematology section for treatment.

When I got the appointment letter it had Alaw Day Unit (oncology) on the top. It was like someone had given me a life sentence. I remember one of my friends, years ago, looking at the death notices in the Daily Post saying 'It's always Alaw Ward, isn't it?' I threw the letter to the back of the cupboard. It wasn't true whatever it was, but the following Monday, when the kids were at school, I got the letter out and read it again.

On 3pm the following Wednesday, I saw the doctor. My auntie came with me. She'd recently lost a friend in Alaw so I felt awful for taking her back again. It is a horrible thing to take people with you, isn't it? Because you're taking them with you on that whole journey, aren't you?

The doctor was lovely. 'You've got non-Hodgkin lymphoma', he said, 'You'll have to have treatment for this, but at the moment we haven't decided how to treat you, because it is a very rare type that you've got'. He asked if I had any more lumps. I told him I was sure the lump in my neck was back. He found it and said he thought it was 10 cm (compared to 3cm when it was operated on).

He did a bone marrow test then and there. It was awful, but the nurse was lovely and everyone was so kind. He told me I needed an MRI scan to see if it had spread, and I'd have to wait for an appointment.

Then I had to go home and face everyone. That was the worst. My husband was just coming off the tractor when I arrived home. 'They think it is cancer', I told him. I just went into the house to my bedroom and cried. You don't want to worry anyone. You protect your children like your mother protected you. I felt I couldn't tell them anything.

The scan came through in a fortnight but it felt like a year – just waiting and waiting.

My doctor told me to phone the minute I had the scan date so I only had to wait a few days to see him. He told me that the lump was still in the neck and one in the chest but it was nothing alarming – and the bone marrow was fine. I met the specialist nurse and she was then with me all the way. They decided to give me a chemotherapy called CHOP.

Treatment

The first one was horrible. The Day Unit was so full. People were everywhere. There was an old gentleman by my side and he was lovely. I felt I was doing something just closing the curtains for him. I felt in the way really – there was so much going on and yet nothing was happening to me. By lunchtime it just got too much. I kept saying I was ok but by one o'clock I couldn't take any more. I was so upset I went out to the car park. I wanted some space on my own for a bit and then my auntie came out to me.

We went to the café and had a cup of tea. In the end it was about 10 to 4 when I was told that they would start my treatment. You think to yourself you've got to do it but you feel so helpless. I went through it 5 more times

I started losing my hair while I was on the ward with an infection. That was awful too. I went to the bathroom and it was just falling out. The nurses had a chat with me and that helped. They were very kind. By the end the lump was going down and I had an MRI scan a fortnight after my last treatment and the doctor said everything was all clear. That was such a relief – but they told me the lump could go away and come back just as quick.

Mindfulness

On my 6th and last chemo, I got very emotional. You look forward so much to the last one and getting back to normal. Then when I got to that day, I got up and started crying. My specialist nurse came up and held my hand. I had my blood test and went to have a cup of tea like I always did. When I started chemo, I started crying again. 'What's the matter with me?' I asked my nurse, 'I should be happy but I'm going to miss this. I don't know whether I'll be alright – it's like having a safety net around you'. She reassured me that I could always phone and then she reminded me of the leaflet about mindfulness. I'd been reading it recently. I came home and phoned for the class quite soon. I thought if I leave it, I might not do it.

When I saw the mindfulness teacher, she asked if I would like to bring someone with me. Ruth, my teenage daughter said 'Do you want me to come with you, Mum?' 'That's up to you', I said. So she came and I was pleased. In the beginning, we'd go up to Ruth's room to do the Body Scan and start to laugh – or I'd snore and Ruth would wake me up and we'd have a laugh. But then we got into it quite well and it became part of our life. I'd look forward to it.

When we did the All Day in the Day Unit, it did bring memories back.* It got a bit overwhelming, but after doing a few practices, I relaxed. I think it was a good thing to go back to that room. It was tough at times but I felt good after it. At first I didn't know if I could cope. The kids were laughing at me 'You won't be able to stay silent!' But I really enjoyed it.

Recently, I had the most horrendous day, so I went and did the sitting practice, for about a quarter of an hour – and after I felt so much better as if something had been lifted from me. The course has helped me tremendously in that way. You learn to do your own practice in your own way. I've been training for the Race for Life and I often walk mindfully and then look up at the mountains. It is nice to stop and do the mountain practice on the beach. It becomes part of everyday life. I try to do something small every day. You feel so much better when you've done it. If you go for a week or two without doing anything and then you do a full half an hour, you notice how much it helps you. You can stand in your own body somehow. It is then that you realize how much your mind plays on your emotions without really noticing what is going on.

I'm so glad that I've done the mindfulness. I think it has helped me cope *after* my treatment and I believe that it will help my chance of staying well and if I believe it, it must help.

* (Sally is referring to an All Day session that participants engage in after week 6, discussed next in this chapter.)

I enjoy the follow ups. It is different to going to the course every week. You come to know the people and have a chat and even have a cry sometimes. You don't want to burden your family. But if I go there, I can sit and practice and have time for me and I feel better for it.

I've got different priorities now – I say 'no' more often. We often don't bother with things do we, we are so busy – and then have a bad day and shout at the kids. Now (since having cancer) I think that I must go and tell them that I love them so much and give them a cuddle before they go to sleep. I've got such a good family.

Got Up Mindfully This Morning

Got up mindfully this morning
My mind was here and there
But I was aware
Til the end of the day

Ruth (Sally's daughter, age 16)
(December, 2005)

Chapter Six
The Eight Week Course

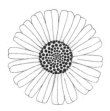

It is not the magnitude of the task that matters, it's the magnitude of our courage.

(Matthieu Ricard, 2003)

Introduction

We are now ready to embark on the MBCT-Ca programme. The participants have been recruited and prepared. They have been told what to expect over the eight weeks of the course – or as much as is relevant at this stage. We now go through the sessions one by one, as they do, gathering some understanding of the building themes and developing mindfulness practice. Most of all, we will learn how the course rests in the hearts and minds of people with cancer, and discover what this offers them.

You will hear many stories and anecdotes that connect you with the experience of the MBCT-Ca participants. These are all quite genuine and took place within the different groups. More than anything, we hope that by sharing their experience, you will get a taste of the course for yourself. You will be listening in to how things unfold over the weeks, and what effect the sessions and home practice has on the participants. Descriptions of the eight sessions of the course, the All Day practice and the follow up class, a month after the last session are all included.

Mindfulness-Based Cognitive Therapy for Cancer: Gently Turning Towards,
First Edition. Trish Bartley.
© 2012 Trish Bartley. Published 2011 by John Wiley & Sons, Ltd.

Week One

In the beginner's mind there are many possibilities, in the expert's there are few.

(Shunryu Suzuki, 1973)

Automatic Pilot

Core theme:

Discovering that we function on automatic most of the time.

We are rarely fully present – but sliding back into thoughts of what has happened or leaning forward into what is to come. In this first session, we start to appreciate that when we are fully present in the immediacy of what we experience, we slow down and notice things more vividly and in more detail. This changes our experience.

Key Tasks for Teachers – Week One

Teacher preparation – a practice of settling and intention before the session starts.

Beginning the course:

- Ground rules
- Brief grounding exercise

Building the community:

- Introductions and action methods exercise

Personal intentions:

- A guided practice
- Intentions letter

The Raisin exercise:

- and dialogue

Week 1 teaching:

- Defining mindfulness
- Exploring the cancer journey and what mindfulness might offer – through the metaphor of Rilke's *River*

Week 1 practice:

- Body Scan and inquiry

Week 1 short practice:

- The Pause

Concluding:

- Week one home practice
- Distributing course materials – workbook and CD1
- Ending – the bells and closing intention

Introduction

The first session arrives. This is the beginning of the course and yet there has been a lot leading up to it. As teachers, we have been connecting and aligning our participants to the course and the learning they will be engaged in, see chapter 5 Starting Out, for discussion of the orientation and assessment process.

Preparing for the class

When everything is ready in the room, we take time to stop and settle. This is probably our most important preparation. Yet often it gets squeezed.

What are we doing in this practice? The mind may well be busy and scattered, anticipating what is to come. We may suddenly remember something. It is so tempting to forgo the practice and jump up and put it right. We practice by staying with the moment, with all that is arising in the mind, and all that is stirring in resonance of anticipation within the body – 'being able to embody the balance of openness and 'groundedness' that participants are invited to experience for themselves' (Segal et al., 2002).

It is also a chance to align ourselves to our intention for this work and with this group. Gently opening to the presence of the people about to gather, we wish them well on the course.

Beginning the Course

When the time arrives, we welcome participants into the room. We offer a very brief outline of the session, even though participants may be distracted. The content of what is said is less important than a friendly grounded presence.

Ground rules

Most teachers offer a few ground rules early on. This helps to build a feeling of safety and trust. We tend to highlight two areas. Others naturally spin off from them.

The first relates to **Confidentiality** – suggesting that what is personal stays with the person it belongs to. What involves our own experience, we can share with friends and family. By encouraging a culture of mutual respect within the group, we are inviting responses that are sensitive and appropriate.

The second ground rule relates to **Participation**. In the course, we learn to focus on becoming aware of our own experience. This allows us to make choices. We now clarify this by explicitly inviting participants to choose their own level of participation at any given time, according to what feels best in that moment. In this way, everyone is being encouraged to take responsibility for their own choices and learning – and for taking good care of themselves.

A young woman Holly, who had breast cancer, joined a new course. She had been tentative during the orientation meeting with her teacher, but eventually shared a fair bit of her experience of cancer and treatment. She said that she was extremely shy in groups and hated having to talk. The teacher reassured her that after sharing her name in the first session, she would not need to say anything if she did not want to. In the event, Holly said nothing at all in the large group throughout the entire course, until the very last session when she quietly told the group that she was very grateful to them and had gained a lot. The other participants had been very gentle with her, including her in their small group discussions. Even though she had said so very little, she was a definite presence in the group.

Arriving in the Body

Before moving into introductions, we guide a short grounding practice. This helps us all to settle.

A Brief Grounding Practice

*Feet on the floor – bringing attention to the contact points
on the soles of the feet between the body and the floor – exploring the
sensations of contact and experiencing a sense of the solidity of the
floor beneath.*

Building the Community

Introductions (brief). Name. What has brought me here? What do I want from the course? Choosing when to speak and how much to say.

As teachers, we all have our own way of facilitating introductions. Suggesting that people first talk in pairs and then share in the whole group can help to reduce anxiety.

We may hear some intense if brief conversations in the pairs during these early exchanges. Some people have a strong urge to share what has happened to them. There may be a need to locate themselves internally in the group. 'Who is worse than me?' 'Who is better?' 'Where do I fit?' There is some curiosity about this, especially at the beginning of the group. This opening round becomes an opportunity to be mindful – inviting people to notice how it feels as they decide to speak. Going round the circle in the time honoured way inevitably increases nervousness, so we invite participants to speak when they want to, in a random pattern.

An action methods exercise

(*Standing up*) 'If this room was a map of the area, (*suggesting one end is north and the other is south*), where do you come from on the map? Choosing to go and stand there'.

This is one of many exercises that can help break the ice. Moving seems to be helpful, as long we remember to adapt around people's physical abilities. This exercise involves people in talking, whilst working out where to stand in relation to other people. The feeling in the room can change quite suddenly after the nervousness of introductions. There is often a rush of laughter and conversation as amusing results on the map unfold with north and south, east and west getting muddled. (It might not be appropriate to use this exercise in areas of significant racial, religious or socioeconomic diversity.)

Personal Intentions

Intention has an important role in the course. By including it early on, we develop a focus and maybe spark an interest in what intention might offer.

An Intentions Practice

Pebble exercise

Settling into a comfortable posture … Imagining that you are standing beside some water – a lake, or a stream or the ocean. The water is very clear and you can see a long way down to the bottom. Choosing an imaginary pebble and tossing it gently into the water – watching it sink very slowly down. Asking yourself – 'What do I most wish for myself from this course?' and 'What do I care about, that this course might support me with?' Not being concerned if answers don't come straight away, just continuing to gently ask – opening to the possibility of something emerging from within you. Eventually the pebble comes to rest…

Source: This exercise is adapted from Jon Kabat-Zinn's practice of a pebble dropping down into a well.

Intentions letter

After the practice, we invite participants to move into new pairs – as the questions are written up on the whiteboard. *'What do I most wish for myself from this course?'* and *'What do I care about, that this course might support me with?'* Those who would like to share in the large group are invited to.

Then participants complete a **form**, which includes some basic questions about hopes for the course and current levels of stress and distress. (These are personal forms which nobody else sees, allowing participants to be more open and honest about their feelings and intentions.) On the back of the form is a **letter**, which offers a space to record personal insights from the intentions practice. These forms and letters are placed by the participants into an envelope with their name on the front. We have developed a bit of a ritual around this – posting all the envelopes into one large envelope and sealing it in front of the group. The teacher then undertakes to look after the sealed envelope and bring it with her to each class. She explains that it will stay

---

sealed and no-one will see the letters until the last class when they will be returned unopened to each of them.

There is value in this process. Participants often forget how things were at the beginning of the course. This is understandable. Most of the learning is based on personal experience. As new skills and responses become integrated, we forget how things were. The letters/forms record the place where we are starting, enabling us to remember and appreciate what we have learnt by the time we come to the end.

Practice

The first taste of mindfulness

The Raisin Exercise (Kabat-Zinn, 1990; Segal et al., 2002)

We guide participants in the experience of seeing, smelling, touching and finally tasting a raisin – as if we had dropped in from Mars and had no idea what this object was.

For the first of many times, we invite a way of approaching things 'as if for the first time'. As teachers, we practice this ourselves as we guide the exercise, bringing a fresh curiosity to the raisin every time.

This is our first mindfulness practice as a group. It is a good example of experiencing something ordinary – and in the immediacy of attention, finding aspects that are extraordinary. Jon Kabat-Zinn created this exercise to cut through expectations; and find an essentially experiential way of introducing what it is to be present and mindful. As he rightly points out 'when you start to pay attention in this way, your relationship to things change....You literally become more awake' (Kabat-Zinn, 1990)

It may be ordinary to taste a raisin, but it can seem a bit odd.

'Felt like we were in church, and you were the priest handing out the special objects!'

'I nearly burst out laughing only everyone looked so serious'.

'We had a good laugh about the raisin when we got home!'

Dialogue

Our first group inquiry follows. It is important in establishing how we work together. We engage in an exercise (or a practice) and then we explore our experience of it. We make this process explicit to the group. 'This is how we will be doing things on the course'.

> Participants learn ...by first having the experience and only afterwards trying to make sense of what it means. (Segal et al., 2002).

As teachers, we embody the same freshness of interest in the inquiry process as we did with the raisin. It is all too easy in the keenness of teaching to rush into explanations of automatic pilot. Instead, on a good day, we gently draw out the stories. We hear about the textures and associations, the likings and the not likings – and the moments of vividly experiencing the raisin. There is always a lot to explore. If we are patient, staying connected and open to the participants and what they are saying, we can count on the learning emerging. What is needed is a trusting, and a focus of attention – connecting one moment to another to trace the links of meaning and learning.

Naomi was in her seventies. She had had a tough time in treatment and things were still pretty difficult. In the dialogue that followed the raisin exercise, she announced that she was never not aware. She was an artist. She knew what it was 'to concentrate and think about things'. The teacher suggested that 'being present' was not quite like that – and immediately regretted it. They spoke on the phone during the week and the teacher was relieved to have an opportunity to start again. 'I keep thinking about the texture of that raisin' says Naomi, 'I've been so wound up this week with all the hassle of hospital appointments. I've sometimes wondered about holding a raisin and trying to get that feeling back'. 'What did it feel like?' asks the teacher. 'Do you know, it is hard to explain', says Naomi, 'but I really knew I was holding that raisin. I could feel the wrinkles and the crevices – and there was nothing else there at all'.

Not everyone has a pleasant experience. Joan had never let a raisin pass her lips. She was told by her grandmother when she was little that raisins were witches warts. Others see their raisin as a cockroach or a bug. Through sharing, they begin to appreciate how the mind affects experience. Many are brought back to their mother's kitchen at Christmas as they smell the raisin. Some get fond of the raisin and feel sad or guilty for eating it. At some point, someone will comment that they often eat raisins a handful at a time and never really taste them. And there is our opportunity to ask, 'Are there other times when we do things automatically, without really noticing?'

Averil attended an 8-week mindfulness course in her local community centre. She was known in the neighbourhood to love her cups of tea. She might have twenty or more a day and had done for years. After tasting the raisin on the first class, she returned the next week in some consternation. She had mindfully drunk a cup of tea — and discovered that she did not like the taste!

Week One Teaching

Defining mindfulness

After the inquiry, we spend a few minutes exploring a definition of mindfulness.

Jon Kabat-Zinn suggests that mindfulness is moment-to-moment awareness.

Mindfulness is paying attention in a particular way....
  on purpose
    in the present moment
      without judgement   (Kabat-Zinn, 1990)

This is written in the course workbook that we now hand round to each participant. (This workbook will guide participants through each week, summarizing the theme of the session, sometimes offering a poem or readings, and clarifying the home practice for that week.) Turning to the relevant page, we ask, 'What was the particular way that we paid attention to the raisin?' Ideas are offered and written up on the whiteboard by the teacher. 'Being curious', 'Slowing right down', 'Doing one thing at a time',

'Focusing on our senses' are examples of what might be suggested by the group.

MBCT for Cancer – A Brief Overview

We then widen out our discussion to look at mindfulness and what it might offer us – both in everyday life and explicitly as cancer patients. We open the workbook again – to read part of a Rilke poem.

> May what I do flow from me like a river,
> no forcing and no holding back,
> the way it is with children.
>
> Then in these swelling and ebbing currents,
> these deepening tides moving out, returning,
> I will sing you as no one ever has,
> streaming through widening channels
> into the open sea.
>
> R M Rilke (1996)

This poem has become important to us on the programme. The metaphor of river works well in relation to the journey of cancer. In dialogue within the group, we explore what the poem might mean, drawing out the metaphor with participants and making links with their own cancer journeys.

Sometimes like a river we amble along. Sometimes things are turbulent, and the river is in flood. Other times we feel stuck, as if damned up with debris. Having a cancer diagnosis is a traumatic experience. It is understandable (to use the river metaphor) if the river water seems to be agitated and in turmoil, or even bursts its banks in flood, or gets bogged down and loses flow of river. How we react to events 'in the flow of the river' determines how we feel about them. Sometimes our habits of mind make things worse. What we learn on the course is how to be able to go more with the flow – feeling the turmoil, the stuckness, the loss or resentment – and learning to be with it, in gentleness.

Looking at the poem may help us glimpse a possibility of seeing things impersonally without blame. There are causes and conditions, but the river is how it is –always changing. This is the beauty of river.

Bringing the elephant into the room

By discussing the poem in this way, we are acknowledging the context of cancer, its relevance to us, and this work we are doing together. Some participants may prefer that we did not. As teachers, we need to be present and sensitive to each person. With most groups, it seems important to gently affirm the courage and challenge of managing a cancer diagnosis and treatment. As we begin to honour their experience, we may notice a change in the 'feeling tone' in the group. Emotions may surface. Some participants may judge themselves hard when they find things difficult. Taking time to acknowledge feelings and responding to them gently – perhaps with a guided breath – is compassionate teaching.

Linking the river with the raisin

The possibility of 'flowing like a river, the way it is with children' may resonate and link back to the raisin inquiry and the notion of 'beginner's mind'. It offers an image for the way mindfulness may help us relate differently to difficulties. We may not know what it feels like 'to flow like a river', but intuitively it sounds good. Thus the power of poetry helps us understand things in a more potent and personal way.

Week One Practice – The Body Scan

We get ready to do the Body Scan, the first of three core practices. Some participants may prefer to sit, because of treatment areas, pain, or mobility issues. Some may be happy to lie on a mat on the floor. Helping people to settle, we get ready to begin.

Our focus in this first Body Scan is to map out the basics of the practice – establishing the building blocks that allow us to 'intentionally move attention around the body' (Segal et al., 2002). The Body Scan is a very significant practice for cancer patients. Detailed discussion of the ways we can adapt

Body Scan for cancer patients is in chapter 7. Cancer patients tend to avoid giving attention to affected parts of the body, except in an anxious intermittent way, which may be more about wanting sensations to go away, Than being present and aware of them. In this first Body Scan, we guide the practice with sensitivity, emphasising gentleness as we move through the parts of the body that are affected by cancer. We will have learnt from participants which parts of the body are affected at the orientation meeting.

Inviting participants to lie down on the mats provided on the floor, or sit in chairs, whatever seems best for them, as we move into the first Body Scan of the course.

The Body Scan Practice

'Settling into the sensations of contact of your body with the floor/ chair, as you briefly scan through from the feet up to the top of the head.....adjusting any part of the body that wants a more comfortable position.....and becoming aware of the detailed qualities of the contact between your body and the floor or chair.......When you are ready, now moving awareness deliberately to the breath breathing deep in the body. Perhaps placing your hands on the belly to guide your attention...and simply resting awareness on the movement of the belly under the hands, as the breath comes in and goes out.....not changing it in any way, letting it breathe exactly as it does, without trying to control it in any way...................We are now going to practice The Body Scan. There is no specific goal to attain. The invitation is simply to follow as best you can, bringing your attention to sensations in different parts of your body and exploring them as I guide you through the practice. Remembering that if you find that you do not want to do something that I invite you to do, always choosing and doing what is best for you. At any time, you may decide to leave the practice and come back to the breath breathing deep in the belly, as you are aware of it now........Now, when you are ready, moving your attention from the belly all the way down to the left foot and then out to the toes of the left foot........noticing any sensations in the big toe – perhaps contact with the sock or stocking, maybe warmth or coolness, throbbing or tickling, a sense of the shape of the toe, maybe teasing out sensations of toe nail or pad of the toe'........(then moving through the different toes, and parts of toes and foot – inviting noticing of sensations, and texture, heat, hardness and softness, contact, inside and outside, and so on).... *'If you find as we do this, that you notice that*

---

some areas don't have much sensation, then seeing if you can explore what 'not much sensation' feels like…………..remembering we are just practising being aware and whatever you notice is fine………..When you are ready, turning to the breath again, and imagining that you can breathe in a different way – bringing the breath all the way down the left side of the body, through the left leg, into the left foot and the left toes, as you are if breathing into the foot and then breathing out from the foot, up through the body and out through the nose. It is as if we are using the breath as a vehicle for our awareness………..On the next out breath, letting go of this focus on the breath and the left foot, and moving up through the ankle to the left lower leg'……(repeating this process through all the different sections of the body – sometimes widening the beam of attention to take in the whole of a limb or the whole of the trunk of the body)…… *'If at any point you notice that your mind has wandered into thinking, or has been distracted by something such as a sound, simply noticing where the mind has got to, and gently and kindly bringing your focus back to wherever we have got to in the body…………………If at any point, we come to an area that holds pain, or discomfort or difficult feelings for you, seeing if it is possible to pause…….perhaps bringing the breath gently down into and around the area, and breathing into it and breathing out from it with kindness and sensitivity……..not trying to change it, but simply to offer this area some kindly attention…..noticing if the mind moves into thoughts about it, and if it does, seeing if you can simply come back to the sensations in the body, wherever you are choosing to focus……* .(continuing through the body, guiding to awareness of sensations in different parts of the body – being especially sensitive, full of care and gentle within the guiding, when getting near to any area that has been affected by cancer, for anyone in the group – ie: breast area, pelvic area for gynaecological, prostrate and testicular cancer, lungs, sternum for oesophageal cancer, stomach, brain and so on)………. *As we come to the end of this practice, expanding into a sense of the body as a whole lying here……….and coming to the breath, breathing into and out from the whole of the body…………………*

Now, if you would like to, gently turning towards any part of your body that has experienced treatment or injury – or feels tender or painful at the moment. Inviting you to bring gentleness and kindness to this part – breathing into it gently, if this feels ok, and opening to any sensations that are present there…………………………………now, when you are ready, coming back to the whole of the body again, bringing any awareness of tenderness into a sense of the whole body'.

As the practice finishes, we invite people to slowly and gently get up, taking time to move, being aware of the body, as we transition slowly back into sitting in a circle.

Body Scan inquiry

We lead a short inquiry following the practice. We will explore things in much more detail in Week 2.

Story

I never promised you a rose garden

If there is time, this may be a good moment to read a story. We often use 'I never promised you a rose garden' here. It is from *Kitchen Table Wisdom* (Remen, 1996).

Week One Short Practice

The Pause

We then guide a simple 'Pause' (Brach, 2003). Practising stopping and coming to awareness of 'What is going on for me at the moment?' or 'How am I now?' reminds us to come back and simply notice. The Pause is part of the home practice for this week (see Chapter 7, The Practices – Short Practices)

Concluding the Session

Home Practice – Week One

Core practice
- **Body Scan** (30) every day

Short practice
- **The Pause** – several times a day

Informal practice
- **Routine Activity** – choosing something that you do every day (like teeth cleaning, having a shower, getting dressed, washing up etc) and doing it mindfully as we did with the raisin
- **Mindful Eating** – eat one meal mindfully

We give out CD 1 and encourage participants not to read past Week 1 in their workbooks – a temptation. There is a discussion around this week's home practice. The mixture of Body Scan practice, short practice of The Pause and informal practices can seem quite a lot. We encourage participants to settle in to finding ways of practising every day. If the questionnaires (Time 1 measures) given out at the orientation meetings have not yet been handed in, this is the moment to ask for them.

Concluding

The Bells

We close the session with the sound of the bells. (Many of us who teach mindfulness use little bells, or a singing bowl, as a way of closing a practice or concluding a session. They naturally invite us into the present moment to hear the sound.) We acknowledge. We then 'come to the breath' experiencing it within the body and the important start that we have made and the significance of the journey we are undertaking together.

Programme

Week 1: Automatic Pilot

Session timing: 2 ½ hours

Welcome: • Brief outline of session	[5 minutes]
Ground Rules: • Confidentiality • Choosing own level of participation	[5 minutes]
Brief **Grounding Exercise**: • Feet on the floor	[5 minutes]
Introductions (brief) (maybe in pairs first): • Name • What has brought me here? • What do I want from the course?	[10 minutes]
Action Methods Community Building Exercise:	[10 minutes]
Intentions Pebble Practice: • What has drawn me to this course? • What do I most wish for myself from this course?' and • What is my intention for myself? • Sharing in new pairs – then large group (brief)	[10 minutes] [10 minutes]
Personal Intentions Letter and form sealed in envelope: • Opened in Week 8 • For their eyes only	[10 minutes]
Raisin Exercise and Dialogue:	[20 minutes]
Mindfulness Definition and Discussion: • What were the 'particular ways' that we tasted the raisin?	[10 minutes]
Poem: • Using river metaphor (Rilke, 1996) to explore cancer journey and the role of mindfulness	[10 minutes]

Body Scan and Inquiry (brief): [30 minutes]
Story – Maybe '*I never promised you a rose garden*'

Guide **The Pause**: [5 minutes]

Workbooks and CD1: [5 minutes]
• Handed out and brief overview of workbook
• Collect Time 1 measures if not already handed in
• Week 1 home practice

Bells and the Breath to Close: [5 minutes]
• The bells
• Coming to Breath

Home Practice	• Body Scan	• The Pause
	• Routine activity	• Eating one meal mindfully

Handouts   Intentions form / letter
Workbooks
CD1s

Resources   Envelopes and large foolscap envelope with sticky
     tape
Raisins in bowl with spoon
Kitchen Table Wisdom (Remen, 1996)
Workbooks
Body Scan CDs
Bells
Mats

© T. Bartley (2012). Mindfulness-Based Cognitive Therapy for Cancer.

Rush Hour

The road is full of traffic
Hurtling onwards
Swapping lanes without signalling,
Changing gear, braking, swerving, accelerating,
Rushing onwards, building tension
In ruthless anxiety to get somewhere else.

Pull off the highway
And park.
Lean safely over the parapet and just watch.
The vehicles thunder past;
Heavy laden lorries;
Zipping sports cars;
Zig-zagging white vans;
Jam packed buses and coaches.

Let them all go by
To their own invisible destinations.

Be still.
Feel.
The sunshine on your face;
The coquettish breeze ruffling your hair;
The murmur of insects busy in the grass.
Savour the smell of dewy moss along the verge;
Relish each season's subtle taste.

Breathe in healing delight.
Only breathe.

Pauline Kenyon (March, 2006)

Week Two

The basic approach to understanding the mind is a process of gradually making friends with oneself.

(Chögyam Trungpa, 1981)

Dealing with Barriers

Core theme:

Noticing the wandering of the mind and learning to come back.

We discover thoughts and judgements just beneath the surface of awareness, but influencing everything. Practising coming back to *this* moment, we learn to be more present and aware – and start to cultivate kindness, curiosity and gentleness towards our experience.

Key Tasks for Teachers – Week Two

Week 2 practice:

- Body Scan and inquiry
- Setting up intention for the practice and the session
- Emphasizing gentleness and kindness in the practice and throughout the session
- Gently turning towards and including areas of treatment or pain

Home practice review:

- Body Scan; routine activity; the pause; mindful eating
- Reflecting on how it was to do the practice

Building the community:

- Continuing to invest in building trust

Week 2 exercise:

- 'Walking down the street' – thoughts and feelings
- The Blob – learning how to map the experience

Week 2 short practices:

- Coming to the Breath
- Reviewing the Pause

Concluding:

- Week two home practice
- Ending – the bells and closing intention

Introduction

Arriving

The start of the second week has a different feel to the first. People have been talking together as they wait. There is a tentative sense of belonging and of being engaged in the same process.

Week Two Practice

Body Scan

Duration: 35 minutes

- Intention for this class.
- Gently turning towards areas of treatment or pain.

The mats are ready on the floor. It is tempting to extend the conversations, but now we start each session with a practice, coming into direct experience of the present as best we can. If anyone is late, there is a place for them near the door.

After a short settling at the start of the practice, we bring awareness to intention. Reconnecting with what we most wish for ourselves, whether it be wellbeing, happiness, balance of mind, health, or whatever comes to mind – inviting us all to remember that intention lies in the heart, we rest there for a moment.

As teachers, we want to make gentleness and kindness explicit in this second Body Scan. This seems especially important for cancer patients. In the first week, we established the basic form of the practice. In this second practice, we have opportunity to touch into sensitive places, inviting kindness and tenderness in on the breath, especially to areas that have experienced treatment or surgery – or have been damaged or injured – or feel discomfort or pain. We may have introduced this in the first week, if it seemed appropriate, but we make a point of doing this now. We are beginning to turn towards and include what is difficult, always with much gentleness – inviting each participant only to do what feels right for them.

'It was nice this week', said Lucy at the end of the Body Scan. She looked a bit surprised. Lucy's face always seemed a little dwarfed by her wig. Her hair had not grown back since treatment and this upset her a good deal. She had been very anxious at her last check up and her consultant had suggested she attend the course.

'It was really horrible last week, when you told us to breathe into the place where we had had treatment. I really hated it', she said with emphasis. 'What did you experience this time?' asked the teacher. 'I'm not sure', Lucy said. She looked pensive. 'There wasn't much there to feel. It just felt ok to try. I think I've always tried to ignore it before', she said, her hand motioning towards her left breast. 'But it felt ok today' she said with a smile.

Dialogue after the Body Scan

Last week's inquiry may have been quite brief. This week we have time to go into things more deeply.

It is interesting to notice how difficult it can be to explore detailed sensations. Participants are not used to talking in this way. Many of them have avoided connecting with their bodies since diagnosis and maybe much longer. Some want to list what went wrong for them, and then move straight into talking about the home practice. Most of them are very keen to hear how other people got on last week. Staying on track with *this* practice as best we can, we invite group members to share their experience.

Liking/not liking

They describe many reactions. Sleep is inevitably an issue, especially for those who are exhausted and still experiencing side effects from treatment. Some people are worried about snoring. Others know that they drifted in and out of the practice.

Christine seemed frustrated. 'When I close my eyes I instantly fall asleep. When I keep them open, I am focused on what I am seeing. I need to close my eyes to tune in, but if I do, I go to sleep. At home I need to do the Body Scan when I am likely to stay awake, but there is no good time to do it because I am so busy and have so much to do'.

How to respond? It is so tempting to seek solutions.

Some participants report feeling relaxed and at ease. With a happy smile, they describe how lovely to it is to settle into the practice, and how calming they found the teacher's voice.

Why is relaxation not a desired outcome? It is not wrong. Feeling relaxed offers much benefit, especially for people who are anxious and facing uncertainty. However, when there is a goal – any goal – other possibilities are blocked out. This reduces the opportunity of being with the experience, whatever it is, pleasant or unpleasant.

> Carol said her whole experience of the Body Scan was very positive. She loved feeling so relaxed. 'It was a wonderful practice', she said. 'All I had to do was control my mind when something came up. I just said 'none of that' to my mind', putting her hand in the air like a stop sign, 'and it worked beautifully', she said, looking very pleased.

So much comes up when we explore Body Scan. Until we get interested in learning how to practise with curiosity and interest (whatever the experience), we probably only want to experience what is pleasant and push away what is unpleasant.

Some participants have problems lying on the floor. It may become uncomfortable for them for a variety of reasons. They may move into intense longing for the end of the practice.

> Susan tended to be quite direct in her comments. She had felt strung out since finishing treatment. She admitted to being pretty sceptical about mindfulness, but was willing to give it a go.
>
> 'I was determined to keep doing it this week' she said. 'But it was SO boring. I was fighting myself to stay put – and I felt desperate to get up and DO something – anything rather than that awful Body Scan', she announced, slightly playing up to others in the group.

'How did you manage to keep going?' asked the teacher, feeling a bit concerned but curious to hear more.

'That was what was interesting. I actually nearly enjoyed two of them!' she said, sounding surprised. 'And then after one that was almost nice, the next one was awful. I realized that I just had to keep going, however it was. I'm quite pleased that I did – and somehow I feel the benefit, although I can't tell you what it is'.

Wanting answers

At this stage, there is not much 'language' to draw on. Participants often find it difficult to describe sensations and 'nice' doesn't go very far. In some ways, things are easier than the first week. There is at least some emerging knowing of what to expect. However, confusion is lurking.

This is when questions may arise – such as 'Why are we doing the Body Scan?' Explanations are sought. Some participants express frustration at not understanding the purpose. They especially want to know how to do it correctly. It is frustrating to be told that 'there is no right or wrong way'. This is no help!

At times like these, teachers and participants alike may all feel a bit unsure. It would be so good to fall back onto solid ground. 'Do this' or 'aim for that' becomes rather seductive. In a parallel process with the group's quest for answers – it is easy for a teacher to fall into the trap of offering them. This keeps us in the role of the one who knows, which may be reassuring, but is not ultimately helpful.

Can we model the richness of the practice, by staying with the experience in the body and acknowledging frustration? Is it possible to invite 'not knowing' into the room? – realizing how challenging this is, especially for people with cancer. Noticing the fear of being with what is difficult, and gently staying with it for a moment or two – then guiding a pause, a brief grounding or coming to the breath might be great practice. Would that we could always remember!

A Mindfulness Teacher's Journal – Week 2

Sitting this morning, I know there is wisdom in the way things unfold. I can trust the process. Remember this.

Last night at the end of the class, I felt dissatisfied. It hadn't quite come together. Something was missing. L spoke for everyone in describing uncertainty. She wanted to know how to breathe. She felt she was breathing wrong. Others joined in to rescue her. (Good omen for how the group will develop – early touch of 'storming' in the group.)

On my way home, the familiar critical voice appeared. A certain stretch of road:

'Ah there you are'.

'It would have been better if you had shut up and dropped into what she was feeling'.

'Yes'.

An ache of regret, the urge to analyze....

And then this morning, on my cushion, the pattern showed itself – the parallel process. Every one of us in the group is the same. We all want to get it right – including me – especially me! We all judge ourselves when we don't. Living with uncertainty and self blame is hard – especially for cancer patients. No wonder we want to shore things up.

Trusting the wisdom of an imperfect process – it is not just me that teaches. Thank goodness!

Home Practice Review

At some point, we shift focus back to last week's home practice.

Wandering mind

Dealing with Barriers – the theme of the week – highlights the central focus of the session. Everyone will have noticed that their mind wandered during Body Scan practices. There may even be the beginnings of recognizing

---

familiar reactions. As we introduce dimensions of mind for the first time, it is easy to get over complicated and jump ahead to later themes.

All minds wander. It is what they do. It is not a problem. Noticing and coming back to wherever we have got to in the body. Staying fairly simple and straightforward seems helpful in week two.

Starting to highlight the way the mind wanders into judging – as a group it may be possible to identify automatic patterns of thoughts that comment:

This is good/not so good/bad/worse than
This is pleasant/unpleasant/awful
I should be doing it this way
I have got it wrong
If I do it like this, it will work out better
I want it like it was yesterday
I want it to go quicker/stop
I want it different

> Melanie was keen to come on the course. Unusually in an oncology group, she was eager to learn to meditate. She had just finished treatment for breast cancer. Her husband had also been ill during this period and she had cared for him, even whilst receiving chemotherapy. She wanted to find some time for herself.
>
> 'On Tuesday, the day after the class, it was so good' she said. 'I stayed awake all the way through and I felt so clear and refreshed at the end. Then I had to miss Wednesday and when I did it on Thursday, I was sleepy all the time. I was so disappointed. I felt as if I had got it wrong and it had done me less good'.

Self-blame is a strong tendency in those who have had cancer. Many people feel responsible for their illness, even though they know that the causes of cancer are varied and not always understood. This may be the first time that participants have become aware of all the negative thoughts bubbling in the mind. The Body Scan slows us down. We begin to recognize how much we judge and blame – how we push away and are at the mercy of thoughts.

> Thoughts can be our best friends and our worst enemies…(they) rise up as enemies. They stampede through our mind in droves, each one creating its own little drama of ever-increasing confusion. (Ricard, 2003)

Physical challenges

The Body Scan also highlights sensations in the body caused by treatment. Numbness and aching joints are common after chemotherapy. Tenderness results from radiotherapy burns. It is a challenge to move up close to these sensations, when the mind is judging and aversive. However, this is the invitation, to see if it is possible to bring gentle curiosity even to pain.

Strangely, pain can almost be easier to explore than numbness, which seems like a blank or a gap. This can be quite distressing – an echo of emptiness. It is almost like a little death – a nameless fear.

Some participants have active cancer. Others fear that cancer has returned. They may feel pain or discomfort in an area, which they know (or think they know) holds a tumour. It takes considerable courage to be willing to visit these areas. The mind may constantly and vigilantly scan and compare, but this is not the same as choosing to dwell there, moving up close, or working round the edges of an area to explore how it feels.

For some it may be too soon. It may be better, perhaps, to pause and gently acknowledge distress, than get busy inquiring after specific sensations – although there is certainly a place for detailed exploration, if a participant is ready to go there.

Kindness and gentleness is powerful medicine. Participants learn this quickly – especially if, as teachers, we can stay grounded and embodied in our own experience whilst still open and connected to theirs. When we tenderly attend to the felt sense within – we can be guided wisely.

Building the Community

Home practice review – small group process

As we are in the early days of the group, we include some discussing in small groups to build trust in the group.

Inviting participants to join with new people, they gather in groups of threes or fours to share last week's experience of routine activities, The Pause and eating a meal mindfully. After a few minutes, we invite them to share small 'nuggets' from their discussions in the large group. It is reassuring to hear others' experiences, especially if they are similar to our own.

After this, participants move into a pair with someone they do not know to look at how it was to do the home practice. What was it like? What helped? How did you get on? Supporting each other to reflect and learn from their experience seems to help them reconnect with intention to practice, no matter what.

As teachers, we know the importance of discussing each participants home practice each week. When we fail to manage this, the group are less likely to complete it.

Week Two Exercise

Thoughts and Feelings Exercise

Walking down the street

- Processing the thoughts, feelings and body sensations that result for participants.
- Writing them in columns on the white board.
- Teasing out the cognitive model and the learning – through discussion.

This exercise by Segal et al., 2002 illustrates the links between thoughts and feelings and body sensations. It shows that the way we interpret an event directly affects how we feel about it – and how it then influences experience (Segal et al., 2002).

It is valuable to keep the scene setting succinct and to the point. Inviting participants to close their eyes, if they are comfortable to do so, we outline the scene:

You are walking down a familiar street. You see a friend on the other side of the road, going in the opposite direction. You try to attract their attention but they don't seem to notice you and continue walking.

There are a number of ways to facilitate this. One is to first ask about the feelings that are present as a result of the scenario. We list these on the whiteboard and then go through them, one by one, asking what happened in each. As the different stories emerge, they are recorded beside the feelings that they relate to.

Here are some examples:

Feelings	Interpretations/Thought
Annoyed	I didn't shout loudly enough/he didn't hear me
Worried	Something might be wrong/she didn't see me
Disappointed	It would have been lovely to talk/she didn't see me
Hurt	What have I done?/I think she was avoiding me
Embarrassed	I must have looked stupid/waving and not being seen

On completion of the scenario, Jennifer immediately called out, 'Well bugger her, I say' and was then rather embarrassed by what she had said. The rest of the group laughed, but she was still engaged in the experience. 'This happened to me', she explained. 'It was the first time I went out with my wig on. I was walking down my town shopping street when I saw my friend. She completely ignored me. I still can't forgive her'.

As the stories emerge, it becomes clear that what we think happened dictates how we feel about it – and this directly impacts on our mood. Indeed it may influence how we feel for a long time, as it did with Jennifer. Equally a pre-existing mood may influence things too. Already feeling low or anxious, we may interpret an event very pessimistically. Yet, we see what we feel, or what we think, as entirely factual, never questioning it unless we learn to.

Sitting waiting for results in clinic, your doctor walks past without greeting you. What might you think?

Asking the group directly (without setting it up as a scenario), they make the link straight away. They immediately say that they would assume that the doctor had bad news for them – and as a result would feel even more anxious. By uncovering the story that lies beneath the situation (that the doctor had bad news), we are able to see 'the stream of thoughts present all the time, just under the surface of which we are not aware'(Segal et al., 2002). It happens so quickly and in no time we are leaping to conclusions and feeling overwhelmed.

The Blob – mapping the experience

Awareness of the way that we interpret events – helps us to begin to disentangle things. The Blob aids this process.

The Blob

Using an example from the previous exercise, we map out the experience on the white board, using the circles of the Blob, to show the way thoughts, feelings and body sensations interrelate and interconnect.

In Williams' 2007, *A Mindful Way through Depression,* John Teasdale teaches about the 'big black blob of experience', he and others write about an undifferentiated 'bad thing', which threatens to overwhelm (Williams et al., 2007). Out of this, we developed a Blob, which rather than threatening to overwhelm, offers us an opportunity to map the separate dimensions within the experience and how they interrelate. Here is how we can do it:

The Blob

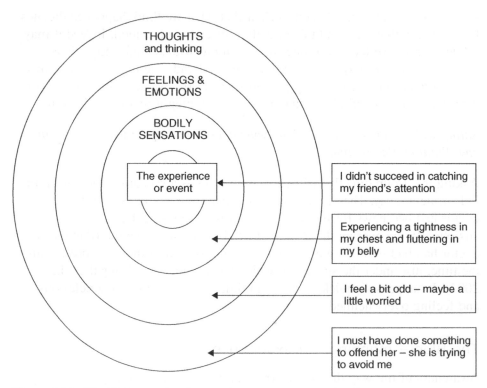

Figure 6.2.1 The Blob, mapping the experience.

The First Ring – invites a noticing and acknowledging of physical sensations. This circle comes first after the event or experience, highlighting the significance of the body and the practice of bringing attention directly to physical sensations. This is the first time that we bring physical sensations into 'Walking Down the Street' exercise.

The Second Ring – identifies the feeling tone within the experience. This might involve a specific emotion or feeling, or just a vague sense of something that is pleasant, unpleasant or neither.

The Third Ring – draws out the thoughts, interpretations or stories we are telling ourselves about the event or experience.

Later we can include a fourth circle that relates to actions and behaviour.

The rather ridiculous name of The Blob offers us a way of adopting a fairly light hearted approach. It is easy to get 'over serious' about the difficult or the unpleasant.

Some participants take to the blob enthusiastically. It lends itself to those of us who tend to analyse experience. Participants later report 'I blobbed it!' when referring to the way they responded to a difficult event.

Mapping the experience

Many people find it difficult to distinguish thoughts from feelings. The blob can help them to do this. It shows the interconnection, and the way the resonance of feelings in the body produces sensations that we can notice directly. We are starting to champion the body and the value of attending to what is going on in there.

The layers of The Blob also help us to be aware of the ways that we add 'extra'. It is like a snowball that with perfect conditions gets bigger and bigger as it rolls along, adding more and more to the original small beginning.

Another useful metaphor is that of a telephone exchange, overflowing with different coloured wires. Seen from the outside, it looks like a gigantic mess. Knowing how to identify the different coloured wires and their patterns, phone engineers can make sense of the whole thing. In the same way, once we learn how to recognize the different dimensions of our experience, (thoughts, feelings and physical sensations), we can start to disentangle ourselves from familiar patterns. We may learn to be able to change the way we relate to events and free ourselves from the expanding snowball that threatens to overwhelm.

In the workbook that was given out on the first week, there is a blob drawn. The Blob is used to record pleasant experiences in the home practice this week. Participants are encouraged to learn how to draw their own, so they can use them in any situation

A poem

If there is time, we might read a poem here. *The Summer Day* by Mary Oliver is very appropriate. Later in the course, we will look at the ways that the experience of getting cancer might offer significance to our lives. Asking what we might do with our 'one wild and precious life' is an opportunity to plant this seed. It resonates with an intuitive sense of validity and inspiration and may also bring feelings of sadness for those who know that their lifespan is limited.

Week Two Short Practice

Coming to the Breath

We now lead a very simple breath practice (instead of 'Mindfulness of Breathing as in MBSR and MBCT). Calling it 'Coming to the Breath, (see chapter 7, the Practices – Short Practices. It also forms the second of the Thread exercises in Chapter 7) we keep it very simple as we guide it. We make a deliberate choice not to get into specifics as to where the breath might be felt. Instead, there is an invitation to simply notice the breath and bring awareness to it.

Some participants have difficulty with the breath. People with lung cancer may struggle to bring attention to their breathing. Now is not an ideal time to get into detailed inquiry, but if a straightforward approach is not enough, we can propose looking at this more thoroughly at the next session or one to one over the phone during the week.

Reviewing the Pause

We guide a pause at some point during the class. It is a good reminder for those who may have forgotten to do it. It confirms the practice to those beginning to bring it into their lives; and it is helpful for us all, especially during times of intensity. With this simple practice, we learn to interrupt automatic ways of reacting, and embed a value in stopping, remembering and simply coming back to the present moment. That is all that is involved.

Story

The jigsaw puzzle

'The Jigsaw Puzzle' from *Kitchen Table Wisdom* (Remen, 1996) tells about a young girl who found the dark pieces in a jigsaw puzzle very scary. So she hid them. Only later when they are recovered and the puzzle is completed, does she realize that they are part of a lovely scene and that the dark pieces are needed to complete the picture. The tale offers another opportunity to acknowledge the context that we are working within. Without reminders of 'the dark pieces' tucked into the process, it can be possible to teach MBCT-Ca to cancer patients and never mention cancer. By finding sensitive ways of turning towards the issues that have brought people to the course, there is opportunity to allow the practice to touch into where we most need it.

Jonathan was in remission when he joined the course. He had just finished treatment, but had been told that he probably only had a few months to live. He was a serious and quietly spoken man, who seemed quietly intrigued by the course. He was sitting next to the teacher as she read the jigsaw story. As she got to the end, she looked up at him sensing his deep engagement.

'I like that story', he said quietly. Jonathan's comment stayed with her. His own life had proved to have some very dark pieces. Would this story help him find a connection to 'something larger?' (Remen, 1996).

Concluding the Session

Endings

As we come to the end of the session, we may want to gather the learning that has emerged. We have covered a fair amount of ground and introduced some new ideas that will take time and practice to integrate.

Summarizing the theme of the week, it is possible to illustrate the way that thoughts can often lie just beneath the surface of awareness – and yet influence the mood and much of what we do. We remind the group that we are inviting a gentle and patient approach to the mind, however many times we wander and wherever we go. We are learning to be tender and kindly with ourselves.

Home Practice – Week Two

Core practice

- **Body Scan** (30) every day

Short practice

- **Coming to the Breath** – several times a day
- **The Pause** – several times a day

Informal practice

- **A new routine activity** – (like teeth cleaning, having a shower, getting dressed, washing up etc) and do it mindfully as we did with the raisin

Exercise

- **Pleasant Experience** (see workbook) – using the Blob

Turning to the workbooks, we review the home practice. Much of it is similar to last week with a daily Body Scan; the Pause and choosing a new daily routine activity to do mindfully. Coming to the Breath is added, linked to a Pause, or on its own, several times a day. We also ask participants to notice a pleasant experience each day, using the blob to record it in detail.

We hand out some coloured dots that can be stuck to things such as the phone, computer, or mirror to remind us to come back and be present.

Concluding

The Bells

At the end, we ring the bells and come back to the breath, with awareness of the body sitting here. Settling into the moment, we bring our intentions to mind and connect with an appreciation for the courage, commitment and learning that we have contributed to the session.

Programme

Week 2: Dealing with Barriers

Session timing: 2 ½ hours

Body Scan: [35 minutes]
- (Intention for this class at start as lie on floor with breath)
- Gentleness key – breathing into areas of treatment or injury

Dialogue: [30 minutes]
- Inquire into the Body Scan just practised
- Then back through the week's Body Scan home practices
- Including The Pause

Review Routine Activities: [10 minutes]
- Eating a meal mindfully in **small groups** of 3Fs
Brief feedback into the large group

Moving into **Pairs discussion**: [10 minutes]
- What was it like getting down to practising?
  Large group feedback (very brief)

Walking Down the Street: [15 minutes]
- Flip feelings and interpretations of event
- ABC model of emotional distress
  (A) a situation happens
  (C) resulting in a feeling which we are usually aware of
  (B) but there are also thoughts and interpretations in
      there, often just under our awareness. C = A + B

Teach **The Blob**: [10 minutes]
- As a snowball
- Use for pleasant experience home practice

Poem: [5 minutes]
- *The Summer Day* by Mary Oliver

Week 2 Teaching if not already covered: [5 minutes]
- Discovering that the mind wanders much of the time
  – back into the past, forward into the future, often
  influencing us just under the surface of our awareness
- Judgement and blame often there
- Coming back with *gentleness and patience*, however many
  times the mind wanders

Guide **Coming to the Breath** short practice: [5 minutes]

Story: [5 minutes]
- *Kitchen Table Wisdom* (Remen, 1996)

Week 2 Home Practice: [5 minutes]
- Give out sticky dots

Coming to the Breath: [5 minutes]
- Closing intention
- The bells

Home Practice	• Body Scan	• Coming to the Breath
	• Pleasant Experience Blobs	• The Pause
	• Routine activity	
Handouts		
Resources	*Kitchen Table Wisdom* (Remen,1996) or story book	
	The Summer Day poem	
	Sticky dots for reminders	
	Bells	

© T. Bartley (2012). Mindfulness-Based Cognitive Therapy for Cancer.

Mooring (in the here and now)

The anchor slips into sand
And I drift slowly
At first not noticing
Away from the place I chose

Pull it up and start again
And it settles among the rocks
I stay where I am
My body is my spirit's boat.

Sometimes in my hurry I set off without an anchor
I can't stop anywhere until I go back and fetch it.

Ann (December 2005)

Week Three

It's not the perfect but the imperfect that is most in need of our love.

(Oscar Wilde, 2001[1893])

Befriending the Breath and the Body in Movement

Core theme:

Learning to work with personal edges and limits, by practising with courage, gentleness and sensitivity – and returning to the anchor of the breath in the body, whenever we need to.

Key Tasks for Teachers – Week Three

Week 3 core practice(s):

- Mindful movement and inquiry
- Setting up intention for the practice and the session
- Emphasizing gentleness and kindness within the practice and throughout the session – noticing how choices are made, when close to edges or limits.
- Sitting practice (if time)
- Introduce briefly

Home practice review:

- Body Scan; routine activity; the Pause; Coming to the Breath

Building the community:

- Continuing to invest in the group process

Week 3 exercise:

- Pleasant experience diary
- Using the Blob to map the experience and draw out learning, emphasizing awareness of bodily sensations

Week 3 short practices:

- Three Minute Breathing Space (Regular)
- Reviewing the Pause and Coming to the Breath

Concluding:

- Week three home practice
- Ending – the bells and closing intention

Introduction

We engage in a lot of practice in Week Three. The title of the week: 'Befriending the Breath and the Body in Movement' speaks to the learning and focus of the session. After the participants come into the room, we move straight into our first practice

Week Three Practice

The mats are out on the floor and we all move straight into standing on a mat after removing shoes and parking belongings. There are chairs around the outside of the room for use at any point during the practice. Participants are encouraged to use them at any time or all of the time. We invite anyone who has pain, mobility problems, or might find it hard to stand for any length of time, to sit in 'mountain' posture on a chair and adapt the movements and postures from the chair. At any point, they are free close their eyes and visualize the movements.

We start by guiding awareness through the body, briefly scanning from the soles of the feet and contact with the ground, up through to the crown of the head. If it is alright for them, participants stand in this 'mountain' posture as they hear the introduction to the practice. Many participants enjoy standing in 'mountain'. It offers a strong experience of grounded and dignified presence. Some adapt it into a core practice and continue to use it long after the course has finished. However, it is important not to leave them standing for too long.

Mindful Movement Practice

Duration: 30 minutes

Let us start this practice by coming into a standing posture.....with awareness of your feet on the floor...whilst keeping the knees quite soft, not locked.....and connecting with the spine rising up through the body. Standing like a mountain, rooted and tall......and as we move into some stretches that I will guide, knowing that in every moment, it is important for you to make choices – perhaps to sit down, perhaps to move, encouraging you all to bring mindful awareness to the way you move

---

into and hold the stretches. Working in each moment with what is best for you and your body, taking care not to 'push through' or do more than is wise, and bringing a gentle and kindly awareness to the body and what is possible for you in this moment.....Now, coming back to your standing posture, if this is alright for you, and bringing awareness to the contact of your feet on the floor... weight of you going down... feeling the solid of the ground beneath you...fully arriving in your feet on the floor........then becoming aware of the spine rising up out of the pelvis... up through the middle of the back... up into the shoulders balanced either side of the spine...on through the neck...and up to the very top of the back of the crown of the head......height going up....weight going down......both grounded and tall.......standing with the dignity of a mountain, rooted to the earth, rising up into the sky.....fully present. Now bringing awareness to the body as a whole and moving in whatever way your body would like to move.......easing out any places that are complaining, having stood for this time.

Note: Please refer to Chapter 7. The Practices – Core Practices section, for guidance around adapting Mindful Movement practice for people with cancer.

We then guide the group into some gentle stretches, encouraging them to be present with their experience by:

- Dwelling for a moment at the edges of intensity to explore their personal limits.
- Returning to the 'mountain' after the movements to feel the effects on the body.
- Bringing presence and kindness into the practice.
- Becoming aware of areas of pain/surgery/treatment.
- Cultivating courage and gentleness towards all experience.
- Learning to befriend the body in movement.

Up to the start of the course, many participants may not have consciously noticed sensations in parts of their body where they have had treatment. It is very common to hear surprise from participants after the practice. 'I had no idea it felt like that. I have never gone there before'. This may already be emerging from the Body Scan practice. However, mindful movement 'builds on the work of refining bodily awareness' (Williams et al., 2007), bringing intensity and dynamic into the process, which increases awareness of sensations and highlights limits.

Dialogue

The inquiry process that follows the practice often brings out examples of both the pleasure and the pain in the practice. Participants may comment on how much easier it is to 'control' the mind with mindful movement than with Body Scan. Teasing this out, it is apparent that the mind has more to engage it within dynamic movement. Some participants who have persistent unpleasant thoughts or background sensations may well find that the mind wanders less. This can surprise those who have been seriously ill.

'I really enjoyed that', said Bill, after we finished. Last week, he had confirmation that his cancer was on the move again, 'it was really good!' He looked unusually energized and bright.

'What was good?' asked the teacher, 'What were you aware of in the body?'

'The absence of pain in my back I suppose' he said, 'there was a warmth there instead, and almost an ease. I found I could do it all, which really pleased me. When we started, I imagined it was going to be really difficult, but I found I could move into the intensity and feel it. I really enjoyed the strong sensations in my body and almost feel more alive now'.

We are practicing new language this week. There is more obvious detail to explore within sensations. This seems to offer more opportunity to describe and be curious about the 'colours' and textures that are there.

For others the experience of the practice can be tough, especially when compared to what they used to be able to do.

Linda looked upset. She had been experiencing ongoing discomfort in her bones for some weeks.

'I nearly cried' she said, 'I started off ok, but I couldn't hold the positions for as long as everyone else. My mind went straight back to when I could have done it and I started feeling more and more upset. I kept hearing you encouraging me to be gentle. This was helpful. I pushed the tears away and lay down and just visualized the stretches in the way you told me to'. She was looking a little more settled as her story unfolded.

'How was it to lie down?' asked the teacher.

'It was ok. I realize now that it takes courage to be gentle. It is not easy. All my life, I think I've pushed through. Stopping and being gentle was quite difficult. It was quite an achievement for me. I'm pleased that I did'.

Later in the session, as the movement CD was handed out, Linda said that she was looking forward to trying the practice at home. 'I bet I can do quite a bit of it, if I take it really gently'.

Others find they struggle with the comparative ease of the practice. People who attend regular yoga classes may dislike the different emphasis and yearn for their usual routine. A commentary may trundle in the background, which includes criticism and wanting, How to work with that?

As teachers, exploring the jumble of experience with participants as best we can, we might acknowledge the almost universal wish for things to be different. We may notice, within ourselves as teachers, how much easier it is to be open with a participant who describes a sense of achievement, than with someone who struggles with the way the practice was guided! In every moment, there is a feeling of liking, disliking, or a gap, which holds no particular reaction. We go straight from moving towards an experience ('ah chocolate cake!') to wanting more of it ('I'd like a second piece'). We go from pulling away from experience ('oh, pain in my back') to wanting it to go away ('if only it wasn't there') – and wanting it to be different.

In the inquiry, there are opportunities to make links between the way we made choices within the practice and the ways we make choices in our lives. Can we cultivate tenderness for the body when we are experiencing intense feelings? Can we start learning to be with strong experience and not immediately pull away? Can we find within us the courage to be gentle?

Last Week's Home Practice

The Body Scan

This is the second week of the Body Scan practice. There is some growing familiarity. Patterns may be emerging.

Participants may be more used to the length of the practice. Some people find that the mind is beginning to settle a little more easily, on some days at least. Others find they are more able to stay awake. With any luck, there is a building routine of doing it, perhaps at a certain time in a specific place. Those who are diligently practicing show themselves at this stage.

Some participants may still feel resistant towards the Body Scan. It can be helpful to explore and affirm the ways that they are managing to stay with the practice, even if only for a few minutes at a time. Paradoxically, those who actively loathe it but persevere, come what may, often do better than those who love it from the first moment. In some ways, we expect this. Those who are challenged but hang on in there, are learning to be with the difficult, a central theme of the course.

Maureen had had a very difficult cancer journey. She said she was anxious even before she was ill. Now she has found it difficult to adjust back to life after treatment. She often felt acutely agitated. She struggled with the Body Scan from the very first time, keeping her eyes fixedly open, and looking quite tense.

'I just had to turn off the CD on Wednesday' said Maureen, 'I could feel myself slipping into this awful black hole. I couldn't bear it. I stopped about two thirds of the way through. After that, I felt really grim for a while, but I managed to get out to my daughters Sports Day and to my surprise, I enjoyed it'.

'What happened the next day?' I asked

'I managed to finish it ok', said Maureen.

Those who find the Body Scan wonderfully relaxing may get much benefit from feeling more relaxed, but are unlikely to learn much about moving up close to what is difficult.

The message of 'just doing it' even if you like it – even if you loathe it – is worth repeating.

As teacher, there will be many invitations to comment on the experience of the participants.

Kenneth said that he had had a tough week. He had felt distressed and upset during his practice. 'I parked it in a box', he said, 'and just got back into my practice'. 'Was that right?' he asked.

Embodying kindness and acceptance seems to be the most helpful response for participants. Acknowledging the experience and reflecting back what has been said, can often be more helpful than delving into the detail, especially if as teachers, we sense an agenda lurking within us.

Participants may find that they are beginning to feel the benefit of dwelling in the body. Jon Kabat-Zinn famously says that there is more right with us than wrong (Kabat-Zinn, 1990). This is very relevant for cancer patients. Knowing this from experience can have quite an impact for participants.

Coming to the Breath

Many of the group find they are enjoying coming to the breath, even if at first they may have felt a bit self conscious.

When she met with me before the course started, Mary described feeling alone and anxious. She didn't share much in the class, so it was difficult to know how she was getting on.

After practising 'Coming to the Breath' for a few weeks, Mary quietly volunteered that she had discovered that her breath was very close to her.

'I almost don't have to remember it', she said. 'It is just there to turn to whenever I need it'. As she said this, she put her hand down close beside her, at the level of her waist. 'It is my best friend, I think', she said smiling a little shyly.

This demonstrates the way that different practices can be integrated into everyday life, and become essentially personal.

Some people find it harder to remember the short practices than the long ones. 'Life seems to overtake me' said Julie 'I am so busy that the day just flashes by, and I find that yet again I've not stopped to pause once'.

Sticky coloured dots given out last week can help, but it often takes time and persistence to build up sufficient momentum to remember to interrupt the busyness.

Small groups

Moving into small groups, participants talk about their experiences of practising the pause and the routine activity. After a few minutes, they are invited to share any special insights with the whole group. The discussion is widened to include a reflection about doing the practices this week. How was it?

Time for a story

If there is time, this might be a good moment for a story. It is probably best to choose a story spontaneously with the group in mind. But some tales seem to call to us on certain weeks. In Week Three, 'Beyond Perfection' from *Kitchen Table Wisdom* (Remen, 1996), highlights a familiar theme of wanting to do well and get things right.

Week Three Exercise

Pleasant Experience

Duration: 15 minutes

Using the blob and asking 'What does it take to simply enjoy the (pleasant) moment?'

- Mapping the experience.
- Finding the connections (e.g. between physical sensations in the body, feelings or emotions and thoughts).

Using the Blob

We have changed the way participants record this exercise in order to help them map different dimensions in their experience. By doing this, they appreciate the way thoughts, feelings and body sensations interconnect. We used The Blob last week in 'Walking Down the Street'. This week, participants have drawn blobs for themselves.

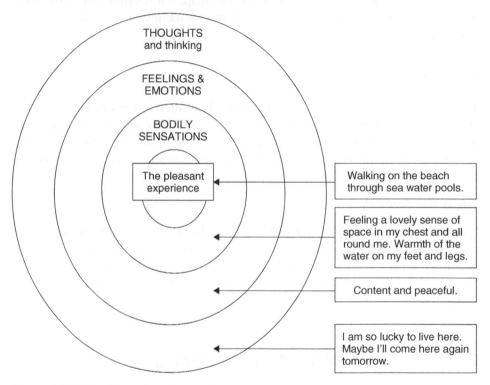

Figure 6.3.1   The Blob, pleasant experience.

As we work through one or two participants' examples, we zero in on body sensations, especially those in the trunk of the body. This is where the most sensitive information is often to be found. We tease out the linkages between the different aspects of experience – and the way the body reflects feelings, which also relates to thoughts.

There is invariably an opportunity to notice how often we want more of something enjoyable. In that moment of wanting more, we are off, away from *this* pleasant moment into an imaginary future experience (or into planning one).

Some find that their pleasant experience was not so straightforwardly pleasant.

Lydia has not been told her prognosis, but she knows that her life will be considerably shortened by cancer. She has two adult children and a younger son aged six. She is worried about the impact of her illness on him.

'I was having a lovely time playing football with Sean. The sun was shining and we were laughing and play fighting as we tried to get the ball from each other. It was brilliant! Then would you believe, in the next moment, I was nearly in tears thinking that I won't see him grow up. I had to stop the game quick and find an excuse to go indoors. I didn't want him to see me crying'.

Those with incurable cancer will often describe the experience of anticipating sadness and loss in the midst of a pleasant experience. Acknowledging the thoughts that underlie the strong feelings, we begin to learn to notice when the mind veers off into the future. On a good day, it is possible to come back – not in avoidance of the future, but in appreciation of staying with and enjoying the immediacy of what is happening now.

Those with low mood may discover there is more to enjoy in small everyday events than they had realized.

Fred said that if anything could have gone wrong with his treatment it did. He had been a very active man, and was forced to retire after his diagnosis. He often feels low.

In the feedback, Fred described one morning when he went to see his chickens.

'I just stood there and watched them' he said, 'I noticed my heart beating regularly, feeling quite good and strong – and my belly seemed warm and comfy. It felt almost good to be alive! I haven't felt like that for a long while', sounding quite bright, 'I decided to come to the breath and just breathe it all in'.

Being asked to notice and record a pleasant experience every day is helpful in highlighting these moments of pleasure. They are so easy to miss, especially if life is challenging.

'What does it take to simply enjoy the (pleasant) moment?' we ask, before moving on.

Week three short practice

First, we guide the Three Minute Breathing Space (Segal et al., 2002) and then we inquire into the experience of it. After this, we teach the shape of it and drawing an hourglass shape on the white board, making a connection in the first two steps with the Pause and Coming to the Breath practices, which are now becoming familiar to participants.

Three Minute Breathing Space (3MBS)

'Bringing awareness to your posture....and the weight of you going down...feet on the floor, contact with the seat...and height of you going up....sitting here, grounded and tall.......Coming into the first step of the breathing space – NOTICING.....asking yourself the question, 'what is going on for me at the moment?' Noticing and acknowledging whatever is there......... maybe in the mind or in the body or in the events around you........and when you are ready, moving to the second step of the breathing space – GATHERING.......gathering the awareness and bringing attention directly to the breath breathing itself deep in the belly.....feeling the sensations of breathing...and whenever you notice that the mind has wandered, just connecting with wherever it has got to , and gently returning to the anchor of the breath in the belly..............and when you are ready moving to the third step of the breathing space – EXPANDING...and expanding around the breath to become aware of the body as a whole sitting here....all the way out to the very envelope of skin.......and a sense of the breath breathing in the whole of the body'

Note: See Chapter 7. The Practices – Short Practices for more guidance on Breathing Spaces.

The Three Minute Breathing Space (3MBS) often becomes a core practice. It skilfully offers all the key steps of the whole Mindfullness Based Cognitive Therapy (MBCT) programme in a sequence that synthesizes the essence, approach and practice in just three minutes. It is deceptively simple. Experience suggests that many people do not practice every step at first.

What seems to help to integrate 3MBS into everyday practice is to be very familiar with the three steps as practices in their own right. By now, through The Pause we have established the value of stopping, noticing and acknowledging what is going on. Last week in Week 2, we introduced the second step of the 3MBS via Coming to the Breath. Many participants will be naturally putting the two together.

The only step that is not quite so familiar at this stage is the third and last step, where we expand around the breath into the body as a whole. This involves connecting to a wider and more spacious awareness, which we have practised in the Body Scan, when we widen the attention to include the whole of a limb, or the trunk of the body or the body as a whole. However, this third step can easily get neglected.

The shape of the 3MBS

As has been suggested, the 3MBS is deceptively simple. By interrupting what is going on and pausing, we are able to connect with our direct experience (Step 1). We then gather awareness and come up close to the breath in the belly (Step 2).

Note to teachers: There has been some debate as to whether the focus of attention around the breath should be in the belly or whether participants should choose their own location (belly, chest or under the nose). Different teachers have different views, somewhat influenced by their own practice tradition. We find that the belly works for us in MBCT-Ca groups. Focusing on the belly offers more possibility of being strongly embodied, deep in the trunk of the body. It also facilitates the placing of the hand on the belly, which helps to connect awareness to the movement of the breath under the hand (helpful if there is any challenge in finding or experiencing the breath). This also supports later practices at times of distress, when it might be hard to remember what to do.

Finally, expanding around the breath, we widen the beam of attention to become aware of the body as a whole – with the breath breathing into and out from the whole of the body (Step 3). We label the steps as we guide the 3MBS. It also helps to draw the shape of this on the whiteboard beside the key headings:

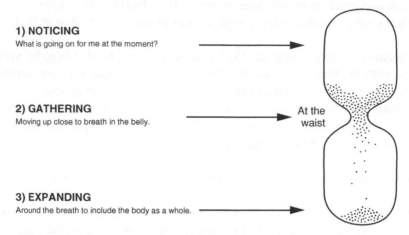

1) NOTICING
What is going on for me at the moment?

2) GATHERING
Moving up close to breath in the belly.

At the waist

3) EXPANDING
Around the breath to include the body as a whole.

Figure 6.3.2   Three steps of 3 Minute Breathing Space (3MBS).

We illustrate the way we start wide at the beginning of the 3MBS. All sorts of things may come to our attention as we stop to notice. These may be aspects of mind or sensations in the body. They may be events around us.

Then in the second step, we gather the attention from wherever it has been, and come to the waist (of the hourglass and of the body). From here, we move up close to the breath fully experiencing the sensations of the breath moving in and out of the belly. If the mind wanders away, we simply notice and come back to the anchor of the breath in the belly.

Then we expand out again, taking mindful awareness out into a sense of the body as a whole. This is a more spacious position. Whilst still somewhat 'tethered' to the anchor of the breath, we move out readying ourselves to go back into our day. This is echoed in the shape of the hourglass going wide again at the bottom.

When to practice?

We need to practice the 3MBS three times a day. By doing this we hope to establish the practice on a regular basis – morning, midday and afternoon/ evening.

It is easiest to remember if we 'hook' the practice to an existing activity, such as getting out of bed, having a drink, eating, or any transition time between one thing and another. We invite the group to move into pairs, with people they have not yet spoken to. Together they help each other to generate ideas and decide when they will practice the 3MBS.

Story

Autobiography in five chapters

We often read 'Autobiography in Five Chapters' here from *There's a hole in my sidewalk* (Nelson, 1994). It is a short piece of writing that describes falling into the same place repeatedly. It seems to resonate with people at this point in the course. Many participants laugh wryly in recognition of the way the story unfolds. Inevitably someone will remark on the fact that it takes three 'chapters' to notice that we have fallen in again and discover there is something we can do to get ourselves out.

Week Three – Sitting Practice

Sitting Practice

Duration: 10 minutes

Brief introduction (if time).

Guide – posture; the breath; and then, the breath in the whole of the body.

Brief inquiry.

In principle, as in MBCT for Depression and MBSR, this is the week to introduce the Sitting Practice. However, there may not be much time. Rather than rush things, it might be wise to leave the practice to next week (Week Four).

Concluding the Session

Home Practice – Week Three

Core practice

- **Body Scan** (30)/**Mindful Movement** (30) on alternate days or **Mindful Walking** (20), if the stretches are too challenging

Short practices

- **Three Minute Breathing Space** three times a day
- **The Pause**
- **Coming to the Breath**

Other home practice

- **Unpleasant Experiences** recorded every day using The Blob

Home Practice

Everyone is encouraged to attempt mindful stretching, if this seems wise, with reminders that we are learning to befriend the body. Sitting out and visualizing the practice is more skilful than pushing through limits. Those who have physical challenges or who are concerned about doing the practice are encouraged to use the Walking Practice. CD2 is given out this week, which has both movement practices on it.

We practice the Three Minute Breathing Space three times a day. The Pause and Coming to the Breath are continued a few times every day. As with last week's pleasant experiences, this week we explore Unpleasant Experience each day using The Blob.

Concluding

Before we finish, we come to sitting, settling the strands of the session and connecting to the breath. The closing practice also gives participants an opportunity to link to their intention for the session – appreciating the commitment they have given to their practice and their learning, and to others in the group.

The Bells

We end with the bells – inviting someone in the group to ring them.

Programme

Week 3: Befriending the Breath and the Body in Movement

Session timing: 2 ½ hours

Mindful Movement:	[30 minutes]

Mindful Movement: [30 minutes]
- Starting with a standing posture (mountain standing), cautioning:
  - dwelling at edges
  - exploring personal limits
  - bringing presence and kindness into the practice
  - awareness of areas of pain/surgery/treatment
  - areas we have been avoiding etc.
- Gentleness is key in befriending the body

Dialogue: [30 minutes]
- That movement practice
- Then back through last weeks' Body Scan practices and
- Coming to the Breath

The Pause: [10 minutes]
- Routine activity (Pleasant exp. later)
- **Small groups'** discussion

Feedback in Large Group: [5 minutes]
- What was it like doing the practice this week?

Story: [5 minutes]
- *Kitchen Table Wisdom* (Remen, 1996)

Pleasant Experience with THE BLOB: [15 minutes]
- What does it take to simply enjoy the (pleasant) moment?
- Mapping the experience and focusing on bodily sensations

3 Minute Breathing Space (3MBS): [10 minutes]
- Guide, inquire then teach shape
- Link with Pause and Coming to the Breath
- Talk with new partner:
  - **When Will I Do This?**
  - Plan and decide 3 times a day [5 minutes]

Poem: [5 minutes]
- Autobiography in 5 chapters (Nelson, 1994)

Short Sitting Practice: [10 minutes]
- Introduce if time

Week 3 Home Practice: [5 minutes]
- Alternating Body Scan and Mindful Movement (new CD)
- 3 minute Breathing Space
- The Pause
- Coming to the Breath
- Unpleasant Experience Blobs

Intention and Bells: [5 minutes]
- Intention
- The bells

Home Practice	• Body Scan / Mindful Movement alternate days • Unpleasant Experience using THE BLOB	• 3 Minute Breathing Space regular – 3 times a day • The Pause and Coming to the Breath • Routine activity (if choose)
Handouts	CD2 (leave walking for now unless it is unwise for a participant to practice mindful stretching)	
Resources	*Kitchen Table Wisdom* (Remen, 1996) or story book Bells	

© T. Bartley (2012). Mindfulness-Based Cognitive Therapy for Cancer.

Who Would Have Thought?

Who would have thought big toe
Is a galaxy full of stars?
Or that the percussion of slamming doors
Would be an interlude of peace?
Softening at the edge of intensity
In the full sun of our attention
Breath by breath
We unfold like flowers.

Katie (April 2009)

Week Four

When we let go of our battles, and open our heart to things as they are, then we come to rest in the present moment.

(Jack Kornfield, 2008)

Learning to Respond

Core theme:

- *Recognizing reactivity* especially within anxious or ruminative patterns of mind.
- *Coming back to direct sensations in the body and the breath.*

Choosing how to respond – by opening gently to experience.

Key Tasks for Teachers – Week Four

Week 4 practice:

- Sitting practice and inquiry
- Posture, Breath, Body as a whole, intense sensations
- Ongoing orientation of gentleness and kindness

Home practice review:

- Body Scan; Mindful Movement; 3MBS (review); the Pause and Coming to the Breath

Week 4 exercise:

- Unpleasant experience exercise using the Blob
- Mapping the experience, noticing sensations in the body, and thoughts and feelings in the mind.
- Recognizing the tendency to fight, fuel, or (want to) fix (3 Fs) – adding extra to trigger aversion and reactivity.
- 3MBS as a responding tool
- Learning to respond with compassion – Thought on a Thread given out
- Attachment/aversion – approach/avoid

Week 4 teaching:

- A vicious circle of anxious preoccupation (Moorey, 2002)

Week 4 short practices:

- The Physical Barometer
- Three Minute Breathing Space as a responding tool

Concluding:

- Ending with the bells, breath and connecting to intention

Introduction

Week 4 focuses on a central tenet of the course: – that of exploring reactions to the unpleasant and learning to respond to them. This can be challenging both to practice and to teach. None of us feels drawn to move up close to what we do not want. Cancer patients, more than most, have experiences, memories, and thoughts that are profoundly disturbing.

Week Four Practice

We start by settling straight into a sitting practice. If there was not time last week to look at sitting position options, we get out stools, mats and cushions and give members of the group the opportunity to try out some different ways of sitting.

Sitting Practice

Duration: 30 minutes

Taking your seat and moving into awareness of:

- Posture – weight of the body going down held by the floor; height going up through the spine gently reaching up towards the space above the head.
- Breath – focusing attention on to detailed sensations of breath moving in the trunk of the body.
- Body as a whole – sitting here with a sense of the breath breathing in the whole of the body.
- Intense sensations – identifying where they are within the body; then offering a choice to move mindfully around them; or turn towards them and explore the sensations; or return to the breath.
- Cultivating gentleness towards all experience.

Note: See Chapter 7. The Practices: Core Practices – for more detailed discussion of the Sitting Practice for cancer patients.

This is the first full length sitting practice. The practice in Week 3 was necessarily brief. We take time to settle into being with the posture and the breath. Now, we come to intensity within the body. Even after a few minutes of sitting still, many participants will have become aware of pain and discomfort – and are probably keen to escape from it. There are parallels here with Mindful Movement practice.

Dialogue

Pleasant and unpleasant experiences almost always appear together in the same practice. It can be interesting to explore this – highlighting the ever changing nature of experience, which like the weather, shifts from light to dark in a moment. Participants may have started to enjoy Mindful Movement and/or Body Scan. Sitting Practice can be quite a challenge and feel very long – a bit like starting from the beginning again. Most of us tend to think that a practice *should* be pleasant, and the mind *should* be steady, for it to do us good. There may be more to dislike than to enjoy in the practice.

As teachers/practitioners, we know the challenge of practising without goal. Wanting more of this and less of that is probably inevitable and natural at this stage. However, we *can* learn to practice with the intention of simply being with experience, gentling to any judgment that arises.

Gradually softening

It is useful to focus in on intense sensations at some point in the inquiry. However, it may be too soon for some, even to work around the edges of intensity. Resistance will soften gradually when the time is right. The body has its own wisdom. Those who have been holding on tight, through an experience of trauma around diagnosis and/or treatment need a gentle and compassionate approach. It can be difficult as teachers not to set up expectations of how things *should* be – presenting responses to intense sensations in a way that includes a subtle (or not so subtle) emphasis on moving into the intensity. For some, moving into exploring the intensity might be the equivalent of unwisely pushing through a safety barrier, put there for good reason. Moving the body around intense sensations or returning to the breath might be a more compassionate practice, which in the end may prove more wise.

Working with intense sensations

Terri found it very difficult to sit still. She had bone metastases and tended to shift her position quite often to manage the discomfort. She had started by sitting on a stool in kneeling position and had then decided to move back to her chair half way through.

'I loved exploring my pain', she said. 'How weird is that! When you invited us to explore the texture of it, I immediately became aware of it like a very smooth grey stone. It was quite big and very beautiful. I was so surprised', she exclaimed, 'Do you think I am odd to see it as that?'

It is hard to accept experience for what it is – simply an experience – even one that is pleasant. We are so keen to analyze things. This can remove the freshness out of experience, a bit like a story told too many times.

It can also be difficult not to judge experience as good or bad, right or wrong. This is a default position for most of us. But by now, participants are getting a little more used to noticing the arising of judgement. Sometimes, in that moment, there is opportunity to simply label it as 'judging' and let it go.

Gwen described her feet as 'antsy and restless' during the practice. She had not long finished treatment and was already back at work. She often looked tired.

'At some point, after struggling with them, I realized just how much I wanted my feet to be different. Almost for the first time, I could see my feet and the horrid way they were feeling; and also the wanting them to be different. I could see the way both parts went together. Rather than judging myself, I could be fairly relaxed about my feet, the practice and me somehow. It made such a difference. My feet eased off a bit, and then got restless again, and I would go back into noticing how much I wanted them to be different – and it was ok. So it wasn't an amazing practice, like some of the others have had, but I feel quite good about it', finished Gwen rather breathless – looking pleased.

Some participants manage to move right into intense sensation with surprising results.

After the sitting practice, James wanted to talk about his back pain. He described it as a constant companion.

'I chose to go into the pain', he said quietly, 'when I got right into the middle of it, I found this deep red – a big ball of red – in the centre of the spine, low down'.

'What was it like, this big ball of red?' I asked him.

'It was glowing at the edges, but it was still', he said, 'at first the pain got worse, but then I went into it and confronted it. It is easier to block it than go into it – but somehow I managed to – and when I did, it just sort of absorbed – the colours changed and the temperature changed. I breathed some kindness in there I think and eventually it was gone altogether', he finished, looking surprised.

We can practice by seeing resistance, aversion, or holding on, a bit like a clenched fist coming out of the solar plexus. As we become aware of not wanting, by noticing tightness in the body, we can open the fist in our mind's eye, and gently releasing the resistance. By opening and softening around the intensity, our experience of it changes and our relationship to it as well. We can be with it.

Mathieu Ricard (Ricard, 2003) describes a teacher of his as if 'outward difficulties would slide off him like water off a rose petal' – a delicious image to inspire.

A Mindfulness Teacher Journal – Week 4

Noticing how often someone catches me in week 4. Taking them to my cushion, I sense that just being with the worry lets my heart open and allows some space for things to be as they are. Trusting.

Sarah fought against getting upset in class last night. She is quite punishing towards herself –and so afraid of being still. She keeps her

---

eyes wide open through all the practices. She was clearly traumatized by her diagnosis. What incredible courage to come on the course and keep coming.

It is too easy to teach the programme with an idea of knowing what is best. With Sarah's terror, learning to get relief from her mind for 10 minutes with the support of coming back and being present with the breath is brilliant. Maybe 'gently' is much more important for her than 'turning towards'.

Later in the day I heard on the radio – 'the silence of absence' and 'the silence of presence' is part of a much bigger story than we might ever dream of – that of finding ourselves. May it be so.

Awareness and wholeness

Occasionally a participant may have a profound experience in a practice.

Jenny looked very peaceful as she came to the end of the practice. I was amused to remember that she had reacted quite strongly when hearing she would be learning to meditate on the course.

And here she was, still sitting on a stool, looking very open and relaxed. 'I felt very whole', she said, 'my body seemed so strong. Out of a general sense of wellbeing, this feeling of awareness emerged. It was like adjusting binoculars into a sharp clear focus. At times I was completely aware of what my mind was doing. It felt wonderful'.

Last Week's Home Practice

Some people are settling into a daily routine. Sara talks about practising first thing in the morning. 'It sets me up for the day. If something is challenging later in the day, I am much better able to cope'.

Others struggle with how little they are doing, or how they would like to do it better. Gillian tried to make a joke out of her movement practice. 'I still wobble loads of the time. I so hope that my balance will improve, but it doesn't seem to, even when I involve the breath'. In every moment, there is wanting and not wanting, pushing away and pulling towards.

Those, who may not be mobile enough to practice the stretches, have been doing the walking practice. Peggy reports that she loves walking mindfully and says that she can really feel her feet connecting with the ground. She has found a practice that she can come back to.

Many participants like the movement practices more than the Body Scan. Leslie comments that she enjoys the act of stretching and then relaxing. She notices herself thinking that she will try to do it better next time, but also tells herself that it does not matter. 'Just doing it is what counts', she repeats to herself, a bit like a mantra.

Asking participants how they experienced the different practices, by Week 4 some people have become more accepting of the Body Scan. Practicing Mindful Movement helps them settle into the Body Scan with a touch less agitation and impatience. This is not always the case.

We remind participants that the course is all about working with difficulty. Is there a way to meet our challenges as opportunities to explore the mind and body? Is it possible to welcome another 'hole in the sidewalk?' (Nelson, 1994). As teachers, we may risk sounding like a gramophone record.

Thich Nhat Hanh likens sitting practice to a glass of freshly pressed apple juice:

> The apple juice became clear after resting awhile. In the same way, if we rest in meditation awhile, we too become clear. This clarity refreshes us and gives us strength and serenity. (Nhat Hanh, 1988).

It is good to be reminded that practice is not a job of work that involves effortful goal. Simply cultivating confidence that the mind will eventually settle, just like the apple juice, we remind ourselves that this is a natural process. When the mind seems turbulent and stirred up, the settling takes longer. Hurrying things will not help. This is hard for those of us who habitually rush!

Three Minute Breathing Space (3MBS)

Last week, participants have been practising the 3MBS for the first time. Some report that it seems to 'work' better at some times than others. Can we see the 3MBS as simply an opportunity to come back to mindful awareness?

Guiding a breathing space again in class helps reinforce the three steps. The last step can easily get lost or missed out. It is the least familiar and may need extra attention.

Guiding and Summarizing

The shape of the Three Minute Breathing Space (3MBS)

1. Starting wide   *What is going on for me at the moment?*
2. Moving to the waist   *Coming to the anchor of the breath in the belly*
3. Coming out wide again   *Expanding to the whole of the body breathing*

Stepping out of automatic pilot and our habitual reactive patterns
Stepping into responding – by coming back to mindful awareness

---

Short practice discussion in small groups

Participants move into small groups at this point for a few minutes to discuss the 3MBS and the other short practices – the Pause and Coming to the Breath. These are starting to become part of everyday repertoire. The small groups support and develop connections that are building in the group. We continue to give time to this every week.

Week Four Exercise

Unpleasant experience

In this exercise, we have an opportunity to understand the way that reactivity increases our suffering. Once we have made the connections, we can begin to spot the patterns, come back, and respond with compassion rather than judgement.

Measured in suffering and pain, the difference between reacting and responding can be huge. In learning to respond, we are walking a razors edge between precision and compassion. Too much vigilance of the precise moment when the unpleasant becomes aversive, and we risk moving into a mind game that is goal directed and prescriptive. Compassion, without understanding the triggers that catapult us into personal booby traps, does not work. True awareness connects us with both the wisdom of the mind that is clear and sharp – and the compassion of the heart that is forgiving and kind. Responding is just that.

The Blob again

Last week participants looked at unpleasant experiences using the Blob again.

Working through a couple of examples, we map out the different layers and the way that they interconnect. As we do this, we zero in on the unpleasant experience as it shows itself in the body, through feelings of tightness, constriction and sometimes heat. We see that by pushing away unwanted experience (felt in the body) fuelled by escalating story lines and negative

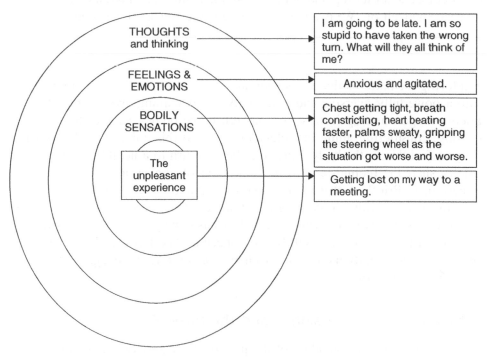

Figure 6.4.1 The Blob, the anxious pre-occupation.

judgement, the unpleasant can quickly become aversion – potentially threatening to overwhelm (especially when we are vulnerable).

The example that follows illustrates the triggers that fuel the aversion, and the shift that opens up once responding becomes possible.

At the weekend, Shirley went to the supermarket. At the cash desk, she queried something and to her surprise, in no time at all, a terrible argument broke out between her and the cashier.

'I was so angry. It seemed so unfair. As the argument was happening, I noticed that my tummy was tight and clenched and I was getting hot, especially in my face. I was probably really red!' she said, looking quite flustered.

'What I noticed afterwards was quite interesting. Every time I told someone about what had happened, and how unfair it was, all the unpleasant sensations and feelings just got stoked up again. Eventually, after a couple of times of telling the story, I realized what was happening. I decided to let it drop and not talk about it again. Then I did a breathing space and felt ok. We had a nice evening in the end and I was fine!'

Exploring the patterns that transform an averagely unpleasant experience into a powerfully aversive and potentially overwhelming one, we direct attention again and again to sensations felt in the body – such as tightening, closing, constricting, fluttering, clenching, etc. At this point, we ask, 'Where do you feel this in the body?' Inviting them to turn to a neighbour, they briefly share the feelings and locate sensations of unpleasant and stressful experiences. Briefly gathering a couple of examples within the large group, we highlight the value of coming to a felt experience in the body – allowing us to realize that we are trying to avoid or push away experience. (Towards the end of the session, this will be introduced as The Physical Barometer practice.) This greatly increases our chance of spotting the triggers and being able to respond differently.

Attachment and aversion – and the three F's

To reinforce this understanding of the patterns of reactivity, we briefly reconnect with pleasant experience, when general sensations of warmth,

---

lightness, openness, flow, and balance are evident. Distinguishing these from feelings of resistance, tightness, and constriction and juxtaposing the two, it becomes evident that pleasant experience is characterized by approach mode (moving towards what we want) whilst unpleasant experience is characterized by avoidance mode (moving away from what we do not want).

Of course, neither stops there. Pleasant experience has the inherent risk of turning into clinging and attachment – (wanting more) – whilst unpleasant experience, as we have been discovering, has the potential to turn into aversion and avoidance (pushing away).

A delicious looking chocolate cake is on the table. We move towards it. 'Ah – that looks good', and start to eat a piece. In no time, thoughts arise about getting a second piece of cake without looking greedy – and the taste and enjoyment of *this piece* is lost in thoughts about the next. A traffic jam is seen ahead on the motorway. Getting tense, 'Oh no – not today of all days', we move into escalating aversion. In both examples, we are no longer mindful of the present experience, but at the mercy of habitual patterns.

Knowing the situation for what it is – whether pleasant or unpleasant – through awareness of feelings within the body, we learn to notice and cut through our personal patterns – by NOT fighting; nor fuelling, nor feeding the story line – but *being with* whatever is there. A participant called these 'The Three Fs'. They offer an easy way to remember how aversion builds and reactions intensify.

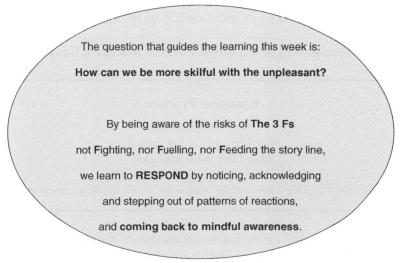

The question that guides the learning this week is:

How can we be more skilful with the unpleasant?

By being aware of the risks of **The 3 Fs**

not Fighting, nor Fuelling, nor Feeding the story line,

we learn to **RESPOND** by noticing, acknowledging

and stepping out of patterns of reactions,

and **coming back to mindful awareness.**

Figure 6.4.2   The Three Fs'.

Three Minute Breathing Space – a way of responding

Guiding a 3MBS, we invite participants to use the regular breathing space as a responding tool whenever unpleasant events occur. It is part of the home practice this week, reinforcing the value of having resources to help us *respond* rather than *react*.

Thought on a Thread – Connecting to our Common Humanity

Just as coloured dots were given out in Week 2, so simple black cotton threads each with a red bead (*Thought on a Thread, www.thoughtonathread. co.uk*), are offered in Week 4. Participants can choose to wear them if they like. The red bead reminds us to pause and come back – perhaps moving into a 3MBS as a way of responding – or moving to another short practice.

The threads invite another important aspect of responding. We share a little of the story of how they are used to introduce simple mindfulness exercises to people in rural Africa affected by HIV & Aids. By connecting in this way, we invite a sense of community amongst those affected by life threatening illness. We link to a shared human experience of suffering. In the end, we all struggle with illness and/or death. By seeing the mindfulness practice community as a link and a means of supporting each other, we can offer compassion to ourselves and others, and connect to our shared common humanity. This consoles us, potentially lightening the isolating claustrophobic reactions to pain, distress and illness – and offering a more spacious kindly awareness that soothes the heart and connects us to others.

If it seems appropriate, we guide a simple kindness practice at this point.

Kindness Practice

May I be peaceful,
May I be safe and protected,
May I live with kindness.

Note: See Chapter 7 in the short practice section for details of all the thread exercises.

We can use these phrases (or personal adaptations of them) at any time. They may be especially helpful when negative judgements arise. Instead of fuelling the experience, kindness facilitates connection and openness – offering another way of responding. Some participants bring these kindness phrases into the last step of the 3MBS.

Week 4 Teaching

Psychological reactions to cancer

At this point, we present a model to the group that we call 'A Cognitive Model of Cancer Distress'. This is the first time that course participants have been introduced to it. Readers of this book have met it before in Part One. It outlines patterns of anxious pre-occupation and speaks to many cancer patients, underlining the themes we have been looking at in this session.

Turning to this diagram in the workbook, we go around the circle. Anxiety resonates in the body and physical sensations result, such as tightness in the chest, racing heart beat, sweating, and feelings of agitation and shakiness (as we found in the unpleasant experience exercise). If this is interpreted as possible illness, and a sign that cancer has returned or spread, then the circle will be fuelled by rumination, negative thinking and vigilant scanning of specific body sensations. This will intensify feelings of anxiety, feed the story line, and result in more pain and tightening in the body. A vicious cycle will thus build.

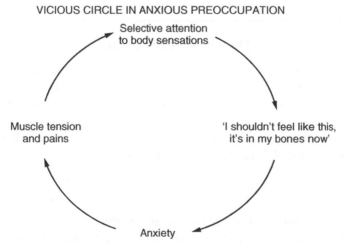

Figure 6.4.3   Vicious Circle in anxious pre-occupation. (Moorey & Greer, 2002)

Inviting comments from the group; 'Have you ever noticed this sort of pattern yourselves?' and the invariable response from the group is; 'Oh yes!' 'What can we do when we become aware of the pattern?' We share ideas that offer us all an opportunity to review the learning around ways of responding.

Week Four Short Practices

We introduce a new practice at this point. This process has already been explored by participants earlier in the session, when they located sensations in the body that became stirred up when stressful or unpleasant events were experienced. The practice helps to identify feelings of reactivity. We invite participants to place a hand on an area in the trunk of the body, where they feel stress. Those who have difficulty finding sensations in the trunk of the body might find sensations in the shoulders or the jaw.

By now participants have explored the connection between not wanting, pushing away and tightness / resistance felt in the body. The Physical Barometer offers a way of identifying (and monitoring) these feelings – like noticing black clouds in the sky that herald a rain storm.

In the home practice this week, the Physical Barometer is tacked onto the Pause and practiced several times a day. We now guide a Physical Barometer.

The Physical Barometer

If you have a barometer or have seen someone consult one, you will know that you gently tap on the glass front. Depending on which way the needle moves, it may be possible to forecast upcoming weather.

We can use our bodies in a similar way to give us sensitive information about the emotional 'weather' arising for us.

Here is how you do this:

1. *Determine some part of the body – preferably in the trunk – such as the chest area or the abdomen or somewhere between the two – that for you is especially sensitive to stress and difficulty.*

---

2. *Once you have found the place, it can be your 'Physical Barometer'. Tuning into it regularly, you may notice different sensations at different times. When you are under pressure, feeling anxious, or frustrated, you may notice sensations of tension, tightness, shakiness, or discomfort. The intensity of these sensations varies depending on the level of your difficulty.*

3. *As you get more practiced at this, you can become aware of quite subtle sensations. These may signal that something is brewing for you, long before you are aware of this in your mind.*

4. *If you wish, you can practice a 3MBS to help you respond to what is happening. Or, you may choose just to monitor the sensations in your 'barometer', moment by moment, and be with them as they are.*

Maureen phoned up her teacher following week 4.

'It was all very well for Shirley last week' she said, sounding fed up, 'She could decide to let the story drop and it did. My thoughts never go away. I can't just decide to drop them. I wish I could, but I can't. When I wake up first thing, even before I open my eyes, I can feel something lurking'.

'Where do you feel it?' I asked her.

'In the pit of my stomach. It is a sort of hungry feeling, but horrid. I really don't like it', she said.

'Can you tune into it that place in your stomach, every time you do the pause? When it feels unpleasant, how could you respond to it gently? What does it need from you?' I asked.

Concluding the Session

We have covered a lot of ground in this session. It can easily feel overfull. Interspersing short relevant practices helps to bring us back and keep the process fresh.

> **Home Practice – Week Four**
>
> **Core practice**
>
> - **Sitting Practice** (30)/**Mindful Movement** (30) on alternate days, or **Mindful Walking** (20), if stretches are too challenging
>
> **Short practices**
>
> - **Three Minute Breathing Space** as a **Responding Tool** whenever an unpleasant or stressful experience occurs
> - **Kindness Phrases** as a **Responding Tool**, especially when judgement arises
> - **The Physical Barometer** linked to the Pause several times a day
> - **Three Minute Breathing Space** three times a day
> - **Coming to the Breath**

The Bells and the Breath

We close with the sound of the bells, coming back to the breath in the body. Reflecting on the session, we bring to mind any moments of learning, pleasure, insight and significance. Connecting with intention that rests in the heart, that supports whatever is best for us, we invite everyone to appreciate any moments of courage, commitment, and kindness that they have offered themselves during the session.

Programme

Week 4: Learning to Respond

Session timing: 2 ½ hours

Sitting Practice:	[30 minutes]
• Starting with posture	
• Intention – then the breath, the body as a whole, and intense sensation.	
• Bringing gentleness and kindness into the practice	
Dialogue:	[20 minutes]
• That practice, especially intense sensations	
○ focusing on the body	
• Then back through last weeks'	
• home practice of Body Scan, Movement practices and 3MBS	
Guide 3MBS and review the shape of it:	[5 minutes]
Small groups for home practice review of::	[5 + 5 minutes]
• 3MBS, The Pause and Coming to the Breath – then share briefly in the large group	
• Pause	
• Coming to the Breath – then share briefly in large group	
Week 4 Exercise:	[Total 45 minutes]
• Unpleasant Experience with the Blob	[10 minutes]
1) **Mapping the experience** – 2 examples from group:	[5 + 5 minutes]
○ Spotting the triggers that turn the unpleasant into the aversive	
○ Where do you feel this in (the trunk of) the body Turn to your neighbour and share detailed sensations. Brief share in large group	
2) **Knowing it for what it is:**	[5 minutes]
○ Compare pleasant/unpleasant	
○ Approach/avoid mode	
○ Wanting/not wanting	
○ the triggers that move into attachment and aversion	
○ *Using feelings in the body to know what is happening*	
○ Not fighting/nor fuelling/nor feeding the story line (**3Fs**)	

---

3) **3MBS**:   [5 + 5 minutes]
   ◦ As a responding tool at times of stress or difficulty
   ◦ Guide 3MBS and brief inquiry
4) **Thought on a Thread**:   [10 minutes]
   ◦ Give out threads.
   ◦ Kindness phrases and brief practice if feels appropriate
   ◦ Compassion as another powerful response. Sense of
     shared common humanity

Week 4 Teaching: [10 minutes]
• A Vicious Circle of Anxious Pre-occupation
• Discuss model and link to unpleasant experience
  learning. How can we respond?
• Recap responding options (see above)

Guide **Physical Barometer**:   [5 minutes]
• Link to the Pause in home practice this week.
• Barometer offers chance to notice feelings of reactivity
  and increase choice of responding

Week 4 Home Practice: [5 minutes]
• Mindful Movement alternate with Sitting Practice (CD1,
  track 2)
• 3MBS (as a responding tool at times of stress and
  difficulty)
• Physical Barometer with the Pause
Give out *Healing and the Mind* DVD (Moyers, 1993). To
  be discussed in week 6

Bells and Breath: [5 minutes]
• Intention to share benefit

Home Practice	• Mindful Movement / Sitting	• The Physical Barometer and the Pause (together)
	• 3MBS and Kindness Phrases (as Responding Tools)	• Coming to the Breath
Resources	Thought on a Threads (see resources section) DVD Healing and the Mind Bells	

© T. Bartley (2012). Mindfulness-Based Cognitive Therapy for Cancer.

The Gift

To pull the metal splinter from my palm
my father recited a story in a low voice.
I watched his lovely face and not the blade.
Before the story ended, he'd removed
the iron sliver I thought I'd die from.

I can't remember the tale,
But hear his voice still, a well
of dark water, a prayer.
And I recall his hands,
two measures of tenderness
he laid against my face,
the flames of discipline
he raised above my head.

Had you entered that afternoon
you would have thought you saw a man
planting something in a boy's palm,
a silver tear, a tiny flame.
Had you followed that boy
you would have arrived here,
where I bend over my wife's right hand.

Look, how I shave her thumbnail down
so carefully she feels no pain.
Watch as I lift the splinter out.
I was seven when my father
took my hand like this,

and I did not hold that shard
between my fingers and think,
Metal that will bury me,
christen it Little Assassin,
Ore Going Deep for My Heart.
And I did not lift up my wound and cry,
Death visited here!
I did what a child does
when he's given something to keep.
I kissed my father.

Li-Young Lee (1986)

Week Five

Have mercy on this pain you have carried for so long.

(Stephen Levine, 1987)

Gently Being with the Difficult

Core theme:

Developing courageous and intention – gently, to be with what is difficult,

by:

- *Stopping* and noticing patterns of mind that signal the arrival of suffering.
- *Locating physical sensations* that resonate within the body.
- *Turning towards and exploring* detailed physical sensations of difficulty.
- Opening to all aspects of experience with tenderness – by breathing into it and *bringing kindness in on the breath.*

Key Tasks for Teachers – Week Five

Week 5 practice:

- Sitting practice and inquiry
- Intention. posture; seeing; breath; body as a whole; sound; and being with the difficult
- Bringing gentle awareness to all experience
- Dialogue around being with the difficult

Home practice review:

- Mindful movement/sitting; Physical Barometer and 3MBS responding; impact of threads on practice
- Reviewing the Pause; Coming to the Breath; 3MBS (regular)

Half way review:

- Recommitting personal intention to the rest of the course

Week 5 exercise:

Using the 'Sea of Reactions' exercise:

- Identifying personal reactions to difficulty
- Exploring detailed physical sensations that arise
- Linking with the Physical Barometer practice
- Responding with an extended breathing space

Week 5 teaching:

- Gently turning towards

Week 5 short practice:

- Extended Breathing Space (Responding)

Concluding:

- Ending with the bells, breath and closing intention

Introduction – A Shift of Focus

Week 5 is the beginning of the second half of the course.

In the first four weeks, our primary task has been to develop a close connection to mindful awareness – both of body and mind – whilst noticing how often we are 'somewhere else', in automatic. We have started to appreciate that there are ways that we all react unhelpfully to events – and each of us has individual and personal versions of these patterns. As the learning builds, there is also a growing realisation that we need to question the assumed automatic validity of our thoughts.

This process deepens as we develop and practice new skills. In week 4, we carefully map the landscape of aversion and the cycles of anxious rumination that relate to people with cancer. Learning how easily unpleasant experience can be fuelled, we begin to see that the very way we try to escape makes things worse. We have some way to go before our knee jerk reactions become skilful responses, but the 3MBS is helping to integrate the practice of responding as a resource.

In the second half of the course, we draw on all that we have learnt to take our next steps. We have reached the point when we ask participants to face the very aspects of their experience that they defend most against. Whatever the focus of the difficulty, it is a considerable step to take – to turn towards and explore the difficult. It seems to imply risk and requires much courage.

> So the practice of sitting is the practice of the warrior, developing confidence to face whatever arises, to turn towards it and use that basic confidence in mind to let down all defences unconditionally. It's a very brave thing to do, also a very mad thing to do, since it runs counter to all common sense notions of self-preservation. But in the final analysis you have no choice – the warrior path of honesty and openness is the only path that is.
>
> (Shikpo, 2003)

In gently turning towards and opening to what is difficult, awareness is brought to sensations in the body – the felt experience of the difficulty. A number of factors already underway may help participants in this. They have been developing openness; a sense of connection within the group; confidence in the teacher; and a growing commitment to the practice. All these factors, and their learning up to this point, support them to turn towards difficult experience. Nevertheless, courage and grounded intention are essential now. Whilst this is challenging, on some level, it also feels strangely wholesome.

As teachers, we draw on our confidence in the practice, the course and the courage and intention of the participants. This session may be a demanding one for us as teachers to hold. It is not easy to open oneself to distress. However, sessions that are challenging, often involve heartfelt learning.

Week Five Practice

Sitting practice

We settle straight into a practice. Sometimes we start with standing in mountain posture, perhaps including a few mindful stretches.

Taking your seat and guiding around:

- *Posture – weight of the body going down, contact with the ground and seat; height going up, through the spine to the crown of the head.*
- *Intention – for this practice and for this session.*
- *Seeing – the shapes, colours, light and dark in objects around you. Noticing how you are drawn to some and move away from others.*
- *Breath – moving attention up close to detailed sensations of breath breathing in the trunk of the body – noticing when the mind wanders, and gently coming back.*
- *Body as a whole – sitting here with a sense of the breath breathing in the whole of the body.*
- *Hearing – allowing sound to come to the ears, experiencing it directly as rhythm, pitch, tone etc – and noticing thoughts that arise about the sound.*
- *Difficulty – deliberately bringing a difficulty to mind; locating the felt experience in the body; turning towards it and exploring sensations (feeling, shape, texture, colour, dynamic, weight, heat etc.), breathing into it and out from it, bringing kindness in on the breath to open and soften to it.*

> • *Breath – knowing that you can return to the anchor of the breath, whenever you need to – and at some point, close to the end of the practice, returning to the breath in the body, and a sense of the body as a whole sitting here.*
> • *Cultivating gentleness towards all experience.*
>
> Note: See Chapter 7. The Practices – Core Practices, for more information about the Sitting Practice. This includes guidance on leading the practice of 'Being with the Difficult'.

It is important to invest in a strong posture at the start of the sitting practice. This is especially relevant when working with difficulty. Spending time and care, we use familiar terms such as 'weight going down', 'height going up', and 'becoming aware of the contact of your feet with the floor, buttocks with the seat'. As we guide the beginning of the practice, as teachers, we invest in our own grounded sense of fully sitting here – really giving attention to direct experience. This is the best possible support we can offer to the group.

Some connection with how participants are settling can be determined through their stillness/restlessness. However, it is also more subtle than that – and is probably realised through an intuitive and almost visceral sense of the group as a whole. Checking in and scanning the group is helpful now and again, as long as this is practised alongside a deep engagement with present experience, especially in the body.

We guide mindfulness of hearing next, before moving to the practice of being with the difficult. Awareness of hearing invites an experience of spaciousness, which promotes openness and may help to reduce the risk of claustrophobia when we approach the difficulty.

We will be guiding 'being with the difficult' practice for two subsequent weeks after this one. It may well get easier as participants and teachers get more joint exposure to it.

Dialogue – Ways of Being with the Difficult

As we inquire of participants' experience, we maintain awareness of the body and what is being felt within it. This supports us to sustain our 'holding' role as teachers. It also supports participants as they explore their experience.

Peggie was keen to talk about 'that funny place between awake and asleep'. 'In fact, I wouldn't have noticed that my mind had wandered if you hadn't commented at the time. I didn't really feel I was in the practice today and I missed it' she finished.

Mark didn't feel very connected either. 'There were things on my mind and there were little aches in my body. When my thoughts went off, I tried to bring them back with gentleness, but I noticed my tendency to just yank them back'.

Jackie found the banging of the doors in the corridor really irritating. 'I kept focusing on it. Grrrr! It meant it was harder to come back – but something happened in the week that was quite upsetting, so I'm not entirely surprised. I could feel some nervousness in my belly and it got in the way of the breath'.

This first practice of directly turning towards the difficult may sometimes seem a little flat. Participants may talk about minor irritations or distractions. This may be unconscious wisdom on their part. More significant issues, such as anticipations of recurrence have potential to overwhelm. As understanding and confidence in the practice develops, so participants will be able to bring more central issues to mind, if this is right for them. We can trust their process.

'There was nowhere to place the sensations in the body. I looked but they were not there', Bethany said. From the very first Body Scan, she had found it hard to connect with physical sensations. It was as if she had none, she frequently complained.

'So how did you experience the difficulty?' asked her teacher.

'It was out there', she said, with her hands demonstrating something moving just in front of her face, 'I could sense a movement and a restlessness and it all seemed to be out there with my thoughts'.

Some participants can connect with a felt experience of difficulty in the body more easily than others. If they are able to share the detail of the physical sensations they felt – then others, who find this more challenging, may gain some tentative understanding second hand.

Kerry said she had a habit of pushing people away.

'I got in touch with a hardness in my chest', she said, 'it felt like a flat board, with straight edges, pushing down a bit in the middle'.

She went on to describe the way it tightened around her breath. 'I had no idea it was there' she said, 'the board completely covered my heart'.

She began to look upset and her eyes became teary. 'When I breathed into it, the board seemed to shrink a bit and my breathing got easier. When I brought gentleness to it and said to myself, 'it is ok for this to be there', it almost faded away', she said sounding a bit steadier.

Lots of feelings may emerge during these explorations that affect the whole group. One person's emotion can ripple round the circle touching everyone else, and helping to connect them all with their own tender places.

Breathing With

Susan was looking rather red and upset after Kerry had shared her experience.

'It is too painful to talk about', she said, looking frightened and very close to tears. She seemed to be holding her breath and the whole group almost appeared to have stopped breathing with her.

When someone is distressed and fearful of being overwhelmed, we might lead a practice of Breathing With (*see Chapter 7, The Practices – Short Practices*). Guiding a responding Three Minute Breathing Space is another alternative. However, sometimes moving into a practice seems to close down the feelings, and appear to give the distressed participant a message about it being best not to be upset.

'Breathing With' allows us to stay present with it all. By placing part of the attention on the breath to steady, and the rest on what is happening around you, it is possible to gain access to some support when things are tough and there is a lot going on. This is just as useful for teachers, as it is for participants.

In situations such as these, we may choose *not* to delve into participants' experience. Taking our lead from them, and tuning into their process, wholly respecting their experience (especially any strongly held defences), we may notice that 'don't know' is a very edgy place to be. It is also a juicy place, full of possibility – 'a gap' in the programme – a space for something else to arrive. In hindsight, it can shape all that follows. It is interesting to notice that these moments, when structures seem to come tumbling down, can be the wisest and most powerful teachings. This reinforces our humility as teachers.

Week Five Teaching

We read *Dragons and Princesses* (Rilke, 1934), to highlight how we have been relating to the difficult. This is read at the end of the first dialogue or at the end of Sea of Reactions (see below) – or both – depending on what seems most appropriate within the process.

We have no reason to harbour any mistrust against our world, for it is not against us. If it has terrors, they are our terrors. If it has abysses, these abysses belong to us. If there are dangers, we must try to love them, and only if we could arrange our lives in accordance with the principle that tells us that we must always trust in the difficult, then what now appears to us to be alien will become our most intimate and trusted experience.

How could we forget those ancient myths that stand at the beginning of all races – the myths about dragons that at the last moment are transformed into princesses? Perhaps all the dragons in our lives are only princesses waiting for us to act, just once, with beauty and courage. Perhaps everything that frightens us is, in its deepest essence, something helpless that wants our love.

So you must not be frightened if a sadness rises before you larger than any you have ever seen – if an anxiety like light and cloud shadows,

---

move over your hands and everything that you do – you must realize that something has happened to you. Life has not forgotten you – that it holds you in its hands and will not let you fall. Why do you want to shut out of your life any uneasiness, any miseries, or any depressions? For after all, you do not know what work these conditions are doing inside you. (Rilke, 1934)

The 'Guest House'

In the past, we used to read Rumi's *Guest House* poem (Rumi, 1995). However, after a number of adverse reactions from participants, we decided to change.

John was struggling with aggressive prostate cancer and was very upset by the Guest House poem. He challenged it at the time and during a phone call with the teacher later in the week. 'I have to fight my cancer', he said. 'If I don't, I'll probably die even sooner. How can I possibly greet it at the door laughing?' he almost shouted, clearly distressed. 'I can't believe you are prepared to read that poem to people in my position'

Attempts to work it through were useless. He was too upset. A little surprisingly, he continued to attend the course. He arrived late to the final session, breathless and rather excited. 'Something amazing has just happened!' he said, interrupting the practice that had just started. 'As I got out of the car, I had this pain in my back. I just couldn't move', he said. 'I stood there paralysed, propped up by the car and thinking that this was it. It must be secondaries. Then I remembered that poem and what we'd said about moving up close to the pain, and I just sort of gave up to it. And it vanished! I can't believe it but it did and then I could move – and here I am!'

It is hard to explain to someone with terminal cancer that the Guest House poem is referring to *thoughts* about cancer – and not to the disease itself. It can seem a fine line. In the light of experience, we decided to forgo Rumi's Guest House and use Rilke's *Dragons and Princesses* instead. It is more gentle and perhaps more in keeping with the focus of the programme.

Coming to the Breath with kindness

Coming to the Breath with Kindness is very similar to Coming to the Breath. As the breath comes in, we invite openness and kindness to flow in on the breath. This allows with it an intention to soften towards experience. Bringing awareness to the centre of the chest, we open to the warmth that naturally radiates from there.

Last Week's Home Practice

We need to link in with last week's practice, having spent time exploring difficulty. Some participants report that their level of practice is slipping. They may be diligently weaving the short practices into their days, but finding the longer ones more difficult to fit in. Hospital appointments, life in general, and even an emerging sense of feeling better, may combine to decrease motivation.

Last week they practised the sitting practice at home for the first time. Many find it a challenge to complete. At the beginning of the course, some may have found it was quite an effort to practise the Body Scan, but they were prepared for this and their motivation was generally high. Then as things develop, the exercise seems to get easier to practise. Mindful movement appears as a welcome change. Now with another static practice, those with persistently high levels of anxiety find it hard to be still. We remind ourselves that we are building momentum in the development of awareness – and consolidating habits in our practice of coming back. Jon Kabat-Zinn has a remark that can be useful at times like these: 'Practice as if your life depends on it.'

Sustaining practice – kindness and discipline model

The kindness and discipline triangle highlights the qualities that we need in our approach to practice – this is an optional process that can be included in Week 4 or 5, if it seems relevant. Sharing the triangle offers us an opportunity to discuss the obstacles to practice that we all experience. Reinforcing the importance of renewing our intention to come back and be present, and put our energy into what we know is best for ourselves, we remember that mindfulness offers an opportunity to start again every day and in every moment.

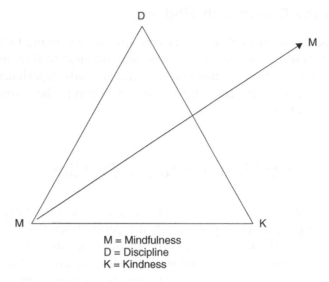

M = Mindfulness
D = Discipline
K = Kindness

Figure 6.5.1(a)   Mindfulness, discipline and kindness.

Mindfulness (M) intersects the line between discipline (D) and kindness (K). It is important to understand that this is not an either/or model – but one that includes and involves both discipline and kindness. However, we all have certain tendencies. Those of us who are strong on discipline might need more kindness. Perhaps some participants, who get into patterns of 'trying hard' might need to invite themselves not to judge too harshly when a day is missed, or a practice is skipped. Here the mindfulness arrow might intersect the line closer to K for kindness.

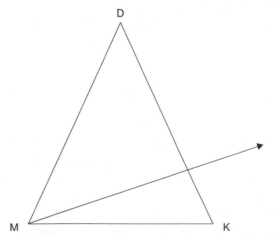

Figure 6.5.1(b)   Mindfulness, discipline and kindness.

Many of us feel that we need to bring more discipline to our practice. Generating ideas within the group might work much better than suggestions, cajoling or hectoring from the teacher. The arrow moves closer to D for discipline to illustrate this.

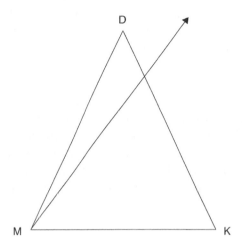

Figure 6.5.1(c)   Mindfulness, discipline and kindness.

All of us need more of both!

Short practices

Short practices are beginning to be consolidated. Habits are forming. Some of them may start to become established routines during the day. Last week, we used the 3MBS as a 'responding' tool and kindness phrases were included. We also practised the Physical Barometer for the first time. Participants inevitably connect to some practices more than others. Indeed, there is no expectation that everyone will integrate every short practice. We encourage people to try each one for a week or so, and then sustain the ones they feel drawn to.

Half Way Review

We invite participants to reflect on their experience of the course thus far – writing two questions on the whiteboard:

- What changes or learning are you noticing at this half way point?
- How can you make the most of the rest of the course?

Participants break into small groups of threes or fours to share their ideas. Some find they notice more than they did – especially in relation to their awareness of nature. Others may be feeling more peaceful and not getting so wound up about things. They may report that they are better able to stop and take a breath before heading into anger or reactivity. Jane said 'I feel I have more choices now'.

Those who feel they are benefitting from the course may move straight into anticipating the loss of it, now that we are past the half way mark. We enjoy something and immediately move into anticipating the loss of it. As teacher, it is tempting to move into talking about follow up classes and ongoing support. It is relevant, but it might be more skilful to stay with the difficult (the anticipated loss) and gently highlight how often we leave before the end.

Mandy had shared something in her small group and was now bursting to tell everyone.

'I had to have a bone marrow biopsy last week', she said. 'The procedure can be quite unpleasant. I planned to do the Body Scan and the 3 minute practice. In fact, I told the nurses to carry on, but not to expect me to talk to them as I'd be doing my mindfulness.

I focussed on my breath and took it in a zigzag up and down my body breathing through my toes! The nurses were amazed. I hardly flinched and I was completely relaxed throughout the whole thing'. She waved her arms about in the air in celebration.

Different participants are at different stages. Those who are struggling with either their practice and/or their current experience might be encouraged to hear how others feel they are benefitting. However, there is an edge between encouragement, irritation and envy, which easily leads to criticism. Nevertheless, this review process is valuable in affirming personal progress, and encouraging and renewing intention.

Week 5 Exercise

Although the sitting practice in Week 5 can be powerful, it is not always possible to develop as much learning around the core theme of the week as we might want.

Reflecting on this over time, it became evident that the task in week 5 involves:

- inviting in difficulty
- turning towards the felt experience of it in the body
- exploring, opening and bringing kindly awareness to this felt experience as best we can with the intention of gently being with it.

In view of this, we changed the title of the week to 'Gently being with the difficult', rather than 'Acceptance, allowing and letting be' – as it is in 'MBCT for Depression' (Segal et al., 2002). The word 'acceptance' tends to feed into what people with cancer think they 'should' be feeling.

The 'Sea of Reactions'

A new exercise is included in this week. The rationale underpinning The Sea of Reactions is to draw out the reactive patterns that habitually emerge when difficulties arise. Then by identifying sensations of difficulty resonating in the body, we make a direct link between physical sensations and our reactions to difficulty.

The Sea of Reactions

Materials:

- Plenty of A4 plain paper (scrap paper is fine with one side blank)
- Thick marker pens

This exercise involves participants in writing their reactions at times of stress and difficulty – putting one word/reaction on each sheet of paper. It helps if the teacher can start things off with a couple of her own examples (eg. Rushing. Irritable) The sheets of paper then go face up on the floor within the circle of chairs. Hand out several sheets of paper and a pen to each participant. We begin by asking the participants the following:

- 'Bringing to mind a difficult situation that you have experienced, write your one word reactions (feelings or behaviours) on the paper in big writing'. *Only one word on each piece of paper*. Continue for a few minutes until everyone has had a chance to write down a number of reactions.
- Placing the sheets of paper (words up) on the floor as they are written – now inviting everyone to stand up and walk on and around the words, having a good look at what has been written (*see below for examples*).
- 'Choose one word that you feel drawn to, that describes what you do or how you feel when things are difficult. It might be one of the words that you have written or someone else's. It doesn't matter'.
- 'Pick up the sheet you have chosen. Finding a partner, sit down and take it in turns to describe the sensations in the trunk of your body when you feel or act like the word on your sheet. Help your partner to get right into the detail of these sensations'.
- Change over after a few minutes.

Some words written in the Sea of Reactions:

blaming	ignoring	frozen	overwhelmed	weeping
angry	trapped	seething	anxious	inadequate
scared	numb	driven	frightened	distraught
alone	brooding	jittery	avoid	frustrated
lost	withdraw	detach	worry	fear the worst
stress	sick	pain	tiny	panic
prickly	anticipation	tearful	irritated	terror
paranoid	guilty	worthless	denial	devastated
restless	agitated	rejected	annoyed	lonely
depressed	resentful	dread	distressed	hopeless

An extended breathing space – responding

After the pairs have finished and have briefly fed back to the large group, we guide an 'extended breathing space' as a responding tool (*see Chapter 7, The practices – short practices*). This includes an invitation in step three to open to, and to be with, whatever is there. 'It is ok, whatever it is, let me feel it.'

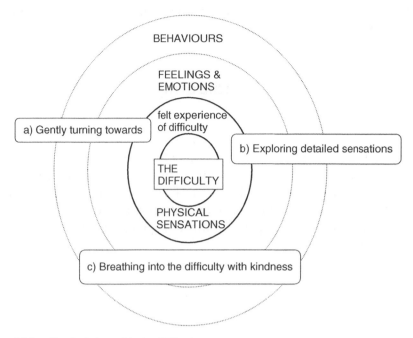

Figure 6.5.2 Gently being with the Difficult.

We leave plenty of time for the inquiry that follows this in order to fully process the exercise and consolidate the learning of the session. If any feelings are still bubbling, we support participants to stay with them, breathing kindness into the body and opening and softening to them as best they can Thoughts are the focus of our session in Week 6.

Week 5 Teaching

Home Practice – Week Five

Core practices

- Body Scan (30)/**Sitting Practice** (30)/**Mindful Movement** (30) or **Mindful Walking** (20) – 30 minutes each day

Short practices

- Extended breathing space – (responding to difficulty)
- **The Physical Barometer** linked to the Pause
- **3 Minute Breathing Space** three times a day
- **Coming to the Breath** with Kindness

MBCT-Ca, we lend DVDs to participants to watch at home. A discussion follows in Week 6.

Concluding

The Bells

It may have been an intense session. Coming back to the sound of the bells, we invite a shared sense of connection with group members in recognition of the support they have offered each other to find the courage to explore the difficult. We close by connecting with our intention and a sense of appreciation to ourselves for spending this time practising and learning about being mindful and aware.

Programme

Week 5: Gently Being with the Difficult

Session Time: 2 ½ hours

Sitting Practice:	[30 minutes]
• Possibly starting with Mountain and a few stretches	
• Coming to sitting posture	
• Intention – then the breath, the whole of the body; hearing; then being with difficulty.	
• Bringing presence and kindness into the practice	
Dialogue:	[20 minutes]
• The sitting practice just done – with a particular focus on being with difficulty	
• Then back through last weeks' movement practice	
Sitting practices; 3MBS; Responding space; and the Physical Barometer	
Read *Dragons and Princesses* (Rilke, 1934), here or later.	
Half Way Review:	[15 minutes]
• What are you noticing?	
• How can you make the most of the rest of the course?	
• Reflect on own and then into small groups	
Include **threads** and what they offered last week	[5 minutes]
At some point in class, when sense of difficulty present;	
Guide **Coming to the Breath in Kindness**	[10 minutes]
The Sea of Reactions Exercise:	[Total 30 minutes]
Write words that describe personal reactions to difficult times – one for each piece of paper and placing on the floor	[10 minutes]
• Choose one word each to focus on (not necessarily your own) and notice impact of these words in the body.	

Working in pairs: [10 minutes]
- Describe specifically to each other what you feel in your body when you remember this reaction (physical barometer)
- In large group – feedback: [10 minutes]
- Then moving into an **Extended Responding Space** bringing gentleness into the 3rd step (going beyond fear into the softness of the human heart)
- Story / Poem (if time) [5 minutes]

Inquiry [10 minutes]

Week 5 Home Practice: [5 minutes]

Short Sitting and Bells: [5 minutes]
- Short sitting and dedication
- The bells

Home Practice	• Body Scan / Mindful Movement / Sitting • 3 Minute Breathing Space / Responding Space	• The Physical Barometer • Coming to the Breath with kindness (if choose)
Resources	*Dragons and Princesses* (Rilke, 1934) *Healing and the Mind* (Moyers, 1993) DVD Paper and large pens Bells	

© T. Bartley (2012). Mindfulness-Based Cognitive Therapy for Cancer.

Why Cry For The Moon?

May what I do flow from me like a river
Sometimes flooding
Sometimes barely moving.

Why rush when the moment is languid?
Why long for stillness when the rushing is current?
Why cry for the moon when the sky is black?

October, 2009

Week Six

Some of the worst things in my life never happened.

(Mark Twain)

Thoughts are not Facts

Core theme:

We are learning to accept that *thoughts are impermanent, empty and essentially impersonal* – though some are charged with strong feelings that can spiral us down in mood.

We practise by *allowing thoughts to come and go, like events in the mind* – held lightly within the spacious container of awareness – and returning to the safe anchor of the breath whenever we need to.

Key Tasks for Teachers – Week Six

Week 6 practice:

- Sitting Practice and inquiry
- Intention. Posture; standing in mountain; breath; body as a whole; sounds; thinking and feeling; and being with the difficult
- Bringing gentle awareness to all experience
- Dialogue around mindfulness of thinking and feeling; and being with the difficult

Home practice review:

- Sitting; Extended Breathing Space (Responding)
- Coming to the Breath with Kindness
- DVD 'Healing and the Mind' (Moyers, 1993) discussion

Week 6 exercise:

- The 'Sea of Reactions' (2) exercise
- Identifying familiar chains of negative thoughts; their effects and how to respond to them
- Generating top 10 negative thoughts list.
- Linking with the Physical Barometer practice
- Extended Breathing Space (Responding)

Week 6 teaching:

- Overview of ways of relating to thoughts and thinking

Week 6 short practice:

- Review Coming to the Breath with kindness

Week 6 home practice:

- Beginning to customize practice
- Short practice CD3
- All Day discussion

Concluding:

- Ending with the bells, breath and closing intention

Introduction

In Week 6, we go deeper into the difficult, identifying the role that thoughts and feelings have in intensifying the cycle of reactions. The focus of the week is on thoughts – and the way they influence experience.

Sitting Practice

We start with a standing posture, investing in a rooted sense of the body standing, present and dignified like a mountain. We are fortunate in North Wales to be surrounded by beautiful mountains. Inspired by their presence, we often draw on the abiding presence of mountain at difficult times.

> Joanne attended an eight week course with her mother in law. In her early 40s with young children, she was in remission, but looked pale and thin. She seemed quite low, but put a lot into her practice, and after three weeks she reported that she was feeling better. Then she had news of a recurrence. She was offered treatment, but would be in isolation for several months, and her chances of surviving were poor.
>
> 'Whenever I feel frightened, I just stand in mountain and breathe', she told the group. 'Sometimes I come back to this several times a day. It helps me get steady'.
>
> Once in hospital, she found she could do the practice lying down. Among her family photos was a photo of the mountain that she could see from her kitchen window. 'I'm ok', she told me, 'Whenever I am afraid, I come back to mountain'.

The sitting practice this week is similar to the one we guided in Week 5. We emphasize physical sensations as we set up the practice.

Including awareness of the experience of hearing, as we did last week, we stress the natural arising and dissolving of sounds in the space around us. We bring attention to the rhythm of sounds and the way they come and go – a door banging, a bird singing, even the background hum of the air conditioning has a rhythm with gaps or changes within the sounds, even if they are tiny ones. In general, we tend not to get too enmeshed in adding extra to hearing. Sounds are not usually experienced as personal – they just happen. This helps to prepare us for the next section of the practice.

When ready, we open to thoughts and feelings – allowing them to come and go within a spacious container of awareness, much like sounds did. No longer relating to them as distractions that take the mind away, we now practise with thoughts as the objects of our attention. This is an advanced practice, and very ambitious for people who have only been meditating for a few weeks. It is also challenging to guide.

If, as teacher, we can connect with a sense of spaciousness, and hold the group as we guide the practice, we can support participants to experience a sense of wider awareness. We use a metaphor to help us – perhaps likening the mind to a vast open blue sky – the sky of mind. This is not intended to be a visualization – but an inspiration that we might open into. Thoughts can then be experienced a bit like clouds that pass across the sky – as they arise and dissolve – come and go.

Inquiry – Thoughts and Thinking

Angela had been quite ill during treatment and was still a little weak at times. Usually a bit reticent, she clearly had something she wanted to share.

'As soon as you said "be aware of your thoughts", all my thoughts disappeared. I got the feeling of a wide blue sky, quite markedly in fact, but I was scuttling around like a rat in a barn trying to find a cloud', she said smiling, 'It was strange when I'm usually so distracted by my thoughts'.

Some people have difficulty connecting to spaciousness awareness.

Janet said she felt uninvolved – almost as if there was no path she could find to walk down.

Julie was ready to drift off. She said she could try to make the sky real by imagining the blue, but she could not feel it within her.

Others find they can touch into thoughts coming and going.

Jane is a young mother with breast cancer. 'To begin with, thoughts wouldn't come – and then I noticed that the clouds were almost queuing up in the corner. Then I was aware of the content of the thought but I didn't feel much involved with them'.

'What was that like?' I asked her.

'It was a bit like a snatch of an overheard conversation', she said, 'when it got louder, I came back to my breathing. Sometimes I had to do this quite a bit – but then I could touch back into spaciousness. I like the blue sky thing!'

Jane's experience highlights how some thoughts are more highly charged. These are invariably the ones with feelings attached. They have the potential to carry us away. Jane was able to notice when this was imminent, and return to her breath as an anchor to come back to.

We have an opportunity to talk about the nature of thoughts as impermanent. If we have not experienced this for ourselves, it is just an idea, but one that may influence the next practice.

There are many metaphors we can use to illustrate thoughts as impersonal, fleeting, empty – such as:

- Clouds passing across a clear blue sky.
- Leaves or twigs floating along a clear flowing river.
- Images on a screen in a large auditorium.
- Weather patterns coming and going.
- Reflections on the surface of a lake or the ocean (used in the lake practice) (Kabat-Zinn, 1994).
- Bubbles floating in the air, popped lightly by the tip of a feather.

They all share the sense of an intrinsic 'container' that holds the image, reflection, cloud etc.

Awareness is not the same as thoughts, although it makes use of thinking, honouring its value and power. Awareness is more like a vessel which can hold

---

and contain our thinking, helping us to see and know our thoughts as thoughts, rather than getting caught up in them as reality (Kabat-Zinn, 1994)

Through this, we can link to thoughts in everyday life – simply as events in the mind – passing, empty, and in many ways insignificant. This might be a good time to refer back to the Vicious Circle of Anxious Preoccupation (Moorey & Greer, 2002), reminding us that even potentially overwhelming and convincing thoughts are not necessarily true – and we have choices in how we relate to them.

Inquiring of the difficulty

It may have been less of a shock to bring in a difficulty this week, but for some it may still be a step too far.

> Catherine was getting a lot from the course. She did not manage to practice the CDs very much, but she was successfully weaving the short practices into her life. She thought deeply about things.
>
> 'I just don't want to look at difficulty', she said, 'I put mine away. I've got so used to getting on with things. I'm not like the rest of you'.

Bringing a difficulty to mind can be hard even when we emphasize gentleness. As teachers, it seems crucial to honour the wisdom of the choices of our participants, even whilst we hold open a door for things to be different. Anything else risks adding pressure to something that should not be forced.

> Liz sometimes felt extremely agitated. She had found her diagnosis very difficult. (She is a shy person who tended to feel anxious at the best of times.) However, she was practising diligently and beginning to experience some sense of settling, some of the time.
>
> 'I didn't want to go near the difficulty' she said, 'I deliberately thought about something else and looked round the room. I was aware of my heart beating really fast and then I remembered to come back to the breath'.

For others, the difficulty may be pervasive and hard to pin down. When there is little direct connection with physical sensations, it is hard to find somewhere to come to. Thoughts move, change, conflate and often take us far away. Yet we often try to stay with thoughts – to puzzle the problem out 'logically'.

Susan had been anxious ever since being told she had cancer. She attended a mindfulness course after her treatment – and was convinced that sooner or later the cancer would return.

'I feel this black cloud everywhere I go. It is just behind me and sort of weighs down on me. Sometimes it feels closer, sometimes a little further away, but it is always there. As I wake up, even before opening my eyes, I can feel it', she said.

She had tried to explore the sensation of 'black cloud' in her body before – without much sense of connection. On this session, Susan was keen to tell her story. 'Do you know something amazing happened last Wednesday? I woke up and it was gone! I kind of looked for it, expecting it to come back but it didn't. It was so surprising – and I had such a good day. But then this morning the cloud was back again – although maybe not quite so black and heavy feeling'.

Some difficulties are persistent and rarely simply disappear. For people with cancer who find uncertainty extremely difficult to be with, it may be that turning towards happens little by little, as courage and confidence develops. Opening happens slowly – like little snatched glimpses, until it is safe to see the whole scene. To move to a place of allowing the 'black cloud' in, is a huge step.

This reconnects with Rilke's *Dragons and Princesses*. So, with this in mind, we practise Coming to the Breath with Kindness or we can lead an Extended Breathing Space (Responding).

Last Week's Home Practice

When there has been a long inquiry after the practice, we invite the group into small groups to discuss their home practice. Increasingly we are looking for ways of passing the baton back to participants, to enable them to facilitate their own learning.

There will be some practices that they like much more than others. Many of them have adapted short practices and perhaps extended or combined them to form their own versions. Only a minority may still be using CDs every day. However, they talk about the way they have developed the habit of coming back to various short practices – probably several times a day – so that when a difficulty arrives, increasingly some are able to recognize it and turn towards it.

Pauline has an active disease, which is progressing slowly. She seems to be enjoying the course, even though she rarely manages the longer practices. However, she loves the Pause, Coming to the Breath, Walking Practice and the Breathing Space, which she does every day.

She talked about a time during the week when she was having a hug on the sofa with her partner. 'It was lovely', she said, 'but then I realized that it may not be long (*that she may live for*), so I did a breathing space straight away and just let it go away – and it did. I didn't build on it or make a story out of it – so it (*the thought*) just went away'.

We continue to look for ways to support participants to do as much practice as they can. Having already shared the discipline/kindness model, we sometimes encourage the group to generate ideas about what helps them practice. This week, a number of good ideas were shared:

- Practise first thing in the morning then I can dip back into it all day.
- Practise in the same place.
- Know or hope it is going to help.
- Apply a bit of 'protestant' guilt!
- Remember that practice helps me deal with times when I get anxious.
- Having more confidence in my practice – remembering the small glow of satisfaction I feel, when I've done it.

We lead an Extended Breathing Space (Responding) with an invitation to practise this time, with the eyes open. Sometimes we might need to do this in the supermarket, or hospital or GP surgery.

DVD Discussion

The group have been watching *'Healing and The Mind'* DVD at home (Moyers, 1993). Participants discuss what they found helpful. Anne mentions that she thought it gave authority to what they were doing. Jill said how funny it was to see people eating raisins just as they had. She remembered how odd she found it at the time, and how it makes a lot of sense to her now. Barbara said that there was nothing new to her on the DVD, but hearing and seeing someone else say the same things in a different way really helped her understand more.

Sea of Reactions – Thoughts

We return to the Sea of Reactions exercise. Last week, we looked at the reactive patterns that tend to emerge when we experience something difficult. This week, instead of looking at how we feel or what we do, we are going to explore the threads of thoughts that arise in our minds at these times. The sheets of paper from last week are placed back on the floor and participants are asked to choose a new word that draws them this week.

The Sea of Reactions (2)

Materials:

- A4 papers from last week with the one word reactions written on them (it might help to thin out the papers, putting the strongest reactions on the floor)
- Pens

Placing the sheets of paper on the floor, we invite the participants to stand up and have a good look. Reminding about the way that our buttons get pressed and things get stirred up.

- 'Choose a new word that speaks to you today. It might be yours or someone else's. It doesn't matter. We are going to work on reactions a bit more in terms of the thoughts that arise around them'.
- 'Pick up your word and find a new partner to work with. Helping each other to pull out the thoughts that go with your word. There might be a train of thoughts that starts somewhere and just keep going'.
- 'Write the thoughts on your paper and we will share them in the group'.

We record the thoughts on the white board as our top 10 negative thoughts – 'Top of the Pops' says one participant – 'Top of the Pits!' says another. We notice the way one thought often leads to another.

Reaction thoughts	
Reaction Word	**Thoughts**
Panic	Is it going to come back? Will it (cancer) get me this time?
	How long do I have? Will I see my kids grow up?
Worry	What will happen next? How will I cope? How will the children cope? Could I have done something different?
Sad	Why has this happened to me? Am I going to die?
Tiny/Alone	There's no way round it, I can't escape.
	Nobody else can do it for me. I am really alone with this.
Guilty	What goes around comes around. I shouldn't have done/said that. I haven't kept in touch with people. It's all my fault.
Angry	Why don't they (doctors) know more about it? I should be able to do this but I can't. Why me?
Devastated	It's the end of the world. I have no future. Have I done something to deserve this?

The group share and discuss their list. They recognise the way that thoughts intensify negativity and increase emotion. Participants spot their patterns. They may notice how often thoughts creep in under the radar. They see how quickly thoughts spiral into an urgency that declares that nothing is right – and everything has to be different – including and especially me. Asked to consider how long these thoughts might affect them – a few hours, a day? Much longer than necessary is the consensus. And what if your mood was already low or you were already anxious, angry or upset? The group know the answers, make the links and can appreciate the implications from their own direct experience.

> The interpretation of events reflects what we bring to it as much or more than what is actually there......We think we can influence how we feel, but ...what

we think is also determined by our mood at the time we are thinking. The idea that **thoughts are not facts**…(enables us to) discuss how the same event can be interpreted differently…and suggests that there is no single truth that our thoughts are telling us…Just because thoughts are compelling does not make them true. (Segal et al., 2002)

In Week 5, tears are sometimes shed as we explore reactions. In Week 6, strong feelings are less common. Perhaps it is getting easier to recognize the patterns and the impact of thoughts on experience.

Different stories and metaphors used during the course may now be remembered – like the snowball that starts small and builds into something huge – or The Blob that has the different layers of experience that interconnect. With luck, someone remembers the 3 Fs from Week 4 that:

- Fight
- Fuel the fire
- Feed the story

A group discussion at this point can draw things out a bit further.

The theme of the week, Thoughts are not Facts, can become a mini mantra for the future. It serves to remind us that thoughts are events in the mind rather than solid truths.

As people with cancer, it might appear that some thoughts *are* facts. Uncertainty is a given. Some participants will be living with a difficult prognosis or an incurable disease. They may perhaps be learning to step off the spiral of rumination, but cancer still remains. Some are confused by this and cannot let go of 'but my cancer is real'. However by Week 6, participants are able to distinguish between a thought train that pulls them into a worst scenario, full of horrifying possibilities – and a developing capacity to hold awareness of the felt sense of a thought (even about their uncertain future) in the body alongside the breath – without fighting it, fuelling it, or feeding the story – on a good day at least.

There are some helpful sections in Segal et al's Mindfulness-based Cognitive Therapy for Depression known as *'The Green Book'* (Segal et al., 2002) to draw from and read out loud to help summarize the group's discussion

The kinds of thoughts we have and their impact on our lives, depends on our understanding of things. If we are in the clear powerful space of just seeing thoughts arise and pass, then it does not really matter what kind of thinking appears in the mind. We can see thoughts as the passing show they are. From thoughts come actions. From actions come all sorts of consequences. In which thoughts will we invest? Our great task is to come to see them clearly, so that we can choose which ones to act on and which to simply let be' (Segal et al., 2002).

Mountain Meditation

As we have already discovered, the metaphor of mountain is powerful. After all the talking, we guide a mountain meditation (Kabat-Zinn, 1994). This offers an almost visceral experience of the essential dignity and grounded presence of mountain. The practice is drawn from MBSR, as is so much of what we do. It is an inspired way of experientially encountering the impermanence of difficulties – of showing how essentially impersonal the weather of our lives is. The 'unhurried dignity of mountain' (Shikpo, 2003) inspires us to realize, in our very bones, that we have an essence and a presence that abides whatever the weather. This is not as a feat of endurance but as an inherent quality within us all.

Concluding the Session

Home Practice – Week Six

Core practice

- **Body Scan** (30)/or **Sitting Practice** (30)/or **Mindful Movement** (30)/ or **Mindful Walking** (20). 30 minutes practice each day of whatever you choose. CD3 (short practices) is also available as an alternative – customizing your practice this week.

Short practices

- **Extended Breathing Space** (Responding)
- **The Physical Barometer** linked to the Pause
- **Three Minute Breathing Space** two or three times a day
- **Coming to the Breath** with Kindness

The home practice is very similar to last week. However, a new CD is given out this week with shorter practices recorded on it, including: a 15 minute sitting practice; the Physical Barometer; An extended Breathing Spaces (responding); and others.

All Day plans

We hold the All Day on the Saturday following this session. There may be some anxiety felt about the prospect of being silent for so long. Practicalities are covered in relation to times, venue and what to bring. During the brief discussion, we explain that the All Day is optional. It is an opportunity to deepen the practice. Other participants may join us who have attended previous courses, both because they enjoy the experience and also because they want to support the current group.

The Bells and closing

There may be a lot to think about at the end of this session. The All Day discussion can stir things for participants. We come back to the sound of the bells, connecting with the intention to be present with kindness to whatever arises. Then we offer appreciation to ourselves and everyone in the group for all we are learning to practise with.

Programme

Week 6: Thought are not Facts

Session timing: 2 ½ hours

Mountain Standing:	[5 minutes]
Sitting Practice:	[25 minutes]
• Starting with posture, then the breath, the body as a whole, hearing, thoughts and thinking, then being with difficulty.	
• Bringing gentleness and kindness into the practice	
Dialogue:	[20 minutes]
• Session practice:	
• Particular focus both on what is difficult and on thoughts and thinking	
Then **small groups** for last weeks' Home Practice:	[10 minutes]
• Movement / Sitting / Body Scan	
• 3MBS and Extended breathing Space (Responding)	
• The Physical Barometer and Coming to the Breath with kindness	
• Pause	
• Barometer	
• Coming to the Breath with Kindness	
Large group **discussion** DVD:	[5 minutes]
(*Healing and the Mind,* Moyers, 1993)	
• Themes and learning	
Return to **The Sea of Reactions**:	[15 minutes]
• Words back on floor (weeding out some not relevant)	
• Choose one word (might be different to last week) and with a partner, add the thoughts that might go with your words.	
• Make them big –including threads or spirals of thoughts	
Process in large group:	[15 minutes]
1. Share thoughts and flip.	
• Develop a list – Our Top 10 Negative Thoughts	
2. Talk about how these affect us (aversion/overwhelm/mood/ body)	
• Are they always true?	
• Look at stories (interpretations)	

- Affect of mood
- Thoughts are not facts – empty like clouds

3. What can we do when these arise?

Extended Responding Space at some point: [10 minutes]
- bringing gentleness into the 3rd step (the softness of the human heart)

Read: [5 minutes]
- Relating to Thoughts 2
    (in *Mindfulness Based Cognitive Therapy for Depression*, Segal et al., 2002)

Mountain Practice: [10 minutes]

Week 6 Home Practice: [5 minutes]
- Sitting/Movement
- 3MBS/Coping Space
- The Pause with kindness
- Physical Barometer

Give out Short Practice CD

Customizing practice

All Day arrangements: [5 minutes]

Breath and Bells to close: [5 minutes]
- Coming to Breath
- The bells

Home Practice	Body Scan/Mindful Movement/Sitting
	3 MBS/Coping Space
	The Physical Barometer and the Pause (together)
	Coming to the Breath with kindness
Resources	*Kitchen Table Wisdom* (Remen, 1996) or story book
	Mindfulness Based Cognitive Therapy for Depression (Segal et al., 2002)
	Large pens
	Bells
	CD 3s

© T. Bartley (2012). Mindfulness-Based Cognitive Therapy for Cancer.

The Critic

Large green warty bits hang off the side of his nose,
and smoky smells come out behind him.

He is creepy and slimy,
slithering around corners
sliding up from under the dark cellar
appearing suddenly and unexpectedly.

'Here I am – thought you'd got rid of me? – eh'
And there he is,
bigger than ever
and just as ugly,
totally without positive possibility.

'What shall I do with you', I plead with him.
'My life would be fine without you.
You bring up hurt and hate
And drop me into places of dark rank emptiness
Like the cellar you slime from'.

'I am the voice in your heart demanding your time,
Showing you dark corners, your secrets and shame.
Without me you would be lost in pleasure,
Sick with the pinkness of satisfaction
Bloated with pride.
You should go on your knees
and thank me for saving you
by showing you the blunders and flaws,
Oh my word you should'.

The farting warty toad stood still
Passion oozing from his eyes
Heart pounding in sincerity
Slime dropping onto the stone floor.

'Kiss me', he said.

March, 2006

All Day

Mindfulness is an act of hospitality. A way of learning to treat ourselves with kindness and care that slowly begins to percolate into the deepest recesses of our being while gradually offering us the possibility of relating to others in the same manner.

(Saki Santorelli, 2010)

Core theme:

To offer participants (past and present) the opportunity of *experiencing the practice at greater depth and in silence – emphasizing gentle kindness* throughout the session.

Key Tasks for Teachers – All Day

- To organize all the practicalities and set up the day.
- To plan a suitable programme and guide the practices.
- To hold the process and the group so that participants can experience the practices in safety.
- Emphasizing gentleness and kindness towards all experience in order to enable them to deepen their practice and experience a day of mindful awareness.

Overview

The day of practice, commonly known as the All Day, is drawn from the Mindfulness-Based Stress Reduction (MBSR) tradition. It is a little like a mini-retreat. It can result in increasing the confidence and deepening the capacity of participants, in their practice of mindfulness.

The Alaw MBCT-Ca All Day lasts for 4 ½ hours, starting at 10:30 and finishing by 15:00. For us, this seems to be long enough. Initially, due to limitations of space, we decided to hold the All Days in the Day Unit of the oncology department. This is a familiar space to many participants, who have received chemotherapy there. We hold the session at the weekend, so the Day Unit is not in use – and all medical equipment such as stands, cold caps etc, are removed – but it is easy to appreciate that the venue itself adds considerably to the challenge for some participants.

Some choose not to attend, or for a variety of reasons do not make it. Others come, but with some nervousness. Some may arrange to meet up with other group members and arrive together. Occasionally, we arrange specific support for a participant who wants to come, but is very anxious – perhaps involving a 'graduate' participant, who sits beside her during the day, who has attended other All Day sessions.

In addition to the challenges of the venue, many participants feel apprehensive about being in silence for the day. Not speaking is a new experience for many of us. Some approach this with interest, curious to know what it will be like. Others anticipate that they will feel anxious and alone, and wonder how they will cope. We take time in Week 6 to prepare for the experience. We talk about the silence and emphasize that the practices will be guided by the teacher (so it is not total silence).

We also explain that there will be stories and poems. However, there will be no group discussion during the session, and we invite participants not to exchange eye contact with each other. We explain that we will break our silence before we leave – and that there is a certain way that we do this. Others will be there at the All Day session who have attended previous other courses – and someone will be available for support should anyone want to talk something through. We discuss what participants might want to bring with them – lunch; drink; extra layers in case it gets chilly; sitting equipment etc.

Setting up the silence

We welcome all participants as they arrive and take our time to help everyone get settled with mats, stools and so on. We introduce those from previous courses to those on the current course, briefly sharing names. Then we set up the silence quite carefully, but not taking too long. We clarify the purpose of the session, mention the arrangements around support and lunch, and then connect to our intention for being there. We emphasize the importance of everyone looking after themselves, by taking breaks when they want to, working with whatever arises, with gentleness, patience and curiosity and seeking support when it might be helpful.

Poems and stories

In preparing for the session, as teachers, we chose a range of poems and stories that we read between practices. It is a lovely process. Guided by a theme of kindness and courage to turn towards, with compassion for ourselves and others, we let the stories or poems choose themselves when the time comes to read them. Visiting teachers have commented that we seem to use more readings than is usual in All Days. However, there is much challenge in just being back in the space where you received treatment – so we deliberately offer plenty of nurturing support through the inspiration of the readings, whilst taking care not to overcrowd the session.

Lunch

This is often the most challenging time for participants. Eating tends to be a social activity and not talking can feel very strange. There is also no guiding voice to offer structure. Rather than specify how long the lunch period will be, we tend to take as much time as the group needs. However, we are careful not to leave participants for too long and ensure someone is 'holding' the group at all times.

Special traditions

It seems important for each teacher to develop his or her own All Day practice programme. This is a time when we can use our creativity and inspiration. We always tend to guide a Mindful Stretching practice followed by a Body Scan. There are usually a number of Sitting Practices, often shorter than we might guide in class – and as the day goes on, we use fewer words and guide less. We also include Walking Practice, perhaps interspersed with sitting, wherever you are. This has a particular resonance for oncology patients, who may find themselves avoiding going near where they used to sit for treatment. Walking allows them to notice this, and experiment with how it feels to go close.

We have a few special traditions, which we have developed over the years. We always have a simple tea and strawberry ceremony, after which we read the story, 'Making a cup of green tea, I stop the war' (Levine, 1987). Graduate participants sometimes lead this. We usually include a loving kindness practice (see Sharon Salzberg, 1995).

Breaking silence

Following MBSR tradition, the silence is broken little by little. First, participants are invited to find a partner, (maybe someone they do not know) and whisper quietly, sharing their experience of the day. After some minutes, we invite two sets of pairs to join up. They may like to talk a little louder, whilst they share the highs and lows of the day. Eventually, taking care not to overrun the time, we come back into the large group and briefly share together.

Safeguarding participants

As teachers, we are keen to have an accurate sense of how each participant is, by the end of the session. We need to connect with anyone who may be experiencing difficulty, before they go home. We tend to turn towards difficulty in the large group, asking questions such as: 'What difficult times did you have?' Further processing of the day can take place during Week 7.

Closing the session

We close the session by returning to our intention. There may be a genuine sense of achievement and inspiration amongst participants. They have survived! We offer to share the learning and benefits of the practice with each other – and especially with anyone coming for treatment the following week. We like to imagine that we leave behind us some good wishes and kind thoughts.

All Day Programme

Courage to Turn Towards with Gentleness
Session time: 4 ½ hours

Programme

10:30   WELCOME
- ○ Availability – silence
- ○ Opportunity to be with ourselves – be aware
- ○ Intention– no need to do it right
- ○ Look after yourselves
- ○ Aspects of positive and negative – try working with them all just the same – curiosity – support available

- Poem/Story
- **Sitting**   [15 minutes]
  - ○ Breath, body > awareness of breathing
- Pocm/Story
- **Mindful Movement**   [40 minutes]
- **Body Scan**   [30 minutes]
- Poem/Story

12:30   LUNCH
- **Walking Meditation:**   [15+ minutes]
  - ○ Guided – getting a little quicker
  - ○ Notice what avoiding
  - ○ Notice what drawn to
- Extended Breathing Space: [10 minutes]
  - ○ (standing in mountain) at some point in the middle of walking
- **Lake**:   [15+ minutes]
  - ○ Using transition to lying down as part of the practice
- Story
- **Sit**/walk/sit/walk

2:10   Green Tea and Strawberries – S Levine story abridged

2:40	• **Loving Kindness Meditation**	
	• **Dedication**	
	• Break silence in pairs – then 4s – then whole group	
	• Share one word that describes how you are feeling now	
3:00	• **Bells**	[5 minutes]

Resources	Story books and Poetry	Lunch
	Green Tea	Strawberries
	Tea Pot	Mats, stools and cushions
	Bells	

**Dychwel at Graidd
y Graig**

Aros
am anadl,
Atal adwaith.
A dewis.

Clywed y sêr
A gweld curiad y galon,
Nofio gwynt y storm
A dychwel at graidd y graig.

**[Translation]
Returning to the Root of the
Rock**

Pause
a breath,
Refrain reaction.
Make a choice

Hear the stars
And see the beat of the heart,
Swim the storm-wind
And return to the root of the rock.

Sarah (November, 2010)

Week Seven

Love is what is left when you throw everything else overboard. The work of love is always going on beneath all other moments, beneath even understanding and consciousness, at the bottom of the bottom.

(John Tarrant, 1998)

Taking Care of Myself

Core theme:

As we approach the end of the course, we start bringing together what we have learnt *to develop an action plan* for ongoing support. We look at what lifts us and what drains us –and we chart an *overview of personal patterns – learning how to make choices that support well being*, now and in the future, in good times and when tough days return.

Key Tasks for Teachers – Week Seven

Week 7 practice:

- Sitting practice and inquiry
- Mountain standing, brief Body Scan from top down; moving to sit; posture; intention; breath; body as a whole; hearing; thinking and feeling; choiceless awareness; being with the difficult, including wanting things to be different
- Emphasizing the spacious container of awareness that gently holds all aspects of experience
- Dialogue especially around thinking and feeling; being with the difficult and choiceless awareness

Home practice review:

- Sitting; Coming to the Breath with kindness;
- Use of short practice CD
- All Day practice review

Week 7 exercise:

- Daily activities review; spiral signature and action plan
- Categorizing activities into nourishing, depleting and mastery activities – exploring how to reduce depleting, and increase nourishing and mastery
- Spiral signature and action plan

Week 7 short practice:

- Breathing Space (Responding) plus action step

Week 7 discussion:

- How have you changed through your illness?

Week 7 teaching:

- Diet (very brief)

Week 7 home practice:

- What can you sustain everyday for a month?

Concluding:

- Ending with the bells, breath and closing intention

Introduction

This session has a different feel to previous weeks. We are approaching the end of the course and it can seem a bit like the end of term. There may be a hint of celebration in the air, and perhaps some anticipation of loss. Whilst wanting to flow with whatever arises, as teachers, we also have to tie up the loose ends. We need to review the tools that we now have available to us, and make plans for ways of skilful responding to whatever life brings. The session programme is rich and full this week, so timings may need some careful attending.

Sitting Practice

This will be the last full length sitting of the course. Finding ways of making the practices our own, we guide a brief Body Scan in standing posture (or sitting for some), going from the top of the head down through the body to the toes. Then, we move from 'standing mountain' into a grounded sitting posture, continuing to guide the basic instructions of 'taking your seat'. People with cancer live with an ebb and flow of uncertainty – not knowing what may come next. Connecting with a grounded sense of the body helps to access an experience of core stability. Then we move up close to the direct experience of the breath, returning to our two cornerstones – the posture of the body and the anchor of the breath – always there to come back to.

Qualities of mind

Throughout the course, we have been cultivating an intention to come back to present awareness. Some participants may try a bit too hard with this. They may get tight or tired – and whatever we do as teachers, in terms of guiding an approach that includes kindness and patience towards the mind when it wanders, participants may still feel that their experience is wrong in some way. At this point, we approach things a little differently and invite a natural resting of the mind, letting it go where it wants – knowing there is a natural tendency of the mind to move – and also to return.

As the sitting practice has developed, we have been learning to expand the beam of attentiveness to connect with spacious awareness. We have been practising this for some weeks. Some participants find they can touch into the experience of spaciousness for a few moments now, without getting lost. They enjoy a natural sense of peace that arises when they practise in this way.

This feels different to a blank experience, when awareness has widened out but is dull and foggy. The metaphor of 'sky of mind' may help some participants to connect naturally with a sense of spaciousness. Others of us might try a bit too hard somehow, to create this – as if pushing the sky out to make it wider!

Awareness has an intrinsic capacity to focus and be spacious. Even when the mind is 'sharp' and focused, there is potential for spaciousness. In the same way, spacious awareness has within it a potential for focus and precision. These two dimensions are present in every moment, as the mind moves into focus or widens out into spaciousness.

At the end of the practice, we guide a short period of choiceless awareness.

Inquiry

Choiceless awareness sometimes appears to mirrors uncertainty, which can trigger anxiety. For some of us, it is almost like an experience of vertigo, when balance is threatened.

Josie looked a bit upset at the end of the practice. She had been very anxious during her treatment and was only just beginning to feel confident within the group.

'I was really disappointed,' she said. 'My practice has been so good this week. I loved the All Day. Then when we moved into the blue sky, I felt lost and scared. I somehow couldn't bear it. It reminded me of when I feel most anxious. I felt so alone'. Josie was close to tears. Her neighbour, reached out to hold her hand.

'What happened next when you felt like that?' I asked her.

Josie looked up, appearing to try to remember. 'I was giving myself a bad time for being so silly, I think. Then I came back to the breath', she said pausing 'and then I kept coming back every time I felt scared. Isn't it funny', she went on, sounding steadier. 'I know what to do and I did it – but in that moment of feeling scared, and thinking I'd lost my practice, everything seemed to vanish'.

By now, members of the group will often reinforce the learning for others in the moment. Josie had not forgotten – and those moments of panic were thoughts not facts.

Ginny looked very happy and relaxed at the end of the practice. She was getting to be quite a keen meditator, even after only 7 weeks. Her cancer was incurable and she was often troubled by anxiety and low mood, but her practice was becoming a refuge to turn to.

'I had a lovely practice. I enjoyed it,' she said. 'I was floating most of the time – drifting away and coming back. I was quite sleepy at times but it was lovely, like being on a boat on the sea, lulled by the waves.'

It might be a good time to ask – what makes a good practice? Aled had an interesting response, which underlines the wisdom in not judging a practice as good or bad. Each practice is what it is.

'I didn't have a good practice', Aled interjected soon after Josie had finished. 'I can't sit properly and don't feel like a mountain – more like a lump – but I can get past all that. I never feel "Isn't this brilliant!" This isn't what it is for me'.

'My practice is not good or bad. It is just a practice. But if I practise in the morning, it lasts me all day. I never get that lovely "Here I am sitting on a stool". For me it is not a thing of beauty – but it produces something that continues to work throughout the day', he finished, sounding satisfied.

As in the previous two weeks, we included 'being with the difficult' within the practice.

Helen was keen to share her experience. She had metastatic breast cancer and often felt restless and uncomfortable. 'I felt so tired and in the middle I had this hot flush' she said, 'I can sometimes breathe in coolness and breathe out heat – so I tried to do that. Then I felt so restless, I just couldn't keep still. I'd move and immediately want to move again. I really wanted it to go away' she said, rushing on, 'then I got a pain in my shoulder, "shall I stand up?" I asked myself. "No I won't", I said, "look at what you are thinking and have another go", I told myself'.

Opportunities to acknowledge courageous practice often come along. Affirming the possibility of starting again, over and over, is something we all need to hear.

Last Week's Home Practice

There may not be much enthusiasm for discussing home practice this week. They are more keen to move on to talk about the All Day. However, last week was the first with the short practice CD. How did they find it? Those with strong motivation and a well established formal practice seem to continue with the core practices – for now anyway. Those who are struggling with the longer practices welcome the new CD.

Annette is busy caring for her young daughter and elderly mother. She is still receiving treatment for breast cancer.

'I really struggle with the long practices', she said. 'But the breath is like a friend. I shut my eyes and notice my thoughts – then I breathe the breath into my lungs – and let it fill my body. At the end, it almost feels like my whole body is inflating. I do this several times a day – can't tell you how many – but always when I notice negative thoughts. I can spot them starting and before they get bad, I do a pause and then come to the breath. This works for me.'

All day discussion

The All Day may have had a strong impact. Sometimes participants are unable to attend. Inevitably they are keen to hear what happened. 'What was it like not to talk all that time?'

Jane had not been able to come to the All Day. Her son had been ill. Several times, Jane said how disappointed she was. 'Was it as if you were there on your own with just the teacher guiding you?' she asked. 'Or did you have a sense of the others even though you weren't talking or even looking at each other?' It was an interesting question and spoke of the strong connection that had developed in the group.

'No', said Sarah. 'We were very much a group all the way through. Even in the middle of the practices, when I had my eyes shut, everyone was there. Actually, I felt we were all helping each other. We were practising together. That was part of what was so good about it'.

John described how tired he felt after it was over. He enjoyed it at the time, but felt really weary the next day. The All Day session is held in the room where he had had treatment.

Gloria had done well on the course. She had been very distressed by her diagnosis, but had kept up a brave face throughout her treatment. 'It was fine while we were practising, I quite enjoyed it. But when we were doing the walking, I realised I was keeping away from the chair where I usually had my treatments. As the walking practice went on, I found I could get closer and closer. I began to think of all the people who must have sat in it since I did. I felt so sad for us all', she reflected.

'When I got home, I just cried and cried', she went on. 'It was as if the sadness was spilling out – and I just let it. Bill (her husband) was a bit concerned – but I told him to leave me alone. I was ok. And I was. I think I cried all the tears that I hadn't let myself cry. I felt so much better after – as if a heavy load had been lifted from my shoulders' she said.

Some might mention how they felt about having others with them on the All Day. This is an opportunity to refer to the community of practitioners, who have attended previous courses. Current participants will join them for follow up sessions. At some point, we practise a Breathing Space (Responding) or Coming to the Breath with Kindness – or both.

What Is Nurturing? What Is Draining?

Daily Activities

1. Make a list of all your activities during a typical day.
2. Categorize them into N for nourishing, D for depleting and M for mastery activities.
3. Explore how to reduce the Ds, and increase the Ns and Ms.

We then move to review everyday life activities (see Segal et al, 2002). Participants categorize their list:

N for nourishing or nurturing – activities that 'lift' us.
D for depleting or draining – activities that lower us.
M for mastery – activities, which are satisfying having completed them (such as paying bills, doing the ironing, defrosting the fridge, etc.).

They then move into pairs to look at ways of reducing the Ds on their list and increasing the Ns and Ms.

Jeremy is an older man, who has become quite frail. He is receiving palliative care and attends with his wife. The course has helped him feel steadier and he has clearly enjoyed being in the group, despite easily getting tired. Though not able to do the movement practice, he has loved watching his wife as she did it. As the weeks have gone by, he has become more and more loving towards her.

'I only have one D and that is shaving in the morning,' said Jeremy. 'It is so exhausting. I have to go back to bed sometimes before I've finished. But I can't bear not to do it myself.'

Jeremy thought for a bit and then became quite animated. 'I know' he said. 'We could move a stool up from the kitchen and I could sit on that while I shaved. That would make a big difference.'

Working with another person can help. Suggestions are made to a partner that on hearing, we can use ourselves. We are learning to apply what we have been practising. When we do things more mindfully, and with more kindness and gentleness, we may not be making vast shifts, but the impact of the activity can be transformed. There are many ways that we can do things differently. By slowing down, bringing awareness to how we feel as we do the activity, we interrupt the pattern and then have a choice to do it differently. It is when we push through, often rushing, and always out of awareness – that we get entangled in the 'knots of our own making' (Rilke, 1996).

This exercise is the first in a larger process.

The action step

We have come to the final development of the Breathing Space. Taking action is an important theme of the session. We guide an Extended Breathing Space and at the end include an invitation to *do* something specific in response. We discuss how we can make choices that offer enjoyment, nourishment and are mindful.

Cancer patients may come to a Breathing Space as a result of worry and anxiety. Choosing a relevant action may not always appear obvious. So with this in mind, we highlight some of the options on the whiteboard as follows:

1. *Mindful and Nurturing:* The first and probably best option is to find something that we can do mindfully that is nourishing or nurturing – that expresses kindness and is enjoyable. Then we choose deliberately to do it.
2. *Letting go*: In some situations, it might be difficult to decide what to do. In reviewing our options, perhaps in the context of something we have

been mulling over for a bit, we may come to realize that there is nothing we need to do. No action is necessary and we can let go of trying.

3. *Trusting Wise Mind*: Sometimes, it is not clear what to do – but we can have confidence that an action *will* present itself, when the time is right. So, we set our intention to trust this inner knowing when it arises.

Spiral Signature and Action Plan

Moving from daily life activities, we look at personal patterns of stress and difficulty. We consider how it might look in the event of (or fear of) a recurrence of cancer.

Spiral Signature (see Fig 6.7.1 below)

1. Turning to the Spiral Signature in the workbook, we invite participants to fill in their patterns on their own – from the early warning signs of stress, down to and including their patterns in the event of severe difficulty – such as a recurrence (or fear of one).
2. Then we share these as a group and develop and expand our ideas.

Note: This is adapted from the Relapse Signature in MBCT for Depression (Segal et al., 2002).

Carole said that she knows she is starting to get into difficulty when she gets busy. She describes how she can get into cleaning the work surfaces in the kitchen frenetically. 'If anyone interrupts me, I am really irritable with them. It is best just to keep out of my way', she says ruefully.

Veronica said she goes very quiet. Inside she starts to feel cold and alone. 'Further down the spiral, I just go to bed,' she said. 'When I was really bad, I went to bed for almost three months. Now I just go for a day. It is different. I know what I am doing and it is a choice rather than something I *have* to do.'

When we were looking for examples at the bottom of the spiral, Lucy talked about negative thoughts.

> 'I start planning my funeral,' she said. 'Later' her voice dropping, 'I lose my thoughts and am just in a very dark place. I have to be on my own then. I couldn't let anyone feel what I am feeling there. But I haven't been there since this course started', she said.

In Week 7, we deliberately bring the topic of recurrence into the open.

'What would you be doing in the event of a recurrence? How would you be behaving if you were worried that a recurrence was possible?'

In the past, participants tended to have established a much more optimistic frame of mind by the end of the course – but not always able to turn to their practice when faced with intense difficulty, such as a recurrence. After noticing this as a bit of a pattern, we decided to strengthen the use of the Spiral Signature to specifically focus on and turn towards recurrence. Whilst still frightening to contemplate, participants have enough confidence in the practice, the group and the process by Week 7 to be able to look at this –and it is vital that they do for the programme to be really effective for them.

Action plan

Generating a personal list of practices

The second part of this process can be a relief after the talk of recurrences. In small groups of threes and fours, participants generate their list of possible practices. These are drawn from core practices (those on CDs); short practices; and informal practices.

This can be fascinating. Participants share how they have adapted what they do. Examples of creativity emerge, especially with informal practices. These clearly demonstrate the ways that mindfulness has been integrated into everyday activity. We learn a lot from each other through this process – confirming the value of our own ideas and hearing many new ones.

SPIRAL SIGNATURE

(fill your patterns – behaviours, thoughts, feelings and
body sensations into the spaces under the numbers
on the right)

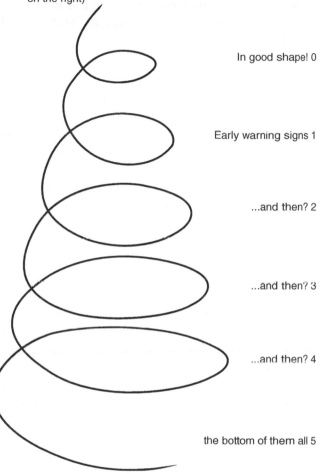

In good shape! 0

Early warning signs 1

...and then? 2

...and then? 3

...and then? 4

the bottom of them all 5

Figure 6.7.1   Spiral Signature.

Action Plan

What actions can I choose to take that will lift my mood, give me energy, give me a sense of mastery/satisfaction and nourish me, *even if I don't feel like doing them* – and in response to the different levels of the spiral signature:

1.
....
....
....
....

2.
....
....
....
....

3.
....
....
....
....

4.
....
....
....
....

5.
....
....
....
....

©T. Bartley (2012). Mindfulness-Based Cognitive Therapy for Cancer.

Here are some examples:

> Feeling the sheets in bed
> Listening to the waves of the sea
> 'Stop making stories – it is just a pain'
> Standing in mountain
> 30 minutes movement to my weird music
> Gin and tonic! Hearing the bubbles
> Making tea
> Looking up at the sky as I walk out of the door
> Letting the kettle boil
> Hearing the sound of my feet on the path
> Breathing
> Coming to my senses
> Feeling the water on my back in the shower
> The peace of wild things

We then ask participants to find practices for

1. Everyday
2. Early – middling stressful times
3. Tough times (such as recurrences)

using core practices, short practices and informal practices.

Here are some participants' examples:

> **Everyday Maintenance**
> - The Pause
> - Coming to the Breath
> - 15 minute sitting practice
> - 3MBS
> - Our own practices – like standing in mountain as the kettle boils

---

Early – Middling Stressful or Difficult Times

- Come to a monthly follow up session (might anyway – but make a point of it).
- 15 minute sitting practice every day at a pre-decided time.
- Breathing Spaces whenever needed.
- Doing a mindful movement practice (or any of the longer practices).
- Reviewing the Physical Barometer and using it every day.
- Noticing spiral of negative thinking, stepping out of it and into favourite short practice.

Recurrence or Fear of Recurrence – or at very Difficult Times

- Come to the Breath with Kindness (and for earlier times).
- Come on another course.
- Thread exercise No.3 every day – remembering everyone who is ill (*see Short Pratices, Chapter 8*).
- Phone a friend – get support – don't be strong and overly brave.
- Contact your mindfulness teacher.
- Standing in Mountain and doing Breathing Space – whenever you feel wobbly.
- Have a cry in the shower – don't hold things in.

We ask participants to develop this further by incorporating ideas that they have heard and liked, as part of their home practice. They will return next week with a completed personal action plan, recorded in their workbook – that includes ways of responding to all the different patterns on the spiral.

How you changed through your illness?

If there is time, and if it seems appropriate, we initiate a discussion with participants about the effects of their personal cancer journey. If the moment was right, we might have raised this last week, as something to think about.

We acknowledge that the course has been largely about helping to develop skills and approaches that reduce the negative impact of cancer and treatment. Now we might explore whether this is the whole picture. We

---

divide into 2 groups – or maybe stay in the large group. As teachers, we simply listen and hold the space. Offering a few questions to get the ball rolling, we then leave the group to explore whatever areas they feel drawn to.

Have you grown as a person?
Do you have different priorities now, since getting cancer?
Have your relationships changed? Do you feel differently towards loved ones?
What about your views on life?

Participants speak of feeling stronger; of appreciating the love of their families more; of wanting to take more time with the things that really matter – such as their children and their loved ones. Some have developed ways of reminding themselves to 'make each day count'.

Sue told the group that she used to be quite ambitious in her job, and tended to work long hours. She was soon to return to work after the end of the course, but now felt it was much less important. 'I now know how important my family is. I want to live my life to the full, however long I've got. Mindfulness will help me do that. This really matters to me now'.

Tony spoke movingly, 'I obviously can't say that I am glad that I've had this experience of cancer but having had it, I'm not going to waste this opportunity to grow in some way'.

'I think I'm a bit more compassionate,' said Beryl. 'I'm a bit more aware of others and their difficulties, whether it's on the news or when I think about people who are ill on the ward – and I send them my good wishes, like we have here in the group'.

The group might like to talk about this for longer, but even a short discussion leaves them with things to think about.

Diet, rest and exercise

It seems important to include something (albeit very briefly) about the basics of good nutrition. Few oncology departments offer much information. When we started these courses, we trawled various books and scanned available research. It is a tricky area with many strongly held viewpoints. We decided to share what made sense to us.

We tend to rely on various books and offer them to the group to look at – perhaps photocopying key diagrams and a few recipes. The Okinawa Program (Willcox et al., 2001) seems to be a useful place to start. A 25 year research study, it outlines the diet, exercise and lifestyle practices of people who are said to have the highest number of centenarians in the world, with correspondingly low levels of cancer, heart disease and stroke. We discuss what we could do to improve our diets. Most people have a sense of the changes they could make. Linking this to the course and more mindful eating can support our intention.

We are keen to avoid putting pressure on participants. We tend to emphasize the value of making small changes that we can sustain. Of buying, cooking and eating food that we enjoy, and know is good for us. If we promote anything, it is a middle path that steers clear of extremes. Then we widen the discussion to include the value of moderate exercise and sufficient rest.

Concluding the Session

Home practice – Week Seven

Practise what you can sustain for a month

Customizing your practice using:
- Core Practices (even if only 5 minutes);
- Short Practices and,
- Informal Practices.

Remembering Jon Kabat-Zinn's advice:

'Weave Your Parachute Every Day. You Never Know When You Might Need It'.

- Complete your detailed Action Plans for next time.
- Write a Poem about your experience of mindfulness.

The Bells and closing

We make plans for our last session. It will mark both an ending and a celebration for the journey we have taken together. We sometimes invite participants to bring tiny quantities of finger food so we can have a bit of a party. As teachers, we bring non-alcoholic sparkling drink. We invite them to write a poem about their experience of the course to bring to the last session. Some of these have been included in this book.

We close the session by practising Coming to the Breath with Kindness. We ring the bells and link with our intention to be mindful and gentle with ourselves – and to appreciate all that we have done in the session and during the week, that supports our intention. If it feels right, we also send kind thoughts and good wishes to those in the oncology ward, down the corridor.

Programme

Week 7: Taking Care of Ourselves

Session timing: 2 ½ hours

Standing Practice: • Body Scan top down (brief) • Intention	[5 minutes]
Sitting Practice: • Starting with mountain • Coming to sitting posture, and then to the breath • Whole of the body/hearing/thoughts • Then working with difficulty • Bringing spaciousness into the practice within choiceless awareness	[25 minutes]
Dialogue: • That practice – with particular focus both on what is difficult and, • On last week's experience of thoughts and thinking – and on spacious awareness	[10 minutes]
Dialogue: • Last week and All Day experience • Body Scan/movement/sitting practice/short CD practices • 3MBS/Coping space/The Physical Barometer	[10 minutes]
At some point in class, when sense of difficulty present	
• Guide **Coming to the Breath in Kindness**	[5 minutes]
Nurture/Depleting/Mastery exercise: • Make a list of a typical day's activities • Categorize N/M/D • Pairs to reflect on how to reduce Ds and increase Ns and Ms • Share highlights in large group	[15 minutes]

Coping plus Action Space:
 • Bringing gentleness into the 3rd step
 • and offering options from wise mind:
    a) mindful and nurturing
    b) no need for action and
    c) action will arise when time is right.
 • Inquiry
	[10 minutes]

Spiral Signature: [15 minutes]
- Look at on own and then flip examples
- Looking at ways we spiral down in group
- Specific focus on impact of recurrence or difficult life events

Action Plans: [10 minutes]
In 3 groups – paper and 3 fat coloured pens
- Onto floor on paper, a practice for:
  1) everyday
  2) early stress times
  3) tough times
- Large group process and share
- Detailed Action Plans home practice into workbooks for
  next week

Discussion (if appropriate):   [10 minutes]
- In what way have you:
  1) grown as a person
  2) developed different priorities
  3) have a sense of significant others – common
     humanity…..

Okinawa Programme (Willcox et al, 2001) **very brief**:   [10 minutes]
- Diet/rest and exercise

Kindness Practice: [5 minutes]
- 3rd thread exercise (if time)

Week 7 Home Practice: [5 minutes]
- Practice what you can sustain for a month
- Customize your practice
- ACTION PLANS for next time
- POEM and week 8 plans
- Give out measures to complete and return next week

Short intention and Bells to close: [5 minutes]
- Short intentions practice
- The bells

Home practice	• Customize – what can you do every day next week that you can sustain for a month	• Poem • Action Plan
Resources	Pens Pens	Bells Measures

My Late Night Visitor

I sit propped up in my bed, comfortable, relaxed.
Pen in hand, I am trying to write a poem.

'Can I get into your bed?'
No pause for my possible reply
Teddy under one arm, pillow under the other
She climbs across me to the other side of the bed.
She arranges her pillow to her satisfaction,
Settles herself with teddy and goes straight to sleep.
We have not spoken a word.

I put down my pen and give in to the moment.
I watch her sleep, I count her breaths.
Have those freckles always been there across her nose?
Her face is beautiful and the more I examine it
The less I seem to know it.
Did my mother gaze like this at me when I was five?
Will my daughter in turn gaze at her daughter when she is five?
I feel a sense of my place in the grand scheme of things
It feels right, it feels good.

She opens her eyes and gives me a steady look.
With a sleepy half smile she turns over and faces the wall.
I pick up my pen.

Liz (April, 2009)

Week Eight

When we stop tensing against life, we open to an awareness that is immeasurably large and suffused with love.

(Tara Brach, 2003)

Going Beyond Fear

Core theme:

Reviewing the journey that we have been on, we realize how far we have come. *Committing to a practice plan* for the next four weeks, *we celebrate the learning* gained as a result of the course and *affirm the significance of the group connection and say goodbye.*

Key Tasks for Teachers – Week Eight

Week 8 practice:

- Body Scan and brief inquiry
- Emphasizing gentleness and self compassion towards all aspects of experience

Home practice review:

- What did you do that you can sustain for a month?
- How will you / did you weave your parachute every day?

Week 8 exercise:

- Reviewing personal action plans
- Intention practice to support putting plans into action

Week 8 discussion:

- Review the course
- Going back through the weeks – maybe paper on floor – refer to workbooks – special highlights for this group – pulling out themes of the course
- Revisit 'Rilke's *River*'. What does this mean to you now?
- Give back 'Intention letters' from Week 1
- What have you learnt? What is different for you now? Discuss in pairs then large group
- Write a letter to yourself with:
  (a) practice commitments;
  (b) anything about what you have valued / learnt / achieved from the course that you want to remember and affirm.
- Give out certificates

Practicalities:

- Measures and DVDs back. Confirm follow up session date in 4 weeks.

Party (optional):

- Sharing participant poems

Concluding:

- Bells, breath and closing intention

Introduction

All endings are significant and this may be especially salient for people who have had cancer. If the group has formed a close bond, as many do, there may be feelings of loss that the course is coming to an end. One of the ways that cancer impacts so powerfully is through its connection to death and dying. This session is an opportunity to be with the 'death' of the group in a way that is respectful and 'allowing'.

As teachers, we seek to be true to whatever this represents for group members, and hold it in gentle awareness. We may notice a strong tendency to reassure. It is so tempting to talk about what follows, in terms of the drop in support sessions. No sooner than the words leave our lips comes the realization that we have veered away from our intention. It happens so often that we remind ourselves of this when planning the final session. Acknowledging the ending is an important opportunity to turn towards feelings with kindness, and allow whatever is there to be expressed. Having done that, *then* we mention the follow up sessions.

Body Scan and inquiry

We return to the Body Scan. This is the traditional practice for Week 8 from Mindfulness-Based Stress Reduction (MBSR). It is a skilful inclusion, right at the end of the course, to mirror the way we started. Participants may choose different positions – on the floor, sitting on a chair, or in the 'astronaut position'. They are probably more at ease with bringing kindness to their areas of treatment or injury. This is familiar territory, after all the times we have practiced being with difficulty. At the end, we discuss the practice briefly. Finishing where we started is intriguing. Offering a perspective on beginners mind – as if for the first time – and beginning again. This is not lost on some participants.

> Ffion found she had breast cancer soon after the birth of her daughter. It was a tough time for her whilst the baby was so young. The course has helped her feel calmer and less agitated. She has developed her practice and longs for the time when her youngster sleeps longer in the mornings, so that she can practice first thing after waking.

'It was like going back to the beginning – but easier!' Ffion announced happily. 'My mind just follows now. It is less effort somehow. But it was much harder to breathe in through the head and down the body to the toes – because there was a bend to get round!' The group all laughed. Ffion had been lying in the astronaut position, on the floor with her legs on a chair.

Just because this is the last session, the practice is not necessarily wonderful.

Jenny sounded a bit fed up.

'There was this loud humming noise all the time', she said. 'I couldn't forget it. I got bothered that I wasn't focused enough. The noise had an impact on my attention in the body. I tried to push it out but then it got even louder. It wasn't until right at the end that I saw what I was doing – trying to get rid of what I didn't want. Strangely that was quite useful' Jenny finished.

Home Practice Review

Last week, the invitation was to practice whatever could we sustain for a month. This is wise advice for those of us who set impossible goals that all too soon collapse! Long term well being for each participant is only as good as her capacity to sustain the practice – whatever shape that may take. Many of us teach participants who are thrilled with mindfulness and the course, but are unable to maintain what they have learnt. They feel better at first but as time passes, old habits of mind inevitably return. Mindfulness too easily becomes a memory of something that was helpful.

As teachers, this task of helping participants find ways of continuing to practice mindful awareness is as important as anything that we do on the course. What matters is not the length of their practice, but how they weave it into their everyday lives.

Here are some participants' plans for the four weeks until their follow up session:

Participants plans for following weeks		
Name and criteria for choice	**Core practice**	**Short practices/ comments**
Susie – plans to mix various practices but stick with one everyday.	15 minute Sitting Practice from CD3 every day.	Loves the Pause and the Breath. Aware of the Physical Barometer most days.
Janet – wants to be realistic. 10 minutes a day. Without the CD so always possible anywhere.	10 minutes own Sitting Practice – breath, sound, thoughts (sometimes) then Coming to the Breath with kindness.	Pause and Coming to the Breath as and when.
Bob – convenient and doable.	15 minute Sitting Practice from CD3.	Frequent Coming to the Breath – Standing in Mountain.
Ruth – longer practices at weekend.	3MBS × 3 times a day – continuing what has been doing for some time.	Breathing Space as and when Coming to the Breath with Kindness.
Peggy	30 minutes Practice every weekday morning before work. Nothing at weekends.	Hard to remember Short Practices except Standing in Mountain. Loves that.
Jennifer	Own version of Breathing Space sometimes 3 times every day for 5+ minutes long.	Notices building negative thoughts – then Pauses and Comes to Breath.
Murray – stick to 30 minutes	Movement Practice (30).	Pause. Coming to Breath with Kindness.

© T. Bartley, (2012). Mindfulness-Bases Cognitive Therapy for Cancer.

Everyone has a different plan. As teachers, we encourage them to adapt and shape their practice in whatever way suits their lives. None of them finish up with a 'text book' practice – whatever that might be. We will be reviewing plans in the group follow up class in a month.

We sometimes tell the story of Pauline, who attended the course some years ago – just to reinforce this.

Pauline finished her eight week course 'wedded' to the Body Scan. At Week 8 she was positive that she would never use the sitting practice again. She really did not get on with it, she said, but the Body Scan had made a big difference to her.

Two years later, she bumped into me in the hospital. She was keen to tell me how much she loves the sitting practice. 'I cannot imagine a day without it now' she said, 'I wouldn't feel right if I hadn't done it'.

We might guide a short practice at this point, – helpful here with all the discussion about future plans.

Action Plans

Having decided on our everyday practice plans, we then turn to the personal Action Plan that is designed part of last week's home practice. In pairs, participants share their ideas. They receive encouragement and fresh ideas from their partner. Sharing in the large group, we may hear ideas that seem especially relevant.

Robin
Robin said that if he was getting low or anxious, exercise was helpful. It was included on his action plan in several places – but he walked not just for mindful movement, but also for the practice of seeing and hearing. It was harder in the winter, as he really disliked the cold and wet – but this was when he was often more vulnerable. His partner in

---

the exercise suggested that he invest in some really good waterproofs. 'What an obvious solution!' said Robin.

Jonathan

From an idea from his partner, Jonathan decided to do a 3MBS before contentious phone calls. There were a number of family crises at present and he dreaded the bad news that came over the phone. It could sink him into despair. 'Such a simple idea – and I am going to put a sticky dot on the phone to remind me', he said.

Judy

Judy has a baking practice. 'I really am aware of the texture, smell, colour and look of the biscuits at all stages of making them – and then there is the taste' she said. 'Baking always cheers me up and it is very mindful'.

Margaret

Margaret said that she was surprised at how helpful it was to stand in mountain. 'It could hardly be simpler' she said. 'I tried it the other day when I was really upset, and it helped a lot'.

Mary

For Mary, it is songs and singing. 'Wherever I am, on my way down the spiral, there's a song that fits', she said, 'first there's the Beatles "Let it be". Then further down when it is tougher – I sing the Leonard Cohen song that goes "There is a crack in everything. It is where the light comes in". I just access the song and sing it – and this gets me back – and the words help too', she said.

We talk about what to do if there is a recurrence – or when things are very difficult. Participants share what they have included at the 'bottom' of the action plan (see Week 7) – in addition to the default practices of Coming to the Breath and/or doing a Breathing Space.

These are some examples of action plan ideas for recurrences or very difficult times:

Action plans for difficult times

Peggy	Get out my workbook and CDs and do the course again on my own.
	Commit to it. Ask my family for support.
Eve	Do a Body Scan – it might be hard but I bet it would help.
Margaret	Phone my friend who has been through this herself and knows about mindfulness.
Judy	Come to the next follow up class – and do Breathing Spaces in mountain 3 times a day.
Bob	Keep up my daily practice and remember I've got through it before.
	Be vigilant with depressing thoughts.
Janne	Phone my teacher and tell her and ask for support.
Mary	Stand in mountain and Come to the Breath with Kindness.
	Look at the mountains from the bottom of my garden. Keep doing this whenever I feel anxious.

When things are difficult, these are the times to turn to the action plans. How are we going to remember:

'What was it we said we were going to do?'

'Is there someone who could remind me to look at my action plan?'

We discuss this, reminding the group how isolating distress can be. Building in times when we get support and kindness from others is also important.

Course Review

We look back at the course. There are many ways of doing this – perhaps using objects or pieces of paper on the floor to represent each week. We are retracing our steps and remembering where we have been and what it meant to us.

Therese referred to the DVD *'Healing and the Mind'* (Moyers, 1993). She said how relieved she had been when a woman on the film said how stupid the raisin was.

'I never told anyone what we did with that raisin', she said. 'What would they think?! That was the daftest time – but one of the best was doing the movement practice in the third week. I felt so clear and well by the end. All the clouds lifted. I hadn't felt like that since before my diagnosis. That feeling gave me hope to carry on, even when it was really hard'.

Returning to the river

We re-read Rilke's *'River'* poem (Rilke, 1996). *What does this mean to you now?*

> May what I do flow from me like a river,
> no forcing and no holding back,
> the way it is with children.
>
> Then in these swelling and ebbing currents,
> these deepening tides moving out, returning,
> I will sing you as no one ever has,
> streaming through widening channels
> into the open sea.

For some, hearing the poem again helps them understand and articulate how they feel. It is similar to a sense of wholeness – to 'flow like a river'. There are many connections to make.

Gwyneth
Gwyneth's job takes her into the countryside. She has only recently returned to work after treatment for breast cancer. She spoke of a river that she knows well and described how it changes – sometimes slow and languid, sometimes almost in flood, with every variation in between. 'Ever since I heard the poem at the beginning of the course, I've been watching that river. I would love to flow like a river' she mused wistfully. 'I'm closer to it since doing this course, but I'm not there yet. But it is a good image to come back to, to help me remember.'

Jim

Jim has been beset with anger and irritation since getting cancer. He talked about what the poem meant to him. 'I think it is all about being more open', he said, 'when I started this, I thought I would learn how to change the bad feelings into good ones. Now I realize that my task is to be friendlier with how I am feeling, even if I feel murderous! The river helps me remember, even if I can't always do it'.

Giving back the intention letters

We now turn to the large envelope containing the intention letters written in Week 1, and open it in front of the group. The envelopes find their way to their owners, who open and read them.

This is an interesting process. Personal shifts and individual changes have been integrated as the course has progressed. Participants may have forgotten specific problems or issues. The letters remind them and enable them to appreciate the changes they have made. They have often needed to be courageous and compassionate towards themselves – and they have needed lots of commitment to complete the significant hours of practice.

They move into pairs once more. Questions go onto the white board to guide their reflections:

- How have you changed?
- What is different for you now?
- What have you learnt that you really value?
- How would you describe the course to someone who was considering doing it?

Write a letter to yourself

This is another valued MBSR tradition. Each participant writes a letter to himself or herself. This might include their experience of the course, of mindfulness and of their everyday practice plans. The letters will be posted back to them in a few weeks time, probably just before the follow up session.

Intentions practice

Inviting participants to link with what they wish for themselves, we connect to a heart intention to practice every day, 'as if our lives depended on it' (Kabat-Zinn, 1990).

> *'Settling into the posture...weight of the body going down....height of the spine going up...... reaching up into the space above the body and experiencing openness and spaciousness around the body.....including the breath in your practice, moving to wherever you feel it most vividly....noticing that the breath connects with the space around you, coming in to you from the space around you and going out into it, as you breathe out............*
>
> *Now, bringing to mind your action plan in a general way..... and then your plans for the daily practice until we meet again..........In whatever way is helpful, come to the heart and to your intention to practice in ways that support your wellbeing...to enable you to come back.....to turn towards what is challenging.....and to bring gentleness and friendliness to whatever you are experiencing'.*

Certificates

We then give out a personalized certificate to each participant. It always brings a smile. The certificate declares that the participant has completed twenty hours of class time and at least twenty hours of home practice – a significant achievement.

Practicalities

We confirm the arrangements for the group's follow up session in a month's time – and collect any post course measures and DVDs.

Party and poems

We might finish the session conventionally – perhaps by going round the group, inviting each group member to say something about what they are taking away. In the Alaw courses, we tend to have a bit of a party. It is simple and low key, but even the mention of a party is greeted with enthusiasm. Participants are unlikely to have celebrated their achievements on their cancer journey. This is an opportunity to do that – and have some fun. They have brought small quantities of snacks, crisps, or little nibbles. The teacher brings sparkling non-alcoholic drink for everyone. As some point, participants read out their poems.

Closing and the Bells

In due course, after the poems have been read, we close the session. Taking our seat and coming to the breath – we link with everyone in the group for the last time. We will be meeting again in a month for the group's follow up session, but this moment marks the end of the course. We invite everyone to notice how this feels – and to connect with an appreciation of all the group has offered, wishing them all well. Widening out, we offer our good wishes to loved ones, who have made it possible to be here, and all those we know who are having tough times. Finally, we play with the possibility that this heart connection and our good wishes can reach down the corridors of the hospital – and touch everyone who lies ill in bed. The sound of the bells closes the course and our final practice.

Programme

Week 8: Going beyond Fear

Session timing: 2 1/2 hours

Body Scan: [30 minutes]
• With lots of gentle kindness

SHORT Dialogue: [15 minutes]
• That practice (brief)
• How was it to do the Body Scan again, right at the end of the course?
• Back into last week's practice
• What did you do that you can sustain for a month

Action Plan: [5 + 5 minutes]
• (part of last week's home practice) in response to spiral signature
• share in PAIRS then in large group

Review Course: [20 minutes]
• Go through the weeks remembering particular moments
• Pull out core themes
• Week 8 is the rest of our lives
• Read Rilke poem – what does this mean to you now?

Give back intention forms: [20 minutes]
• What have you learnt? What is different for you?
• How would you describe this to an interested friend?
• In new **PAIRS**
• Whole Group sharing

Weaving your parachute every day: [10 minutes]
Write a letter to yourself including your practice plans and anything that you value/want to remember about the course and what you have learned

Intention practice: [5 minutes]
• Support for putting plans into place

Certificates: [5 minutes]

Practicalities: [5 minutes]
- Follow up group session, Measures back, Books and DVDs in **Poems** and Party

Short sitting with Dedication and Bells: [5 minutes]
- Dedication
- The bells

Resources	Rilke Poem (Rilke, 1996)	Pens
	Paper and envelopes	Bells
	Intention letters in large envelope	

© T. Bartley (2012). Mindfulness-Based Cognitive Therapy for Cancer.

Heading Home

Over mountains,
a cloak of rolling clouds
for the noble standing
of the Nantlle kings.

At their feet,
the silken surface of lake,
with ripples spread
like drops of kindness
from the heart
of the lovely Baladeulyn queen.

And in the wide clear openness above,
a lone circling buzzard -
calling.

We hold freeze framed,
these sights and sounds,
a teaching in the body mind.
Etching in us, intent -
to come back.

Trigonos,
North Wales, (December, 2010)

The Follow Up Class

Keep it simple and stick to the present moment.

(Ajahn Chah, 2004)

Gently Turning Towards

Core theme:

Reviewing the last month of practice and participant's action plans. Keeping the session focused on *supporting the intention to maintain a daily practice* of mindful awareness – and *bringing kindness into every day*.

Key Tasks For Teachers For Follow Up Class

Sitting practice

- (plenty of spaces without guiding) and brief inquiry

Last month's practice review and refining plans

- What did you do? What obstacles did you encounter to practising what you planned? How do you come back?
- Recalling all the practices that we have learnt – from the core; short and informal practices.
- Sharing the 4 Movements of MBCT-Ca – Intention; Coming Back; Turning Towards the Difficult and Kindness
- Reviewing and refining individual Action Plans and Daily Practice Plans
- Intentions Practice to support personal practice commitments

General monthly follow up information

Closing process

- Bells and Closing intention

Introduction

We meet again a month after the end of the course to review how things have gone. The follow up class has an important summarizing function, highlighting the bones of the eight week course. In essence, we focus on reminding participants what they know and helping them to bring this into a commitment to sustain a daily practice.

We often find that as teachers, we have some apprehension before the class. Have the participants continued to practise? Will any of them turn up? Are they all still well? Walking down the corridor to the waiting area, it is easy to be aware of thoughts about who might or might not be waiting – and they are invariably wrong.

Helping to remember

Last night three members of the group were missing. One had sent apologies for lateness to another group member. The other two were surprise absentees – but as we settled to practice, they arrived a little breathless – and there we were, a complete group again.

This was commented on, as we finished.

'I felt comfortable once everyone was here', said Janet. 'It was as if the circle was joined up again and we were all safe'. As she spoke, she looked round the group. She was met with nods of agreement. The group had formed a strong bond, which had been important to them.

We include the follow up session in order to support ongoing practice; help them review what they have done; and look at what needs more attention. It is easy in the pleasure of reconnecting to get sidetracked – and in view of the limited time available (only one and a half hours), it is sometimes a bit of a challenge for the group to stay focused.

The Practice

- Standing in mountain, maybe a few stretches.
- Sitting practice with a focus on the breath and the body.
- Very brief inquiry.

We start with a mountain standing posture, followed by a few simple stretches. Then we come to a sitting practice. Once established in the posture and with the breath, we guide very little. After all, the participants are practising independently now.

A brief inquiry follows. There will probably be a strong pull to talk about how it has been since the end of the course.

Review of Last Month's Home Practice

We then invite participants to move into small groups of 3s and 4s, to review their practice since the end of the course. We write questions on the white board to help them stay focused:

- What did you do? Did you practise as you planned?
- What obstacles did you encounter to practising what you planned?

There is usually much to discuss. Many of them will have had some awareness of the others as they struggled, failed and started again with their practice. They will be keen to hear how everyone got on, hoping they were not on their own in not doing all that they planned. This is where rich sharing can take place. They have learnt to affirm each other and offer reassurance – and in doing so can hear and receive reassurance themselves. When the volume of conversation in the room begins to drop a little, we return to the large group, to share a few choice 'nuggets' from their discussions.

Steven attended the course with his wife who had breast cancer. She had found the whole experience of diagnosis and treatment very troubling. He had a long history of depression. When they heard about the course, both were keen to attend.

Steven started telling us about the 'mood' that descended on him over Christmas. It was very familiar to him. 'As soon as I felt it starting, I practised straightaway for just 15 minutes. I repeated this several times over the following few hours. Do you know that my mood and that awful aggression that comes with it, faded in just a few hours? It usually lasts for several days. I couldn't believe it.' Steven looked very pleased. We were congratulating him as Jane broke in with 'But sometimes we just have to live with the difficulty don't we? That is what you keep telling us. My barometer never changes. The knot is always the same, always seems tight and I do so want it to go away'.

Jane had been hounded by acute and persistent anxiety after having breast cancer. She was not yet 40 and had found the whole experience of diagnosis and treatment miserable and very distressing. She had been very conscientious on the course, following instructions to the letter. Her workbook was full of additional notes and she seemed to put a lot of effort into the course – maybe trying a bit too hard at times.

We agreed with her gently. The group seemed especially sensitive towards her in that moment. It was unusual for her to speak with such passion. She relaxed as she heard the reassurance from the group and quietly commented, 'Maybe I could be more kindly to the knot in my chest'.

Recalling the practices

We place three large sheets of paper on the floor:

1. Informal everyday practices.
2. Short practices.
3. Formal practices.

We then discuss what we regularly practise in each category – and what we might turn to at times of difficulty. This is similar to what we did in week 7.

There are overlaps between categories, but this does not matter. The exercise is simply a device for sharing and consolidating ideas, which will be much more productive than 'teaching'. It also offers an opportunity of remembering other practices that we have learned over the course.

Informal everyday practices

Examples of creativity often emerge as we share:

Beth

Beth was in her early 50s. She was much affected by the side effects of chemotherapy treatment. Her feet hurt and her joints were stiff and painful. She shared an experience of looking out over the cliffs on the coast at the end of the day, when the sun was going down.

'I was so moved by the beauty of the shadows and the light that I walked much further than I would normally have done. It was very special somehow. I wasn't bothered about taking exercise. I just enjoyed bring there and seeing everything. Stan (her husband) was happy too, because we walked together much further than usual. Often he has to walk on his own. Thinking about it afterwards, I realized that being really present with everything around me on that walk, brought us closer together somehow'.

Mike

Mike had been very sceptical about the course – but he had been conscientious with his home practice. He longed to be less anxious and wanted to 'get back to normal' after his cancer diagnosis (which was incurable, and likely to involve long periods of remission). He described how his favourite practice was to stop, go outside and look up at the sky – especially when he felt wound up and tense.

'If the sky is overcast, I remember that there is a clear blue sky behind the clouds', he said, 'sometimes I have to stand for a bit to get into that sense of the clear blue of the sky – but when I do my mind starts to open and clear. Once I feel more settled, I bring my attention to my feet on the ground and I move into standing like a mountain and experiencing the space of the sky all around me. I always feel steadier after. This really works for me and it doesn't take long'.

It is interesting to notice how helpful these individual practices become. They may not follow the way as teachers we might guide them (as in Mike's example – we might have taught him to come into mountain standing first). However, it becomes apparent that the very process of personalizing the practices embeds them in a powerful way.

As we discuss this, participants may come to appreciate in a new way that we can turn any activity into a practice. It might be a routine activity (such as taking a shower), a special time (such a watching the birds), a habit that is established (stopping and pausing every time the phone rings), or a disciplined commitment (listening to the clock every time it chimes the hour).

Short practices

By now, certain short practices have become habits. The Pause is usually a favourite, as is Coming to the Breath and Coming to the Breath with Kindness. One young woman shared that her breath was 'just here', gesturing beside her body, a bit like a very faithful pet always beside her. She barely needed to shift to connect with it.

Some participants connect strongly with the 3MBS and often make it their own in some way. We might guide a breathing space to remind those who are not so practiced with it. The Physical Barometer has a mixed following. Those who still struggle with connecting to their body sensations may not have used it. Some people incorporate the Physical Barometer into the first step of a Breathing Space. They may also use it as a practice in its own right, when unpleasant or difficult feelings are present. One woman calls her Physical Barometer her foghorn.

Formal practices

It may be surprising to find how few participants use the longer practices once the course is over. MBCT-Ca does not attract people who are interested in meditating *per se*. Their motivation is around a wish to reduce their personal patterns of suffering. Many of them may practise very diligently while the course is running, but only use the short practice CD or even their own personal versions of short practices after it has finished.

Some participants return to the longer CDs (especially the Body Scan) during periods of difficulty. The factors that enable participants to continue to practise during crises are not well understood and would benefit from research. We need to learn more about the mechanisms that connect people to practice.

Four MBCT-Ca movements

After discussing the practices, we place Intention; Coming Back; Turning Towards the Difficult; and Kindness – Four Movements that are central to MBCT-Ca – written on large pieces of paper, one by one on the floor next to the practice sheets. There is no need to offer much explanation. We simply describe them as the key underpinnings of the course that come together to support the practices. Even though this is the first time we name them in this way, most participants are very familiar with them already – and may gain much benefit from seeing them written down. Connections can be made in simple direct ways that can be very insightful. (See the next chapter, chapter 7, for a presentation of The Second Circle – Mindful Awareness and the Circle of Practice. This offers a diagram of MBCT-Ca and include the four key 'movements' explored here.)

---

1. Intention

There is a proverb that goes: *'If you think small, the result is small. If you think vast, the result is vast. It all depends on your intention'*.

We have been learning to connect with our intention – finding it within the heart – and discovering that it offers us strong support for our practise. We start by cultivating a wish for all that is best for our health and wellbeing – best for us as individuals, and best for those we care about. Then we commit ourselves to connect with that intention regularly, in order to align our actions and our practice to it.

---

2. Coming\Back

Coming Back is the movement of mind that shifts from automatic pilot to direct present awareness.

What and where are we Coming Back to?

Here are some examples from participants' discussion:

- Breath   *'I like the idea of the anchor that secures me to the present'*

    'I'm coming back to being more alive and aware when I'm connected to the breath'.

    'When I notice my thoughts building and getting black, then I come back to the breath and my thoughts lose their power somehow'.

- Body   *'I come back to my feet on the floor – works every time!'*

    'I come back to my whole body, right out to the surface of my skin'.

- This moment   *NOW*

    When I do walking practice, I love saying HERE and NOW as I pause and turn. I can really feel that'.

- This place   *HERE*

    'I sometimes concentrate on being on this very spot on the floor'.

---

3. Turning Towards The Difficult

If Coming Back is the basis of all our practice, how do we turn towards the difficult?

What is involved in this?

Here are some examples of participants' responses:

'I sometimes think I need to do another whole course to be able properly to put this into practice. I can do it when we are being guided in class, but it is so hard on my own when I get worried about something big, like what if the cancer comes back'.

'If I'm practising regularly and sort of in tune with myself, then I notice my barometer –and as soon as it starts to wind up, I can do a breathing space, or come to the breath, or maybe just breathe into it (the sensations in the barometer). If I can catch it early enough, then I can somehow relax around it. But if it has already got going, it is much harder and I might just as easily get busy and run away from it '.

---

4. Kindness

Kindness is an intention and joins with Coming Back and Turning Towards.

How can we remember to practise bringing kindness to our experience?

Here are some examples of participants' responses:

*'I like doing Coming to the Breath with Kindness. Sometimes, it feels like there is a ripple that spreads
around my body – and I like imagining it going into my mind too'.*

'I wish I could be more kind – I try to be kind to others, but I should be kinder to me'.

'I'm remembering a bit more than I used to – especially when I practise, but now we have finished the course, I'm afraid that I'll just slip back into bad habits again'.

Session practice (2) – a new intention

We then lead a short intentions practice. This allows participants to commit to their practice intentions. They have discussed what they do and looked at the themes that underpin them, now we invite them to bring a specific practice plan to mind that will support them over the next few weeks and months. It might be the same as what they have been doing since the end of the course – or it may have changed, perhaps influenced by ideas in the group.

At the end, participants share briefly with a neighbour, and then turning to their workbooks, and record their new practice intention at the back of the book on the page provided

Monthly follow up sessions

We give out letters inviting participants to join the regular monthly follow up sessions. These are open to anyone who has attended a mindfulness course on the unit. Dates for the whole year are listed. Members of the group are encouraged to come soon. They can attend regularly or infrequently, as they wish. The informality of the sessions is emphasized.

Goodbye to The Group

Although we have already said goodbye in week 8, there are bound to be further farewells to say in this last meeting. Group members may well meet again at follow up sessions, or at All Days, but they will never meet again in this configuration. This is significant. There may be some sadness. Some may want to hug and initiate an exchange of phone numbers or emails.

In openly acknowledging this ending, we have an opportunity to embrace the loss and turn towards what might otherwise be avoided. We have been on a significant journey together and have touched each other's lives. In connecting with people who have similar feelings and experiences, it has been possible to share fears and learn alongside one another. A sense of connection and good wishes for others is how we finish, as we ring the bells in the group for the last time.

Programme

Follow Up Class (one month after the end of the course)

Session timing: 1 ½

Practice: • Mountain Standing, maybe a few stretches and then sitting with a main focus on the breath and body Not too much guiding	[20 minutes]
Inquiry: • The class practice and then back over the month • In 3s and 4s – What did you do? Did you practice as planned? What obstacles did you encounter? How do you come back? • Share nuggets of these discussions in the whole group	[20 minutes]
Exercise – 3 Sheets on the floor: 1) Informal Everyday Practice 2) Short Practices 3) Formal Practices Discuss and share what they do and what might do if in difficulty	[15 minutes]
Teaching – 4 Movements: 1) Intention 2) Coming Back 3) Turning Towards the Difficult 4) Kindness Probably need to briefly teach intention and then discuss other three, posing questions for the group	[10 minutes]
Intentions Practice: • In light of reflections and discussions – what are your personal practice commitments • What are personal practice commitments? Share with neighbour and record in work book	[5 minutes]
Handouts: • Follow up sessions • Give out letter with dates and details	[5 minutes]
Bells: • Ending and the breath • Finishing with sharing benefit of course with group and wider	[5 minutes]

Resources   Bells   Follow Up session handouts
                 Work Book

Friends

Fear and a frown were my friends
Never letting me down, always present
Tears instead of laughter
Sorrow instead of joy
Blinkered to all the goodness still inside.

Quietly the breath carried on – just waiting
The same breath I always had
Staying with me through the year
Patiently hoping I'd notice
Something so deep had not changed at all.
I follow the breath, I try to control its pace
It is uneasy so I let it work alone
Sometimes deep and slow
Sometimes short and shallow
When I am lost, it knows just what to do.

I am different, I know myself better now
I acknowledge my fearful friends
The breath welcomes them in
Treats them with kindness
The breath, and kindness, my new best friends – and you

Liddy (December, 2009)

Chapter Seven

The Second Circle: Mindful Awareness and the Circle Of Practice

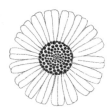

Introduction

Now that we have encountered the MBCT-Ca programme in detail, we are ready to turn to the next circle diagram. Earlier, we read about the first circle, the Circle of Suffering, which draws a cognitive model of cancer distress that develops from reactions to cancer diagnosis and treatment. This second circle moves us from the experience of being a cancer patient to the learning that develops as a participant on an MBCT-Ca course. We call it the Circle of Practice as it focuses directly on the intervention of the eight week MBCT-Ca course and the movements participants make as they develop their practice of mindful awareness.

It is apparent on looking at the diagram that the overall markings used in this second circle are lighter compared to the first. This represents the possibility that participants have less claustrophobia, heaviness and constriction. Openness is beginning to develop.

We meet Jane, David and Sheila again in this chapter (see chapter 1). They are three cancer patients who joined the eight week MBCT-Ca cours that was running in their North Wales oncology department. They brought different perspectives with them in both their approach to and adjustment of cancer

Mindfulness-Based Cognitive Therapy for Cancer: Gently Turning Towards,
First Edition. Trish Bartley.
© 2012 Trish Bartley. Published 2012 by John Wiley & Sons, Ltd.

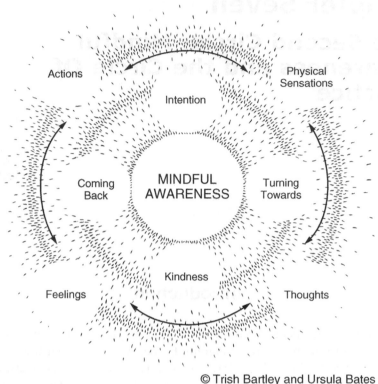

© Trish Bartley and Ursula Bates

Figure 7.1 Circle of Practice – Mindful Awareness.

and treatment. Their experience of the MBCT-Ca course will help to illustrate some of the ideas that we discuss here.

At The Centre

Mindful awareness

The practice of Mindful Awareness is what we develop on the MBCT-Ca course. This is a lifelong practice, but even after eight weeks some connection is possible, with dedicated commitment to home practice.

As in the first circle, what lies in the centre strongly influences the whole circle. As our mindful awareness practice deepens, the mind settles. No longer so identified with our immediate thoughts and feelings, we begin to develop the capacity to see thoughts as simply thoughts – and human experience as part of the tapestry of life. It requires courage for participants with cancer to practise with an internal sense of uncertainty. Mindful awareness enables them to open to experience, whether pleasant or unpleasant. They are developing a capacity to be detailed, precise and focused in their attentiveness and also to be able to cultivate a wider, more open and spacious, 'panoramic' awareness (Trungpa, 1995).

Middle Ring

Four movements

1. Intention
2. Coming Back
3. Turning Towards The Difficult
4. Kindness

Four movements underpin the entire MBCT-Ca intervention. The articulation of these four movements is influenced by Shapiro's model of mechanisms of mindfulness that uses three axioms of Intention; Attention; Attitude to describe 'the moment by moment interwoven and cyclic process of mindfulness' (Shapiro et al., 2006). Another significant inspiration comes from Self Compassion (Neff, 2003), which draws on the practice of mindfulness and kindness, and a perspective around common humanity.

In the first movement, we gather into intention. Then in the second, balancing between attention and wandering, we come back to the breath and the body. Turning towards whatever is difficult is the next movement. Then finally, we open to kindness. To sit, to balance, to move with courage and to experience connection are the great gestures of every living being and are life itself.

1. Intention

Our intentions are closely linked to our motivations. Connecting to intention is central to the support of the development of mindful awareness practice. By cultivating helpful intention at the very beginning of the MBCT-Ca course, we connect back to it at the start and the end of each class. This links each participant to their own personal vision of wellbeing. Starting from what drew them to a mindfulness-based course – their experience of cancer and treatment – they are invited to connect with a deeply felt wish from the heart, for what is best for them. (In the first circle we refer to 'people with cancer; in the second to 'participants'; and in third to 'practitioners'.)

Intention is dynamic and evolves as practice develops (Shapiro et al., 2006). It is therefore a key source of support for a personal commitment to the course. 'When kindness, generosity, love and wisdom motivate our intentions, then happiness follows' (Goldstein, 2002). The opposite is also true. So we learn to look after our intentions with care, by practising with kindness and a commitment to be present.

Intention helped Sheila stay with the course and kept her on track with her practice even when she felt like running away and hiding. Her traumatic experience at diagnosis was still very raw. Yet underneath, she knew that mindfulness had something to offer her. So even though she was often right at the edge of what she felt she could manage, she stayed with her practice and attended every class, because she had made a clear decision to do that. Connecting with her intention kept her true to this commitment. Without it she would have given up.

2. Coming back

From the start of the course, we learn to recognize and step out of automatically reacting and step into an experience of present awareness. This starts with the raisin exercise. The invitation is there to see the wrinkles of the raisin, to touch the texture of it, to taste the flavour – and in that moment of seeing, touching or tasting, we come back to our direct and immediate experience. In that moment, we are present.

Through the practices that build on the course, and by connecting to sensations in the body and/or the breath, we learn to 'come back' to ourselves. Jane had no trouble learning to come back to her body. She found she could become interested in the detailed sensations that she could feel in her back, or her feet or wherever she placed her attention. Increasingly, she realised that as she did this, she felt more settled. It became easier to notice when her mind wandered off into thinking or worrying, and she found she could bring it back to wherever she had got to in the practice. In everyday life, she learnt to come back to her feet on the floor and to her breath, when her thoughts or feelings started to trouble her.

'Coming Back' is short hand for the movement that returns us to mindful awareness – that enables us to come back to being present and aware. The participant begins to feel a sense of being grounded, held and contained by her experience of 'coming back'. Perhaps, her troubling emotions lose their intensity and her mind grows in flexibility and stability and finds other ground to stand on. She is no longer so identified with the thoughts and feelings as they arise in her mind.

At first this 'coming back' seems to be an act of will – bringing the mind back when it has wandered away. Later it seems that awareness almost brings itself back. Coming Back links with 'Attention' in Shapiro and colleagues' model of Reperceiving (Shapiro et al., 2006). They draw out three axioms, Intention, Attention and Attitude. However, a subtle difference in emphasis unfolds with the model of 'reperceiving'. The natural dynamic of the mind is viewed here as intrinsic and unproblematic. Staying present and learning to attend to one object for a long period of time is not a focus of MBCT-Ca. Like pressed apple juice settling in a glass, the process of clearing and steadying the mind is natural and needs no determined effort (Nhat Hanh, 1988). Time, intention and a certain discipline of practice allow the mind to settle. Seeking to deliberately stay mindfully present has the risk of resulting in tightness and fatigue – a bit like a cat sitting at a mouse hole waiting to pounce – always on guard and never able to rest. Instead, connecting with the intention to be present, and relating to the mind with gentleness and kindness, we come back.

3. Turning towards the difficult

People with life threatening illness have two levels of trauma. There are actual medical experiences of intrusive procedures and treatment. Then there are cognitive and emotional difficulties in assimilating their experience to their normal worldview. Some become stuck in a rigid, tense, superficial coping. Most, after an initial period of shock, actively set about trying to integrate their old worldview, with the world they now find themselves in. This is an uneven process, with traumatic material often returning.

Jane started to find the courage to turn towards the experience of her mastectomy. To begin with, it 'freaked' her out – but with practice and intention, she learnt to move her awareness around the edges of the area, and gently come up closer to the physical sensations. She learnt that it was not the sensations that were 'freaky', but the thoughts that her mind added. Before the end of the course, she was beginning to be able to breathe into the area. She still felt unhappy with how it looked and sad at the loss of it, but she was more able to bring kindness to her distress, rather than blame or judgement.

Implicit therefore, is the practice of stopping, noticing and acknowledging the difficulty that has arrived. The participant seeks out the feeling of this within the body and then turns towards the sensations, exploring around the edges or moving right into them. The breath supports this process, using gentle attentiveness towards whatever develops.

David could understand the principle of turning towards. It made sense to him, but as he found it hard to locate the physical sensations in the trunk of his body, he found it difficult to practise. Then he was invited to explore that very feeling of difficulty – of not getting it right – of wanting to feel the sensations, but not finding any. He discovered a dull tightness in his chest. When he explored this and breathed into it, he was surprised to find that the sensation grew in size and intensity. Then after a while as he continued, he sensed it gradually ease and open. He felt more secure after this, and was impressed with the effect of the practice.

Turning Towards provides the container in which the difficult can be experienced and integrated. Of course, this is counter-intuitive. The automatic tendency of all beings is to push away, resist and avoid what is difficult and unpleasant. Turning Towards is *not* about getting distance from the experience, observing it objectively, or witnessing it from a safe place. It is the opposite of turning away. A degree of courage, trust, confidence and even surender is required. Turning Towards is the medicine, once adequate grounding and the practice of Coming Back is established – which enables a practice of allowing, letting be, opening and softening to the pain of sickness and misery, that ultimately transforms our suffering.

4. Kindness

Kindness towards oneself, ones struggles and mistakes, is essential for change. Kindness is usually associated with an attitude extended to others. Here it includes an approach to self and links to self compassion (Neff, 2003). So often, behind our external rigidity and critical dualistic thinking lies a lonely deprived notion of self that believes it is not good enough. Kindness as 'ground' (often expressed as love) is a basic tenet of the all spiritual traditions. In mindful awareness, kindness is the ground in which our practice grows.

Kindness relates to acceptance and an active openness to what is here, now. Letting go of the tendency to compare, cling to and desire, what we perceive is good – and reject, avoid and push away, what we perceive as bad – requires a radical shift. The intention to open to experience, ultimately leads us to become more receptive to kindness. For the person with cancer, who has often been socialized to fight their illness, this is a significant and challenging change. It takes courage to be kind – and choose to support one's own wellbeing. Habits of pushing through or being driven by old uncompassionate ways easily deplete and drain.

Sheila found it helped to practise with kindness, by connecting with the feelings she felt when one of her children had hurt themselves. How she was with her children and how her mother was with her, helped her to develop kindness towards herself. It was not an easy process for her, but she got some glimpses of it. Jane found it helped to bring attention to her heart and let the breath move kindness from her heart around her body. She liked to feel the warmth and sense of flow. She believed it was helping her be more forgiving towards herself, and less judging. David learned about kindness through coming back. He noticed how often he judged himself when his mind wandered. Having made the connection, he decided to practise bringing his mind back kindly, every time he noticed the judgements. It was a bit like training a puppy, he agreed – encouraging the puppy rather than chastising it.

The practice of kindness requires a turning towards experience, and accepting all that experience brings, both pleasant and unpleasant. Kindness invites in essential heart qualities, and inches the participant closer to befriending their experience and connecting with others like them. The more kindness is practised, the more natural this movement seems to become.

Outer Ring

Thoughts, feelings, physical sensations and actions

The outer ring holds four dimensions of experience: thinking, feeling, body sensations and actions (or behaviours). These are the basic materials of our practice. They are what we use to map our experience – moving away from the 'big black blob' of experience (Williams et al., 2008) that threatens to overwhelm – into a capacity to differentiate the separate yet interconnected aspects that make up experience.

Summary

This then, is the second circle diagram, which underpins the essence of the MBCT-Ca programme. On the outside are the dimensions of experience. The practice of mindful awareness is at the centre and surrounding it are the movements which develop the practice. Not surprisingly, this second circle is called The Circle of Practice.

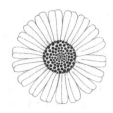

Personal Story

Derek

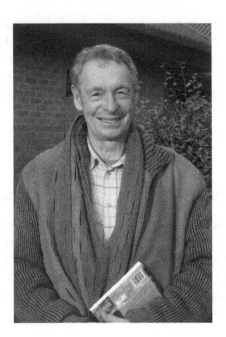

Derek is Welsh. He is retired and now in his late sixties. He has two grown up children and is very happily married to Mairwen. Derek is a keen musician and plays and composes music regularly with his friends. He was diagnosed with a rare cancer in 2007 and after major surgery, attended a mindfulness course in 2008.

Mindfulness-Based Cognitive Therapy for Cancer: Gently Turning Towards, First Edition. Trish Bartley.
© 2012 Trish Bartley. Published 2012 by John Wiley & Sons, Ltd.

Diagnosis

In 2007, I started feeling ill. I was treated for colitis, but there was more going on. So I went in for further tests. After a lot of deliberation, they found a very rare cancer, which affects the lining of the abdominal cavity. It was not very invasive, but it bungs you up with a lot of cysts. It was quite a shock to know I had cancer. In some ways I was quite philosophical. I felt that I'd had quite a good life. These things happen, so why not to me. I was more upset about my wife and worried about the effects on her. Both her parents had died of cancer and she had nursed them to the end, so I felt pretty sad to think she had that to face.

Treatment

Basingstoke was the lead hospital for this condition. We had a bit of a wait, but went down before Christmas. I was feeling pretty knackered by then. They told us about this particular operation that was quite extensive and involved peeling off all the internal lining of the abdomen. We wanted to think about it for a few days, but we said yes, we'll go ahead. They said they had a vacancy before Christmas and explained what would be involved.

Anyway, I had the operation but apparently there was some haemorrhaging. Mairwen was called in and was told that they did not know if I would pull through. I had nine hours of surgery on day one and three hours on day two. My kids were summoned. I was out of it and having weird dreams in intensive care. By day four, I was beginning to come round and rallied quicker than they had expected. I spent four weeks in hospital in Basingstoke and then back in Bangor where I became a day patient. I felt uncomfortable for weeks after and a bit slow in the mornings – but all in all, not too bad. I was told after the surgery that I probably had at least three years – although after that, the cancer tends to come back. But I haven't asked any more about that. When I was on the mindfulness course, I had a recurrence (in October 2008). I was put onto this particular drug, and the doctors have been very pleased with its effects so far. The cysts have shrunk and I'm feeling pretty well most of the time.

What brought me to mindfulness?

I was in a bit of an anxious state after all that time in hospital. I had lost a lot of weight so I was in touch with a dietician. I told her that in general I was not feeling very bright. She suggested that I might consider joining a mindfulness course. I suppose I was a bit depressed. Mairwen was very good. I would sit there in my chair at home, not feeling like moving and she would say, 'Come on, let's go out. It will do us good'. My sleep was affected. I would wake early and I sometimes felt very restless. I was not sure that I was going to get much better, and didn't feel like bothering too much. I wasn't down all the time, but in a given week, there were periods most days when I would feel pretty low.

Mindfulness

I'm quite interested in things about the mind and mood – in emotions and things that are not easily quantified. I thought that there was a good chance that mindfulness would be useful. Having cancer is a unique experience and you don't know exactly how anybody else feels about it. A lot of people on the course empathised well. I liked that. I thought that was a good thing to do. We could actually take a step forward by doing the course. It showed me that you can still be yourself, having come through what we had all experienced.

There was a planned progression and structure to the course. You could take things from it and adapt them to suit yourself. I did all the CDs regularly during the eight weeks. After, I didn't stay with the longer practices, but moved to the short ones and did them pretty regularly. Recently, I decided to go back to the shorter ones again and do them a bit more – like topping up.

When I was in hospital in Basingstoke, I started to understand aspects of love a bit more – it was very powerful. I received loving comments through cards and messages from family and friends. There were all these people offering kind thoughts in a very genuine way. This was quite a positive side to having a serious illness. It was a bonus to have experienced it. I felt strongly that there is a lot of goodness in the world.

It was a similar sort of feeling on the course – being in the same boat and being pleased for each other. It was a good thing to feel like that.

I left the course in December 2008 and have come back to quite a few follow ups and All Day sessions since then. I find it is a positive experience to be immersed in it – I don't know people socially – but there is a supportive feeling amongst those of us who attend. I like being part of that. I come to All Day practices for myself and for everyone. I like being part of it. We've had a few laughs too. Doing a walking exercise in one of the All Days, there were lots of visitors peering through the glass door. They must have thought – 'Look at them. They are in a bad way in that ward!'

I seem to have particularly latched on to the sayings. I do a breathing practice to start and then repeat various phrases to myself. I do this most days. It sort of encapsulates my aims for myself in relation to others. I vary it slightly from time to time:

> May we be peaceful
> May we accept what needs to be accepted without anger
> May we direct gentle kindness to each other
> May we make sound choices
> May we, in a troubled world, appreciate the many good things around and in us

It is a bit like a prayer. By using 'we' – it extends things. There is a slight focus on me and Mairwen, but the intention is for ourselves and for others.

I think I am a lot more tolerant of little niggles. I can take it or leave it – I get a bit annoyed with practical things sometimes, but I'm a lot more laissez faire with something that is not very important. I'd stand up if there was a big injustice – but before doing mindfulness, I'd have got much more wound up about all sorts of things. There is a certain mellowness in me now.

I'm interested in the way people think about religion and God and things like that. I'm not religious myself, or follow any particular faith. When people talk about God, I say I hope you are right. It would be marvellous if everyone could be healthy and live in peace. I just say my phrases to myself – I'm a humanist I suppose – and believe good things should be encouraged.

My practice has offered me the chance to be thoughtful in a positive way. As a biologist, I've always found aspects of nature and the living world quite remarkable. Mindfulness has allowed me to feel more positive about my life. It is quite hard to know what would have happened if I hadn't done it. We are both pleased that I've found something that helps.

The power of kindness is very powerful in itself.

Chapter Eight
The Practices

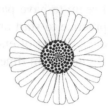

This immediacy of knowing – right now – of the breath, a sound, some movement, points to the innate wakefulness of our minds. We learn to become familiar with it, and trust it ... It is all within us: we are what we are looking for.

(Joseph Goldstein, 2002)

Introduction

In working with people with cancer, we often need to adapt and develop the practices that we use on the programme. The first part of this chapter looks at the core practices of Body Scan, Mindful Movement and Sitting Practice. It explores them within the framework of the movements of Intention; Coming Back; Turning Towards and Kindness that we have been looking at in the last chapter. After this, we move on to describe the short practices that we use in the MBCT-Ca programme.

Mindfulness-Based Cognitive Therapy for Cancer: Gently Turning Towards,
First Edition. Trish Bartley.
© 2012 Trish Bartley. Published 2012 by John Wiley & Sons, Ltd.

The Core Practices

Each moment can be fresh, each breath a new beginning, a new letting go, a new letting be ..... Why not trust your experience in this moment just as you would trust your foot to find a way to keep you balanced as you move over rocks?

(Kabat-Zinn, 1990)

Introduction

Each core practice is introduced at a specific point in the eight week course. They build sequentially. Participants first experience them in class, guided by their teacher, then they practise them at home with the use of CDs.

As the teacher guides each practice, she experiences it herself in her own body and mind. Awareness of edges, limits, wandering mind, wanting and not wanting and much more, will be present for participant and teacher alike.

30 Minute practices

In MBCT-Ca, the core practices last for 30 minutes, which is less than the traditional 45 minute practices in MBSR and MBCT. This was chosen partly in response to the low energy of participants, many of whom have just finished demanding treatments, and partly because of the number of short practices in MBCT-Ca.

Body Scan within MBCT-Ca

The words remember and remind ... imply connections that already exist ... for instance when we 're-member' to pay attention, to be in the present, to be in our body ... we remember our wholeness (Kabat-Zinn, 1990)

In the Body Scan, we learn 'intentionally (to) move attention around the body.' (Segal et al., 2002). In the orientation meetings, we tell participants that they will be doing a lying down practice at the end of the first session. They then practice the Body Scan every day at home for the first two weeks and every other day for the third week.

Implications for people with cancer

We invite participants to choose whether to lie on the floor, or sit on a chair – or move part way through. Many may be physically able to lie down, but may have difficulty or feel anxious about getting up. We will have talked about this at their orientation meeting. We have mats to provide a clean surface for those lying down – and blankets and cushions to add comfort.

The Body Scan is a very significant practice. When illness strikes, especially one that is associated with pain, uncertainty, and possible death, people with cancer may become vigilant about sensations in the body. However, this awareness is not mindful or practised with a view to being with sensations. Instead, it is motivated by a desire to push them away and tends to involve anxious rumination. In the Body Scan, we are invited to 'find a way to re-establish contact with the body, whether what comes up is pleasant or unpleasant.' (Segal et al., 2002).

When working with people with cancer, as teachers, we take much care as we guide into different parts of the body. We need to know about participants' treatment sites, levels of pain or discomfort, and areas of active disease. We also want to have a sense of how much fear each participant is experiencing.

Our task as teachers is to find ways of 'holding' the practice, so that our participants are able to attend to their body with gentleness and courage. It can be a slow, tender process. It requires us, as teachers, to stay grounded and embodied in our own experience; aware of individuals and how they are; whilst also in touch with the wider group process.

Body Scan practice overview

- **Settling into the sensations of contact** of the body with the floor/chair; and the quality of this contact.
- **Moving up close to the breath**, breathing itself deep within the belly (perhaps with hands resting on the belly to guide the attention).

- **Moving the attention** from the belly all the way down to the toes of the left foot – and then guiding in detail through the different toes, and parts of toes and the foot – **inviting noticing of sensations**, and also of texture, heat, hardness and softness, contact, inside and outside, and so on. Noticing areas of not much sensation and inviting an interest into what *that* feels like.
- Imagining that we can breathe in a different way – by bringing the breath all the way down the left side of the body and into the left foot and the left toes, as if **breathing directly into** the foot **and then breathing out from** the left foot, and up and out through the nose – using the breath as a vehicle for awareness.
- Repeating this process through different sections of the body.
- Sometimes **widening the attention** into the whole of a limb or a larger part of the body, always inviting attention that is gentle, kindly, compassionate and curious.
- Remembering that **there is no goal** other than to notice sensations in the body as best we can, and be present with them.
- At times, reassuring our participants that **it is normal for the mind to wander**. It is what minds do. Whenever we notice, we gently come back to the body and the sensations.
- At the end of the practice, inviting participants (if this feels alright for them) to gently turn towards any part of the body that has experienced treatment or injury. **Bringing kindly attention** into this part – breathing into it gently, if this feels ok, and opening to any sensations present there.
- As the practice finishes, inviting people to slowly and gently get up, taking time to move, being aware of the body, as we transition slowly back into sitting in a circle.

Common reactions to Body Scan

At the start of the course, many participants feel anxious and stressed by recent events. Energy may be low. Some are sleeping badly and feel exhausted. Drifting off to sleep during the practice is not surprising or unwelcome, although it may provoke a sense of guilt. As the weeks pass, it seems to get easier to experience more of the practice. As teachers, we balance the need for rest, with inviting the possibility of waking up to the practice.

Some participants love the Body Scan from the very first. They relate to it as a relaxation practice. The challenge is to help them explore sensations. Why are we so keen *not* to focus on relaxation as an outcome? It can be very healing and helpful. However, if relaxation is the goal, we block out being present to other possibilities.

Many loathe the practice from the start. They may find it hard to stay with it and become resistant and agitated, irritated, or connected with distress. It may be difficult to move up close to, or be aware of much sensation in the body. If these participants can keep doing it – without expectation, many find that whilst they may not actively enjoy it, they do become aware of some benefit, even though it may be hard to express what that is. In the orientation meeting, we have promoted the value of diligent practice. As a result, many participants are well prepared for challenges that may arise and seem to manage pretty well.

Body Scan and The Four MBCT-Ca Movements

1. Intention

Intention underpins the start and close of Body Scan practice, reconnecting our participants to a commitment to their own wellbeing. This supports the possibility of goal-less effort and befriending experience however it is. Through intention, we bring the heart into the practice as an ally.

2. Coming back

Coming Back is shorthand for the dynamic of mind that wakes up out of its automatic wandering – and returns to a here-and-now awareness. This involves both a 'coming back' and a 'lingering there' (Kabat-Zinn, 1990).

As practice develops, the capacity to come back into the focus of direct sensations naturally evolves. The breath is then included, becoming a vehicle for awareness, before letting go and shifting focus to another area. This is repeated over and over – focusing in on specific detailed sensations, lingering and exploring, bringing the breath down into the area and then letting go and moving on.

Body Scan also invites coming back to more spacious awareness of (say) the full extent of a limb. In this process of 'up close', precise attention, and wider more spacious awareness, we learn how to relate to the wandering mind. Sleep may have entrapped us (perhaps for much of the Body Scan) or a protracted scenario may have enticed us away. Parts of the body may have been missed. When we 'wake up', we are invariably at the mercy of the judging mind, which condemns us for not being present. The practice invites the mind to come back whenever it wakes up – and be present with things as they are, with kindly attention.

3. Turning towards

We invite participants to move awareness to a treatment area or place of injury at the end of the Body Scan. We would NOT invite participants to turn towards the site of their disease – or use the word 'cancer' as we guide practices. Referring to 'treatment areas' or 'places of injury' seems to avoid aversive reactions and invite gentle awareness. Inviting a kindly breath down into the area, we practice turning towards and being with it.

Even at this early stage, we are starting to practice 'turning towards' with kindness. This is significant for people who tend to avoid the very places that most need their attention. Many are surprised at how little sensation is there – or how resistant they are to turning towards it – or perhaps how healing they find it, when they do. We guide this in a way that invites gentle curiosity and care – so that those who do not want to explore these sensations always have a supported choice not to do so.

4. Kindness

Kindness is a central ingredient in the practice. For those who have had traumatic physical experiences, the body may be an unfriendly place to linger. Up to now, attention may have been glancing, avoidant, and resistant. This is very different to mindful awareness, developed over the weeks of practising the Body Scan, which has a fresh, curious and gentle quality. As the practice matures, it often becomes a favourite, even for those who are at first quite challenged by it. It offers us the chance to befriend in kindness the very place where we have been absent for so long.

Mindful Movement within MBCT-Ca

Goodwill and warm curiosity towards our feelings will put us in greater touch with the full experience of our lives (Williams et al., 2007)

We first practise Mindful Movement in Week 3 session and then at home with a CD, alternating with the Body Scan and then the Sitting Practice for a number of weeks. Both Body Scan and Mindful Movement facilitate awareness of the body, albeit in different modes. Both develop a more grounded inhabiting of the body. It often comes as a relief to do a moving practice after the static encounter of the Body Scan. Even those with advanced disease, or who have had recent treatment say that Mindful Movement is easier 'to be with'. The mind appears to wander less.

Implications for people with cancer

Every MBCT-Ca group has people who have a range of physical abilities. Some participants have significant physical limitations. Then there are those who are keen to extend into stronger poses. We practise in a way that encourages all participants to work with their limits in any given moment.

Remembering how easy it is to push through in keenness to do more, we establish that the purpose of the practice is to be aware of sensations of stretch and intensity in the body, and to make choices moment by moment around those sensations. We may move into them, dwelling at the edge of intensity, exploring and breathing into it. We may sometimes choose to move away from the edge, whilst respecting what is right for each of us in each moment. We are learning what it means to respond to intensity mindfully.

Whilst some people may try to do too much, others may be understandably tentative and fearful around surgery or treatment sites. As teachers, we encourage our participants to practise by choosing skilfully how far to go, how long to hold each stretch and importantly how to be gentle. Some participants may choose to sit on a chair doing what they can – or closing their eyes and visualizing they are doing the practice. Others manage some postures, perhaps the standing stretches, but may find the lying down ones too arduous. We take care to notice when participants have chosen to sit out or take a breather. This offers an opportunity to affirm the skill in making wise choices to everyone in the group.

It is vital for us to know about participants' cancers, treatment areas, places of pain, and issues like stoma or ileostomy bags. Whilst this is important when guiding the Body Scan, it is even more relevant now, whilst guiding mindful movement practices.

We tend to guide different postures for different groups. The 'standard' mindfulness routine often starts with strong stretches – arms above the head. This is unsuitable for breast cancer patients. It might be better to move into other postures first, perhaps returning to stretching upwards later, once the practice of working gently with limits is established.

We continue to remind and encourage our participants, throughout the practice, to hold for as long as feels right to them; or choose not to do the movement at all; and to congratulate themselves for choosing to come out of a posture early. We include stretches or twists with the awareness that some will find them challenging – taking care to guide them in a way that invites very precise awareness in each moment; offering lots of choice; and encouraging gentleness. As one participant wisely noticed, 'It takes courage to be gentle'. We seek to offer safe challenge, so that participants learn to make mindful choices, especially in the context of intensity. If we guide the entire practice very gently, there is no opportunity to work with limits.

Mindful walking

A Mindful Walking Practice is included on the second track of the movement CD. This is a valuable practice and helpful as an alternative movement practice for those not able to do the mindful stretches.

Mindful stretching practice overview

- Offering different options from very beginning – having a chair to move to – perhaps choosing to sit, **imagining** the movements.
- Guiding briefly into a **standing posture**, awareness of the soles of the feet and contact with the ground, up through to the crown of the head.
- Whilst participants are in standing posture, **introducing the practice** – including some caution around not pushing through edges and limits; and encouraging the making of kindly choices and practising without goal. **Not leaving participants standing for too long** – especially at the beginning of the practice.
- Moving out of stillness and responding to any parts of the body that want to move – **moving mindfully**, attending to the body as it would like you to.
- Returning to standing posture; exploring the contact between the feet and the floor – 'weight going down', and the movement of the spine up through

the body – 'height going up'. Use terms such as **mountain standing** (or **sitting** for those on chairs) – grounded, tall, present and dignified.

- Then guiding **choice of postures** appropriate to the group – some standing – including twists and balances, if appropriate – some lying down movements.
- **Breathing** freely and fully during the movements, bringing the breath into any areas of intensity; dwelling there with full awareness of edges; and gently choosing when to come out guided by the sensitivity of the body in each moment.
- At the start of the lying down section, guiding into fully relaxed lying pose (do <u>not</u> refer to this as the corpse pose), awareness of contact of the body with the floor – 'weight going down' onto the ground – awareness of full length of the body – **lying mountain**.
- Pausing between each posture to come back to mountain standing or mountain lying with **mindful awareness of effects** of last posture/s within the body.
- Whenever moving into a new position, using the transition as part of the practice, inviting awareness of the whole body and the experience of moving.
- Probably finishing in lying mountain posture fully **letting go and relaxing** into the contact of the body with the floor, scanning through the body for effects of the postures. Breathing deeply through the whole body.

Mindful Movement and The Four MBCT-Ca Movements

1. Intention

At the start of each practice, we invite participants to connect with their personal vision for their own wellbeing, and to commit their intention to practice bringing gentleness and awareness to each movement.

2. Coming back

Coming back over and over to awareness of the moving detail of experience in the body – whether it be noticing when we automatically push through an edge – or when we learn to come back to 'just this much' in the body – using the breath to support awareness of whatever is arising.

3. Turning towards

Intensity in the body. If it seems skilful and wise, gently moving the mind into it, breathing, and opening into and around the intensity. When discerning the edge of a limit, coming out of the posture and easing back to awareness of the body as a whole, standing or lying.

4. Kindness

Is integral to this practice. We practise to befriend the body exactly as it is – learning to bring gentle awareness to the places of intensity in the body – and judgement within the mind. With kindness and compassion for ourselves, especially in the context of illness and treatment, we make wise choices.

Sitting Practice within MBCT-Ca

Introduction

The Sitting Practice further develops what we have started in Body Scan and Mindful Movement. It offers an opportunity to tune into the moving reactivity of the mind. Within Sitting Practice are many individual practices that train the mind in developing different aspects of mindful awareness.

This includes:

- Inviting the mind to be attentive to detailed, precise, and close up experience (such as the direct sensations of the breath expanding the muscles in the wall of belly as the breath comes in)
- Inviting the mind to open into more spacious awareness, holding experience within a wider container (such as expanding into awareness of the body as a whole sitting there, with the breath breathing in the whole of the body)

Sitting practice is introduced in Week 3 or 4, and then guided at the start of all subsequent weeks (in slightly different form) until week 8. It is practiced at home with the CD1:2 used in Week 4, alternating with Mindful Movement.

We spend time 'taking our seat'. This offers a strong foundation that we can come back to. It establishes a safe container that holds experience as it arises.

Posture

Weight going down, awareness of the solid of the floor beneath you. Height going up, awareness of the spine moving up out of the pelvis through the body, towards the space above you. Arriving in the body. Awareness of the space beyond and around the body. Finally – inviting the heart and chest to be open and the belly to be soft. Present. Dignified.

Even after we have become familiar with Sitting Practice, we continue to take care in fully arriving in the body at the start of each practice.

Stools are available. However, sitting on a chair is just as good, and may be better for those with stiffness or pain. We invite people on chairs to sit slightly away from the back of the chair, if this is possible for them.

Implications for people with cancer

The Sitting Practice can be demanding. It is another relatively still practice, after the welcome dynamic of Mindful Movement. For those still impacted by trauma, the gaps of silence and the 'internal' focus may be too difficult. As teachers, we support an approach that encourages gentleness and appreciation of the personal challenges involved.

Practices guided in class may be easier than those practised at home, due to the support of the group and the teacher's 'holding' presence. In Week 6, a third CD (Short Practice) is given out, containing a 15 minute sitting practice. Participants seem to get on well with it, often continuing to use it long after the course has finished.

Some people have trouble with awareness of the breath. As teachers, we may anticipate that people with lung cancer may have difficulty with the breath, but many manage well, often successfully finding their own ways of adapting. Whatever the issue, it will be possible for everyone to find an anchor within the breath, the body, or with sound. However, we may need to use opportunities within the dialogues to help those experiencing difficulties with their breathing to find their 'anchor'.

Sitting practice structure – overview

- Arriving in the **posture** of the body.
- Directing awareness of **the breath** breathing deep in the trunk of the body, wherever sensations are felt[1].
- Gently noticing the **wandering of the mind**, which is bound to happen – perhaps distracted by thoughts, sound or sensation in the body – and coming back to the breath with kindly awareness.
- Expanding into a sense of the **whole body** and the breath breathing in the body as a whole.
- Becoming aware of **intense sensation** within the body and exploring options of choosing to move mindfully around it, or turning towards it to explore detailed sensations, or returning to close-up attention on the breath. At some point, returning to a sense of the whole body breathing.
- Expanding to include experience of **hearing** – of sound arising and dissolving in the space around.
- Relating to **thoughts and feelings**, no longer as distractions, but as the focus of awareness – as events in the mind that arise and dissolve – held in the wide container of spacious awareness.
- Opening further to connect with **choiceless awareness**, held within a spacious 'sky of mind' – being present with whatever arises, moment by moment – be it the breath; the body; specific sensations; sound; thoughts or feelings. Coming back to focused awareness of the breath breathing at the end of the practice.

Being with the Difficult Practice

Implications for people with cancer

We guide this practice towards the end of the Sitting Practice in Week 5 and the following two weeks. Establishing a reasonably settled practice

---

[1]There is some debate as to where to place the attention to experience the breath. Some traditions invite a focus just under the nostrils. This facilitates concentrated mindfulness of the breath and can be very calming. We tend to invite practitioners to become aware of the breath 'deep in the body', wherever they feel it most vividly. This usually promotes a more embodied relationship to the breath and is 'further away' from the apparent source of thoughts.

experience before embarking on Being with the Difficult section, we invite participants to bring to mind something that is outside their here-and-now experience.

We guide this with care and sensitivity. Whatever cautions we offer in relation to the wisdom of choosing a moderate difficulty, it is worth bearing in mind that some participants may choose their fear of recurrence. This holds a strong charge and has a risk of overwhelm. Conversely, we also notice that many participants keep well away from choosing any challenging issue, especially at first. This may be less of a conscious choice and more of an intuitively wise one.

Being with the Difficult

Introduction

Depending on the robustness of the group, it may be skilful to start the approach to this practice quite gently in Week 5 – encouraging participants to choose difficulties with increasingly more charge over Weeks 6 and 7 – as they become more confident in the practice and their own capacity to turn towards the difficult.

Exercise

Having established the breath as a safe place to come back to, we now move to a new step in the practice. Inviting you to bring to mind a current difficulty – not choosing the biggest, but perhaps one that has some level of charge for you ..... Noticing how it looks to you ... Not getting into the story line, but bringing it to mind ......

Now sensing where the resonance of this difficulty is making itself felt within the body. What sensation is present? Seeing if you can locate this precisely, perhaps in the trunk of the body .... then inviting you to gently turn towards it. Moving up to the sensation of difficulty in an open, friendly and curious way – or maybe choosing to work around the edges of it – or perhaps deciding to explore it from a safe distance ..... What is the shape of the sensation? ... texture? ... colour? How does it look to you? How does it feel – moving or pulsing? Is it getting stronger or changing in some way? ..... gently exploring it and bringing kindly awareness to it. We are not trying to change it – but simply to practise turning towards and being with it.

> *When you are ready, inviting you to breathe into it and breathe out from it .... using the breath as a vehicle for your awareness ..... noticing how this feels ...... and bringing tender and kindly awareness to whatever is there .... knowing that at any time you can come back to the breath .... exploring, turning towards the felt sensations of difficulty, opening to them .... saying to yourself, 'it is ok, whatever it is, let me feel it.*
>
> *When you are ready, coming back to the body as a whole sitting here and the breath breathing in the whole of the body ..... you may be aware of the difficulty still resonating within you or it may have changed .... gently breathing the breath in the whole of the body.*

Sitting Practice and The Four MBCT-Ca Movements

1. Intention

Intention is included at the start of the practice and returned to at the end. By now, participants are familiar with this. Intention invites the heart into the practice, helping participants to be open, friendly, curious and kind – supporting their wish for wellbeing.

2. Coming back

Coming back to the anchor of the breath in the body enables participants to relate to the wandering mind that otherwise may lead them to places of reactivity. Awareness dawns that 'coming back' is not so much an effort of will, but a natural movement of waking up and returning to direct experience. There is a memory – intention in its truest form – that knows to come back to the immediacy of the present moment.

3. Turning towards the difficult

Turning towards the difficult – is developed further within the Sitting Practice. From the first, we turn towards intense sensations in the body, and acknowledge and explore them. From Week 5, 'turning towards' moves centre stage. The 'difficult' is invited in, to be explored in the body, breathed with, and offered kindness and compassion. Without compassionate awareness, 'turning towards' might be brutal – but in reality it is 'turning away' from difficulty that waters the roots of suffering.

Kindness

Kindness is central to all practice. Awareness entails kindness – just as kindness always involves openness and awareness. We are relearning some basic and wise qualities of mind and heart.

We now move on to look at the short practices in the programme. We summarize these in the next section and then describe in more detail, those that we have developed specifically for the MBCT-Ca intervention.

The Thickening Stillness

Silence rolls in like mist
across the shores of our short history
boundaries erected in haste
cease to be.

A pause, a glimpse, a heartbeat
leap out, then fade away
breath slowing, deepening
sighing release.

An inscape revisited
a nakedness re-touched
and in the depth of the fire
and in the depth of the earth
only this:
compassion
And clear light.

"But you said.." and "she said.."
"and you did" and "he did"
fading and retreating
and in the thickening stillness
healing begins.

Stewart Mercer (2002)

The Short Practices

Paying attention to the world around you, rather than wishing to alter it, changes everything ..... I began to enjoy the afternoon and the breeze on my skin.

(Gwyneth Lewis, 2002)

Overview

People with cancer want to live in ways that will help them access steadiness and peace of mind, and support them to manage uncertainty. They want time to live their lives and focus on what is most important to them.

Some are still getting over the effects of treatment – experiencing aches in the body, adjusting to the psychological impact of cancer and its treatment, dealing with long term implications such as early retirement, return to work, change of self image, different energy levels, and much more. Some will need additional treatment in due course. Coping with recurrences, treatment choices and the likelihood of a shortened life span are immensely challenging, especially at first.

It is therefore unlikely that many participants will choose to sustain the longer core practices on a regular basis. Instead, in moments each day, they come back to their own mix of short practices that they have adapted and integrated into their everyday lives.

For this reason, we have developed a number of new practices for MBCT-Ca, whilst continuing to rely on the value the Breathing Spaces.

The challenge of guiding short practices

It is tempting to imagine that shorter practices are easier to guide than long ones. The reverse is probably true. In a very short time, as teachers, we need to get ourselves into the practice, grounded and embodied, in order to guide the group effectively. There is little time to manage this. Often, we choose to take time to settle *before* starting the practice. This allows us, as teachers, the opportunity to come back and arrive into ourselves – allowing us to be strongly in the experience of the practice as we start to guide it for our participants.

MBCT for Cancer Short Practices

This section outlines all short practices within MBCT-Ca in the sequence that we introduce them on the course. Those that I have developed are described in detail below. Short practices from MBCT for Depression (Segal, et al., 2002) or MBSR (Kabat-Zinn, 1994) are also listed. Brief notes are included that refer to the ways that we have adapted or developed practices for people with cancer.

Table 8.1 Outline of all Short Practices.

Practice	Original Source	Introduced	Duration
The Pause[‡]	(Brach, 2003)	Week 1	Less than 1 minute
Coming to the Breath[‡]	Adapted from MBSR – Mindfulness of Breathing (Kabat-Zinn, 1990)	Week 2	Variable[**]
3-Minute Breathing Space (3MBS) (regular)	MBCT (Segal et al., 2002)	Week 3	3 minutes
Standing In Mountain[‡]	MBSR – Mountain practice and mindful movement (Kabat-Zinn, 1990)	Week 3 onwards	Variable[**]
Breathing With[‡]	MBSR (Kabat-Zinn, 1990)	When needed. Not in home practice	Alongside difficulty
Physical Barometer[‡]	MBCT-Ca (Cited in Williams et al., 2007)	Week 4	Less than 1 minute
Breathing Space (Responding to Difficulty)	MBCT for Depression (Segal et al., 2002)	Week 4	3 minutes +

(Continued)

Table 8.1   (*Continued*)

Practice	Original Source	Introduced	Duration
Extended Breathing Space (Responding to Difficulty)	MBCT for Depression (Segal et al, 2002)	Week 5	5 minutes +/–
Coming to the Breath with Kindness[‡]	MBCT-Ca – drawn from loving kindness practices	Week 5 and whenever needed	A few minutes
Thread Exercise 1: Grounding[‡]	MBCT-Ca	Week 4	Less than 1 minute
Thread Exercise 2: Coming to the Breath[‡]	MBCT-Ca	Week 4	Variable*
Lake Practice*	MBSR (Kabat-Zinn, 1994)	All Day	20+ minutes
Mountain Practice*	MBSR (Kabat-Zinn, 1994)	Week 6	20+ minutes
Loving Kindness Practice*	Many sources and inspirations including MBSR (Kabat-Zinn, 1994)	All Day	20+ minutes
Thread Exercise 3: Kindness Practice[‡]	MBCT-Ca	Week 7, and also when appropriate	A few minutes
Breathing Space (Responding) plus Action Step	MBCT for Depression. (Segal et al., 2002)	Week 7	3 minutes ++

[©]T. Bartley, (2012). Mindfulness-Bases Cognitive Therapy for Cancer.

[‡]Discussed on the following pages.

*These three practices are strictly speaking not Short Practices – since each lasts for more than a few minutes.

**Variable suggests anything from a few seconds – to a more extended practice of a few minutes or more.

The Pause

This simple practice (adapted from Brach, 2003) helps us to come back and reconnect with the present moment.

Begin by **stopping** what you are doing – and asking yourself one of the following questions:

- What is going on for me right now?
- How am I feeling right now?

Keeping this very simple, you might want to adapt the question to make it your own.

Practising this several times a day helps develop the habit of interrupting automatic reactivity, stopping and coming back.

Possible applications

- *Routine Activities.* We might choose to practice the Pause every time we do specific tasks such as: at mealtimes; while we open email; while washing up; when we go outside.
- *Specific Times.* We might choose to practice a Pause whenever we notice we are feeling: speedy; anxious; stressed; irritable; or upset.

Developing the habit of pausing helps to interrupt and notice automatic patterns. Introduced in Week 1 and practiced for the first three weeks on its own, we then combine it with other short practices. At first sight, it seems too short and simple to be of much use. Yet it becomes a key practice for many participants, enabling Coming Back many times a day. It opens the door to a 3MBS practice – and maybe to a choice to do something nurturing. As the initial movement in the first step of the 3MBS – The Pause becomes the crucial action that disturbs the mindless 'underbrush' of thoughts and emotions – and offers the beginning of choices to be free of them.

Coming to the Breath

The breath is an anchor to come back to – a place of safety – enabling participants to step out of 'mindlessness', where habitual patterns dwell – and step into mindful awareness.

1. *'Shifting your position to become aware of your feet on the floor ... the feel of your body in contact with the chair ... holding you ... Weight going down ... Then, when you are ready, connecting with a sense of your spine rising up through the body, holding you upright ... tall ... dignified ... Height going up'.*
2. *'Becoming aware of the fact that you are breathing ... Letting the breath breathe itself – not interfering with it in any way ... Simply feeling the sensations of the breath deep within the body'.*
3. *'If at any point, you notice that your mind has wandered away from the breath ... into thinking, or distracted by a sound, or perhaps drawn to a sensation in the body, remembering that this is not a problem – it is what minds do ... And as soon as you realize that you have wandered away, gently coming back to the anchor of the breath ... to the sensations of the waves of the breath breathing in and breathing out'.*

Coming to the Breath is essentially a simplified Mindfulness of Breathing practice. We noticed that participants found Mindfulness of Breathing, a silent unguided practice, difficult to manage so early on, in the course. Anxious thoughts seem to crowd in. We simplified the instructions and let participants decide how long to practice – guiding it for only a few minutes in class. Awareness of the breath is essentially simple (see Core Practices, this chapter) effective and natural – always there to come back to.

Standing In Mountain

People with cancer can experience waves of anxiety that incapacitate them and can be potentially overwhelming. Standing in Mountain offers access to the experience of feeling grounded and more settled. This promotes emotion regulation.

Before we start it is important to note that standing for any length of time can be challenging – so we invite participants to sit in mountain, whenever they feel it might be best, or sitting from the start – taking care of themselves and bringing kindness to their choices.

This practice can be done anywhere, at any time. Other short practices can be added to it – such as Coming to the Breath or a 3-Minute Breathing Space

Exercise

'Standing, (with your eyes open or closed) ... feeling the contact of your feet on the floor beneath you ... exploring these points of contact ... the quality of the contact ... the texture and focus ... then when you are ready, moving up through the body, checking that the knees are soft ... the pelvis is slightly tucked ... the spine is aligned and tall ... the chin is slightly tucked ... with awareness of the spine rising up through the body, all the way to the top of the back of the crown of the head ... Once you have established the posture, bringing to mind a mountain and feeling yourself standing like a mountain ... the base of you rooted and grounded, at one with the crust of the earth ... the height of you like the peak of the mountain, rising up into the sky above ... feeling the whole of your body standing in mountain ... Then if you would like, opening your eyes, if they have been closed, and letting your gaze fall softly on the floor or ground in front of you ... feeling a strong sense of grounded presence mountain ... breathing deeply in the belly of the mountain, strong ... grounded ... tall ... abiding. Remembering that you can come back to mountain standing at any point in your day.*

Breathing With (Kabat-Zinn, 1990)

This practice (adapted from Kabat-Zinn, 1990) is for times such as waiting in a Follow Up Clinic, when more complicated practices might be challenging to do.

Breathing With might also be used in class when someone in the group is distressed. Breathing With can help to steady and ground emotion and distress, allowing us to be able to continue to process and turn towards whatever is arising.

---

*'Inviting you at this point, to come to the breath ... not turning away from anything that is arising for you ... but simply **breathing with** whatever is there with your eyes open ... Reconnecting with the support of the breath – sometimes in the background ... and sometimes in the foreground as an anchor to come back to, whenever needed'.*

*'Also bringing awareness to the contact of your feet on the floor – feeling the solid of the ground beneath you – and **breathing with** that'.*

*'Whenever you notice that thoughts and feelings have taken you away again – returning to **breathing with** whatever is arising – not pushing it away – but using the breath to support you to come back to this present moment, over and over'.*

The Physical Barometer

We introduce this practice in Week 4 in connection with the Unpleasant Experience process. It offers an immediate 'read out' on the levels of stress or difficulty being experienced. People with cancer find that anxious or depressing thoughts can easily be triggered. The Physical Barometer brings awareness to feelings via sensations in the body, often before reactivity has normally been registered. Regular tuning in to the Physical Barometer facilitates an early response to situations, before aversion sets in or threat overwhelms us.

If you have an old fashioned barometer or have seen someone consult one, you will know that you gently tap on the glass front. Depending on which way the needle moves, it may be possible to forecast upcoming weather. We can use our bodies in a similar way to give us sensitive information about the emotional 'weather' arising in us.

Here is how you do this:
1. *Determine some part of the body – preferably in the trunk – such as the chest area or the abdomen or somewhere between the two – that for you is especially sensitive to stress and difficulty.*
2. *Once you have found the place, it can be your 'Physical Barometer'. Tuning into it regularly, you may notice different sensations at different times. When you are under pressure, feeling anxious, or frustrated, you may notice sensations of tension, tightness, shakiness, or discomfort. The intensity of these sensations varies, depending on the level of your difficulty.*
3. *As you practice this, you can become aware of quite subtle sensations. These may signal that something is brewing for you, long before you are aware of this in your mind. If you wish, you can practice a 3MBS to help you respond to what is happening. Or you may choose just to monitor the sensations in your 'barometer', moment by moment, and be with them as they are.*

Coming to the Breath with Kindness

Starting with guiding Coming to the Breath practice and when settled onto the breath ....

Exercise

'Now, inviting kindness to flow in on the breath ... using the breath as the vehicle for kindness ... and letting it circulate throughout the whole of your body ... filling every corner, crevice, and area of pain or discomfort ...... kindness emanating from the heart flowing into the whole of the body mind like a soft breeze'.

Coming to the Breath with Kindness is an uncomplicated practice. The step of bringing kindness in on the breath is really just a movement that includes an intention to open and soften to places in the body and mind that are in pain or distress. We use the breath as a vehicle for kindness, in a similar way as in the Body Scan, when we use the breath as a vehicle for awareness. This practice is similar to a loving kindness practice, only much shorter and more simple. People with cancer tend to blame themselves. Learning to practice with kindness floated in on the breath develops a gentle approach to the judging mind.

This practice is often incorporated into everyday life. 'I noticed I had moved into nasty judging of myself for that, so I came to the breath with kindness.'

The Thread Exercises

Introduction

The threads are connected to Thought on a Thread – a project that links with a community support HIV & Aids NGO in South Africa – 'connecting our compassion to support practical local action'. (See Resources section at the back of this book for information about where to order threads).

Red beads tied onto simple black thread are the little bracelets that we give to participants in Week 4. They tie them onto their wrists if they would like.

Initially they function as reminders to practice the Physical Barometer. The third thread exercise can be used as a way of connecting with the others in the group, after the eight week course has finished – and those beyond the group who are suffering.

---

1. Contact with the ground .... Exploring

Feeling the feet on the ground and exploring detailed sensations in toes, balls of the feet, and heels. Noticing texture, contact, pressure, pain (if there is any), ease, and weight. Doing this for a few moments – maybe linking it to a daily activity (such as getting out of bed, or finishing eating). We can also practise this when awake in the night, by bringing awareness to the contact of the body with the bed.

2. Hand on the belly .... Breathing

Placing the hand on the belly and bringing awareness to the breath moving under the hand. Doing this for a little while – noticing when the mind wanders to something else (which is quite normal and not a problem) – and having noticed, gently returning to the breath and the hand on the belly. Doing this regularly and whenever we feel stressed or anxious.

3. Touching the bead .... Connecting

Touching the red bead, linking into the heart and opening to the possibility of sending kindness to ourselves. Breathing kindness from the heart around the body. Not forcing this, just opening to the possibility. Repeating one of these phrases if you would like – or adapting your own:

> *'May I be safe and protected'*
> *'May I be peaceful'*
> *'May I live with kindness'*

We can also link into the heart and think of others, who are ill or having tough times. Wishing them well wherever they are:

> *'May you be safe and protected'*
> *'May you be peaceful'*
> *'May you live with kindness'*

It is best to do this exercise for oneself first, before moving on to do it for others.

Breathing Spaces Notes

Adaptations within MBCT-Ca

The 3-Minute Breathing Space (3MBS) (Segal et al., 2002) is introduced in Week 3 and practised three times a day for the rest of the course. On first acquaintance, the 3MBS appears to be straightforward. However, it encompasses and condenses much of the course, and will probably take several weeks to be able to practice effectively. When this has been learned, it becomes a core practice for many participants.

The 3MBS and the other short practices are very important for MBCT-Ca participants. As already mentioned, few of them practise the longer core practices after the end of the course (except the 15 minute sitting practice on CD3). To help the learning of the 3MBS so that it becomes a well integrated and accessible practice, we introduce some of the steps of the 3MBS as separate short practices. For example:

1. The Pause is introduced in the first week and is part of home practice for the rest of the course. This encompasses the bones of the first step of the 3MBS
2. Coming to the Breath is introduced in Week 2 and practiced at home for the rest of the course. This replicates the second step in the 3MBS.

This just leaves the third and (probably) hardest step. We have already practised this in the Body Scan and also in the Sitting Practice, when we expand into a sense of the body as a whole. Making explicit links with previous practices reminds participants that their existing learning can be transferred to the 3MBS. Linking 3MBS to existing activities helps us remember to do the practice.

We introduce The Breathing Space (Responding) in Week 4. It follows exactly the same form as 3MBS – but we practise it whenever challenging, difficult or unpleasant experiences arise.

The Extended Breathing Space (Responding)

We introduce this in Week 5. Like the Breathing Space (Responding) above, we practise it whenever we need to, in response to what has arisen that is challenging or difficult. As with the other Breathing Spaces, it has the shape of an hourglass or egg timer – starting wide with the first step, moving narrow into the waist at the second and going out wide again with the third step (see this diagram in Week 3). It is an extended version of 3MBS with a more detailed step 1 and an extended step 3.

---

1. Noticing and Acknowledging

In the first step Noticing and Acknowledging – *We practice the Pause – 'What is going on for me at the moment?' We then extend it, by noticing and acknowledging what thoughts are present ... what feelings are current ... and then coming into the body, what physical sensations are there? Turning towards and including the Physical Barometer and tuning into whatever is there – be it subtle or strong.*

2. Gathering

In the second step Gathering – *Coming back to the breath, with the option of placing the hand on the belly, emphasizing the anchor of the breath and the belly moving under the hand – as we come up close to direct awareness of the breath. Remaining with the breath in the belly for as long as we choose, anchoring to a sense of the present moment, breath by breath.*

3. Expanding

In the third step Expanding – *Expanding from the breath to a sense of the body as a whole and the breath breathing within the body. Then, opening up a space of awareness beyond the body and the breath, to include whatever is there – and breathing with it all with kindness and gentleness. Saying to yourself, if you want to, 'It is ok. Whatever it is, let me feel it'. We can extend this last step for as long as we choose. If thoughts and feelings are there, we may choose to label them ... 'thinking' ... 'worrying' ... and then returning to the breath and the body as whole and breathing with it all.*

A number of significant movements are held within this third step. First, we turn towards whatever is there and are gently present with it, in the wider space of awareness. We practise this whilst still in contact with the stabilizing anchor of the breath, there to come back to at any time. Lastly, as the practitioner finishes the practice and returns to her everyday life, she is bringing present mindful awareness back with her.

The Breathing Space (Responding) Plus Action Step

An Action Step is included in Week 7 and this completes the development of the Breathing Spaces. The last version of the practice starts with the Extended Breathing Space (Responding). Then as it comes to an end, we invite our participants to reflect on what action to take in response to difficulty or challenge, which has wise and kind intention.

We sometimes offer three options at this point:

1. Doing something that is mindful and pleasant – nourishing and uplifting
2. OR – Maybe no action needs to be taken. Sometimes situations are such that the skilful and caring action is to let the situation go – and not take any action.
3. OR – It may be that it is not immediately clear what action to take. In this event, you might choose to trust your inner wisdom to guide you – cultivating the intention that you will take action and know what to do, when the moment arises.

WHAT IF?

Two small words
What if?
Two small words
What if?

What if?

STOP!
PAUSE!
BREATHE!
FEET ON THE FLOOR!

Mind starts spinning
What if?
Stomach is lurching
What if?

Knots all inside
What if?
Body shaking

Mind slowing
Knots undoing
Stillness growing
Panic fading

What if?
Feeling sick
What if?
Panic grips
What if?

What if?
If what?

Jane (May, 2011)

Following Next

Having explored the short practices within MBCT-Ca, it is appropriate that we now turn to an outline of a mindfulness-based intervention for people receiving palliative care, since it predominantly uses short mindfulness-based practices. This next chapter is written by Ursula Bates, who has worked in hospice and oncology settings using mindfulness-based approaches for many years. She has refined her intervention for people receiving palliative care so that it can be flexible and responsive to the needs of her participants, who attend open day hospice groups, as they approach the end of their lives.

First, we meet Bridget who cared for her husband through his illness. They both attended an MBCT-Ca course in North Wales in 2009, the year before he died.

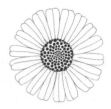

Personal Story

Bridget

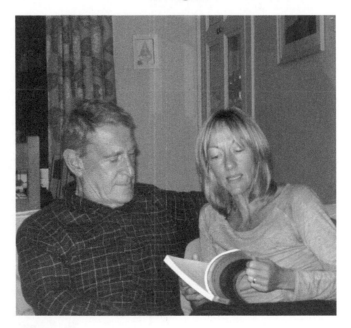

Bridget, 52 and a vet, was in partnership with her husband when he was diagnosed with incurable cancer. She cared for him for two years and was beside him when he died in July 2010. They both attended a Mindfulness course in February 2009.

Mindfulness-Based Cognitive Therapy for Cancer: Gently Turning Towards,
First Edition. Trish Bartley.
© 2012 Trish Bartley. Published 2012 by John Wiley & Sons, Ltd.

The Beginning

When Geraint was diagnosed, I wanted to reach out for skills that might support us through the process. When we were offered Mindfulness, I jumped at the opportunity, and hoped it would give us strength.

Both his daughters also had cancer. The sorrow that caused him made me angry – my usual response to emotional stress. The 'Intentions' letter, written at the start of the course, has stood the test of time:

> *'I hope you grow in wisdom and find a way to walk beside this family with love and selflessness. I hope you find ways to ease his life and cooling waters for the heat of your rage. I hope you find strength to live alone and have no regrets for the way you share this time.'*

The course

I was amazed at how much any awkwardness was diffused in the first session. The group was lovely; I felt invested in their future, not needing chapter and verse of their lives, but with a huge sense of wishing them well. Listening to the voice on the CDs always recalls the warmth and the positivity of the sessions.

Challenges

My anger didn't go away. It would build, cyclically, and last for a few days. Then I would be good and lovely, for some time. Though Geraint saw this pattern, he was often in bed and that gave me the chance to compose myself before I went to him. Many times I was able *not* to say things that were on my mind, and I attribute that to mindfulness. This saved me so much guilt.

'Wobble', you said in class, 'that's what we do'. It helped us to accept that though our intentions were good, in the circumstances we might well be expected to wobble at times. We were quite kind to ourselves and each other if we didn't get things right.

Living with fear

His prognosis was utterly real to me – in my mind, hope never predominated. I was obsessed with how to give him a fitting funeral. On her first visit, the senior district nurse detailed how they would help me, if he chose to die at home. I saw him bedridden in a special bed here, a prolonged deterioration, liver metastases, pressure sores – the images never left me. It is a choking cancer, so I expected he would die horribly. Throughout his treatments – and he was often very ill – I just thought, 'You ain't seen nothing yet. Wait till the end stages. You must soak this up. Put your shoulders to the yoke'.

Every day I woke with the knowledge: 'One day you will not be here. One day I will do this alone', but the main thread of this three-stranded plait was just 'What do we need to do now? Bring cheer or comfort?'

When Geraint had chemo, he slept badly and was noisy. He woke me all the time, and then I was tired. But if I was beside him, I could just put my hands together and go back to sleep. If I tried to find sleep in the other room, I would wake at three in the morning and all the fears would be there – the dying man, the bed, the choking – and I couldn't get off that hamster wheel of fear. So, once he was diagnosed, I slept beside him, all the way to the end. At least I still had a husband to lie beside.

Mindfulness and what it Offered

What do I know about how I would be now, without mindfulness? But there were many positives: it absorbed Geraint in a way nothing I could do, would. When we could not do well with the day, with the illness, with the challenges, with the mind – we could do a practice. Geraint described this as taking the top off the waves. It levelled you, steadied and grounded you. I saw the practice CDs like little stabilizers. And if we hadn't had a practice, what would we have? You can't just ramp up the anti-depressants on a bad day, can you?

Our last Turkish holiday

I was so angry that the precious last holiday in Turkey was almost annihilated by paradoxical anxiety (a side effect of his medication). I should have known what it was. We are in the most beautiful place in the world, on our boat. The sun comes up over the mountains like a flaming sword on the waters, and it could not be lovelier. Geraint is in paradise, but he cannot get out of bed. He is curled over. Two things make it bearable. One is to get him over the stern of the boat into the cold water for a swim, and the other is to do a 15 minute practice, sitting on the bunks. It is tough on my back, but it doesn't matter – and between the practice and the cold water, he would get going – and by lunch, he would be okay.

The funeral and after

I can trace the different phases after he died. In the first two weeks, preparing for the funeral, I was uplifted. He had suffered horribly, but he had also been spared a great deal. I was so grateful for both of us. I felt very strongly that I had loved Geraint and been loved, and I was proud of both of these things.

After the funeral, there was a profound sense that he was not there anymore. All those things that I did – his cardigan in the bed, his photo beside me, and every day opening sympathy letters, saying to myself 'how kind' and 'how lovely', – yet I was really onto the next phase. 'I am alone now. I have to make something of this next life'. I went to look after a friend's place for a week and I felt quite neutral, calm, as if it were a retreat. But, packing up to leave, I felt very depressed. It was a grey day and everything drained out of me. I just wanted to press a button and exit this single life. I was depressed all that weekend – inert – couldn't get out of bed. But the sun shone on Monday and I put on my bikini and lay on the lounger. The sun was hot on my body and I thought, 'Ah, but you don't want to die today, do you?' I wanted to find a new life and a new partner.

I've used mindfulness when I've woken in the small hours. I just lie there and do a sitting practice – it calms me and I often sleep again. If I go away, I take my mindfulness CDs and my Pema Chödrön (1997) book. I don't usually open the book or listen to the practices, but they are there. What I turn back to now, when I am stumbling, is the sound of your voice taking me through the short sitting practice.

Mindfulness and Love

I remember near the end, we were in the bathroom, sitting there with a degree of intimacy that we hadn't needed to go to before – but none of that mattered. Now there was just the bleeding and the vomiting and the dying to do. There was no dignity, and no hope left anymore. There was just love and by the end of it, that was all there was.

We were very fortunate; it was a long marriage, and although it was very tempestuous and raw in its early years, in its last fifteen years it grew in love. The key change was in Geraint's tolerance. Once he realized that my fury and reactivity wasn't personal, and said 'You tell 'em, Bridge', – it just enabled love to be there.

I guess I see mindfulness as facilitating the love that was there. It doesn't create it, does it? But it can free you from minding if you fail to cope with all the challenges, the fears and the future – and then you can stick with pure love. We were so different, but we thought so much the same. We were fortunate, weren't we? 'Love Geraint – Love Bridgie' – that was most of our conversation in the last few days. That was all that needed saying.

Chapter Nine
Mindfulness in Palliative Care

Ursula Bates

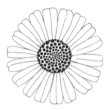

You matter because you are you, and you matter to the end of your life.
We will do all we can not only to help you die peacefully, but also to
help you live until you die.

(Dame Cicely Saunders, 1965)

When active treatment and cure is no longer an option, quality of life –
including physical, emotional, spiritual and existential aspects – becomes a
prime goal for the patient, carers and family members. This chapter explores
the application of a mindfulness intervention in an open group in a day
hospice setting.

Blackrock Hospice serves an area of 250,000 people, in Dublin, Ireland. It
provides home care, day hospice and in-patient service and annually delivers
a palliative service to some three hundred patients and families. The day
hospice opens three days a week where patients receive nursing care,
physiotherapy, hydrotherapy, psychosocial and complementary therapy.

The Mindfulness Groups

A mindfulness group meets each morning from 11.10am–12.00pm and is open to
all patients. Most "day patients" come once a week for the 12 week program,

Mindfulness-Based Cognitive Therapy for Cancer: Gently Turning Towards,
First Edition. Trish Bartley.
© 2012 Trish Bartley. Published 2012 by John Wiley & Sons, Ltd.

with an option of a further 12 weeks. A range of psychological distress is reported in the literature on palliative care with some 20% of patients having significant levels of anxiety and depression (Breitbart et al., 1995).

Day patients attending the mindfulness group have a wide variety of metastatic, malignant, and non-malignant terminal conditions. Attendance varies widely, due to poor health, medical appointments or transport difficulties. Therefore in any one session, there may be several new members, some established members and a few who are on their second admission to day hospice. Group sessions are 45 minutes long. Over 12 weeks, participants will attend 9 hours of mindfulness, which is about one third of the standard 8 week MBSR course.

Most patients choose to stay for 24 weeks so gradually their practice deepens. The groups meet in a bright day room facing the garden. They sit in supportive chairs. We include only very gentle upper body stretching in the mindfulness classes because of participants' physical limitations. Interruptions, while kept to a minimum, are inevitable, as patients need to leave for individual appointments. We include the interruptions and nearby sounds from the busy unit as part of our practice from the beginning.

All groups are taught by an experienced mindfulness teacher and attended by psychology interns. We often have visitors, such as medical doctors or a student on placement, as the hospice trains a wide range of disciplines in palliative care. The psychology intern participates in the class, prepares the material, maintains records in the medical chart and keeps ongoing group notes. These record the practices, poems, stories and themes of each group, which are helpful in ensuring that key themes are not overlooked in the constant flux of a changing group membership.

Often, an established group has to move back to the beginning to include a new member. We talk of this as going back to core practice and encourage everyone to work at his or her own pace. We find that a new member integrates and is supported by the depth of concentration in the others. While this constant shifting is not ideal, it reflects the challenge to use what is available here and now – even when this is far from perfect.

MBCT-Ca and the pattern of suffering experienced by cancer patients, with its key maintenance factors of distress, rumination, avoidance and trauma guides the treatment of palliative patients. Cognitive behaviour therapy has been adapted for older patients (Sage et al., 2008) and used extensively and effectively with cancer patients (Moorey & Greer, 2002). Qualities such as courage and compassion are essential in negotiating the journey towards death. These qualities are as important for teachers, who themselves need to develop the capacity to accompany participants into unknown and uncertain liminal spaces.

Assessment

All patients attending day hospice are assessed on intake. Information about their physical symptoms, emotional distress, family needs and patient goals is available to the multidisciplinary team. On the basis of their intake assessment, and in discussion with the Nurse Manager, patients are invited to participate in the mindfulness group. Most are encouraged to attend for a taster session and to withdraw if they feel it is not suitable for them. This inclusive system has led to good ongoing attendance by male patients, who are generally slow to take up therapy services. In 2008, 27 male patients and 39 female patients attended group, with an average age of 74 years.

James was 43 years old and had multiple myeloma. He lived on his own and had limited social contacts. At first he was very reserved and refused all services. On assessment, he revealed a life-long history of social anxiety and withdrawal. He had difficulty with his diagnosis and in expressing his emotions. Mindfulness was explained to him and he was encouraged to explore it for a few sessions, whilst seeing an individual counsellor for support. In the end, he attended the mindfulness groups for over a year. He was quiet but always attentive in the group. He came to the ward for his final weeks and used the body scan and mindful breathing to the end of his life.

A small number of people are not suitable for classes, mainly owing to serious agitation, moderate to severe hearing loss, and ongoing serious psychiatric difficulties.

Aidan, 51, was recently diagnosed with multiple sclerosis. He found the mindfulness group emotionally overwhelming and was tearful afterwards. He had not spoken openly about his deterioration and when engaged with the breathing exercises, he became engulfed in his own unexpressed grief. He decided to go for individual counselling, knowing he could rejoin the group when he felt able to engage with the work.

The purpose and nature of the group, is explained at the start of each session, as well as the importance of active participation and practice. Practice is encouraged but optional, and exercises and tapes are distributed. However, the emphasis is on participation in group. Older group members often take on the role of supporting the induction of new member.

Sean, 75 years old, had been so shocked by his palliative status that he had spent some six months in bed waiting in terror for death. Now he became the one who often welcomed new members into the group.

'I thought I was dying', he said. 'It was hard coming in for a respite stay on the ward. Fergus (the physiotherapist) sat by my bed every day and gradually got me to walk. Then, coming to group, I began to understand that I was experiencing panic attacks. Now, I still get them but I can steady myself with my breathing and I can tell people around me what is happening. This is a place you can talk about what is going on inside, and not take to the bed like me'.

Key Tasks for Teachers – Palliative Care Group

1. **Before starting** – Review each participant with the Day Hospice manager. Visit the day room to assess the energy level of the group.

2. **Getting started** – Offering a brief overview of stress in chronic illness and the purpose of the group.

3. **Intention** – Guiding a personal intentions practice
4. **Sitting** – Establishing a mindfulness-based breathing practice
5. **Coming back and turning towards the difficult**
   - Grounding exercise
   - Practice – following the themes and sequence of the exercise for the 8 weeks MBCT-Ca
   - Inquiry
   - Poem or Story.
6. **Kindness** – Supporting kindness for oneself and others

Each session follows an established structure, which has a theme embedded in it. This helps build the security of the group. With fragile, elderly patients, this predictability enables them to orientate to the work of the group.

Intention

> Intention is a commitment when spoken from the heart brings tremendous power for good (Bartley, 2003).

Jon Kabat Zinn (1990) reminds us that the attitude with which we undertake the practice is like the soil. Good soil is loose, open, damp, warm – full of a range of decaying matter and organisms. So when we ask people to commit to being present and be aware in the hospice setting, we are often asking them for a radical change in orientation towards themselves and their own state. In my teaching I think of this as calling to an emergent potential that people may not be consciously aware of – but which is there nevertheless.

As I sit in the room I see people with ambivalent and mixed intentions, who have a potential to move in the direction of mindfulness, but who do not yet have any conscious awareness of what they want, or what might unfold. So I ask them to consider choosing to be here, in this place, at this time, together.

This brings up anger and bitterness as well as acceptance and relief. Questions such as "Why me?" get aired and discussed in the group. Stories of serious disappointment with treatment, physical vulnerabilities, feelings about being abandoned and being a burden are shared.

In choosing to come back to be present, some sense of freedom returns to what has been a disempowering experience for many. As each week passes, the choosing becomes more intentional, as people decide to turn up to the work and to themselves, however they are in the moment. Courage deepens with each choice.

Coming Back

Coming Back to the present requires participants to engage with their bodies. They are being asked to turn towards experiences that they have often disassociated from. This was the way they coped with medical investigations and treatment. Grounding is a step by step way to re-engage – offering the mind a physical anchor to come back to. Patients with post traumatic stress symptoms benefit from basic grounding, to regain a sense of control.

Grounding can be practised in stressful everyday situations, such as:

- moving from sitting to standing
- fear of falling
- when feeling anxious.

Participants repeatedly tell us about a gap between the mind and the body. They feel in spirit about 35 years old, yet need to constantly adjust to a failing body. They anticipate moving as if much younger, and then often find themselves off balance.

Patients share many difficulties with short term memory and coping with daily activities. Using mindfulness, to keep coming back to the moment, leads to interesting discoveries about how to find ways to manage. Inner wisdom begins to emerge through a compassionate attention to the needs of the body.

Claire, who was distressed by losing her keys a number of times, used the grounding exercise to steady her mind and support her memory.

I held the door keys in my hand and felt the metal and the coldness. Then I looked at the bowl in front of me and gently put them inside and focused them in the bowl. I took a few slow breaths. The next morning when I woke up I could picture them in the bowl.

Grounding Practice

Take a moment to get yourself settled on your chair. Closing your eyes, if that feels comfortable for you. ... Noticing where your feet are ... feeling the texture of your socks against your skin, the temperature of your feet, are they hot or cold? ... bringing your awareness up along your body ... noticing the gentle pressure of the chair against the back of your thighs ... bringing your mind into that sensation – and noticing the temperature of your legs and the texture of your skirt or trousers against your legs ... moving up your back and feeling the pressure of the chair against your back – the sensation of hotness or coldness – the feeling of the cloth, rough or smooth ... noticing what your hands are touching – and the texture and temperature against your hands.

Gently taking a moment to tune into your body ... Do you notice any tensions in your legs or back? If you need to gently move any part of your body, then doing what you need to do slowly and mindfully ... Gradually assuming an upright and dignified posture.

Sitting Practice

Most patients are on pain medication, which dulls their acuity and induces periods of drowsiness. I frequently ask these patients to talk to me about their experience of meditation practice during illness. Most recall being unable to engage in formal practice. They rely on short practices and external aids such as pictures of a teacher, or saint, audio recordings and resting in a sense of trust knowing that others are practising on their behalf.

So with palliative participants a range of objects of attention and very small goals are essential. Lucia McBee's adaptations for frail elderly patients are useful in clinical day care settings (McBee, 2008).

Short sensory attention practices:

- Using an object as a focus of attention. *The day hospice room has several painting/plants which I use as a focus of attention. Guiding the patients in looking at the painting or plant in detail noting all the variations of colour that they can see.*
- Guiding participants to focus on what is directly in contact with their hands and experience it all fully as possible through touch.
- Mindfully eating a raisin or orange and fully experiencing it through all their senses.
- Listening to sounds in the room and around us.

All participants need be able to sustain mindful breathing for even a short period before moving to the last four sections of the 8 week course, to help them learn to contain and work with arising distress.

Turning Towards The Difficult

In palliative care groups, common difficulties arise such as falling asleep, agitation, and emotional distress.

As a teacher, I have to be mindful of participants falling asleep and include this in the practice. In group, we speak of 'Now I am drifting into sleep – Now I am coming back', being gently curious. Over and over as one approaches death, the mind will experience a range of different states, such as: drifting, dreams, loss of clarity, and a gradual withdrawal from this world of phenomena. Working with the movement of these states is important for participant and teacher.

Slowly trust deepens that the group is a place to be both aware and unaware – to be able to tolerate altered states, whilst trusting that the inner self endures and is held by the group and the universe. It is this gradual development of trust that assists the person in moving towards death.

The opposite also occurs where a participant becomes agitated, and needs to be supported directly to be able to become calm.

Practice of Supporting an Agitated Participant

- Establishing the main group in a breathing practice and asking them to continue to rest on their breathing.
- Asking the agitated participant to keep her eyes open, and look at you or at an object; teacher's breath matching her breath at the same pace and in the same body place (upper chest or stomach) as the participant is breathing.
- Continuing the pacing and then say to the participant, 'On the next out breath, I am going to place my hand on your hand'.
- Then, 'On the next **in** breath I am going to gently squeeze your hand'.
- Continuing gently squeezing their hand on each in breath. Gradually allowing your own breath to return to its normal pattern. Slowly pace your hand movement to reflect any change in the patient, gradually matching it to your own breathing rate. Gradually the participant begins to match your breathing pattern.
- Encourage them just to follow the movement of their own breath.

There is a wide range of intense affect in these groups. Anger, despair, demoralization, impotence, uselessness, envy of those who are well, guilt and self blame, shame and a sense of exposure, loss of independence because one needs help with bodily functions are all present. Catharsis is not directly encouraged or discouraged in mindfulness. The patient is invited to observe with a gentle and open awareness, any feelings that arise and if possible, to welcome them in.

In group, as strong feelings arise, I will support people to experience them in the moment. As calmness returns, through inquiry, I will try to explore where the feelings are held and name them – 'So in your stomach there was a heavy feeling. The word that comes to mind is despair – How would it be to be present to it, soften towards it and allow it space?'

The group is a safe place to explore such feelings and generally what one member experiences resonates with the others. Yalom, in his seminal article on group therapy with the terminally ill, noted that the threat of death is such that 'most psychotherapy patients and most therapists will not stare at death very long, before they lower the blinds of denial' (Yalom & Greeves, 1977). In the face of such anxiety, the defences of denial, depression and avoidance are activated. So careful building of the capacity to sustain a sitting practice, and the support of the group is essential in enabling participants to manage the balance between defence and experience.

Poetry and Story

Forces are manifest in poems that do not pass through the circuits of the mind (Bachelard, 1994).

All our patients have been journeying with serious illness for an average of three years, and many have been in very difficult medical situations. Caroline Garland describes a traumatic event as one in which:

The mind is flooded with a kind or degree of stimulation that is far more than it can make sense of or manage (Garland, 1998).

Participants have internal experiences for which they have no words. Poetry offers images and language that awakens the imagination, from which a depth of understanding can flow. Finding an image or expression of emotion that matches the internal experience allows it to be shared in the group. This enables the mind to digest the distressing material. As a result, the participant is able to expand his or her capacity to bear difficult emotions.

Bachelaed (1994), in his exploration of the poetic imagination, speaks of the reverberations of even a single poetic image:

By its novelty, a poetic image sets in motion the entire linguistic mechanism … (*and*) places us at the origin of the speaking being (Bachelaed, 1994).

One participant with oral cancer, no longer able to speak, gestured excitedly to the group when we read from Rilke,

> So you must not be frightened if a sadness rises before you larger than any you've ever seen, if an anxiety like light and cloud shadows moves over your hands and everything that you do. You must realize that something has happened to you'. (Rilke, 1934)

Pointing to herself, she wrote on her notepad 'SADNESS', gesturing with her hands to a sadness bigger than herself.

When we have a group of cognitively fragile patients, *'Favorite Poems We Learned in School'* (Walshe, 1998) is a useful resource. Many Irish children have learnt them off by heart, and they remain with us until the end. In one group, Kitty, who was gently fading and could no longer read, was delighted to recite out loud *Trees* by Joyce Kilmer. To her joy, the whole group joined in. We encourage participants to bring in their favorite poems and stories which we then share in group.

Poetry and Story in the palliative group have been the main voice of the shadow side. Feelings of despair, darkness and impotence have emerged most strongly when mediated and contained by image and rhythm.

Kindness

These are some of the ways that kindness is practised and embodied in group.

- Beginning with positive warmth to support people coming into the room.
- Listening in the inquiry for self criticism. Beginning to name it as a mental attitude with gentle curiosity.
- Wondering out loud about other ways to be present to judgement, labelling it watching it, a gentle 'Ah there I go again'.
- Turning towards kindness.
- Reading the poems on *'Two kinds of intelligence'* by Rumi (1995) and *'Kindness'* by Naomi Shihab Nye (1994).

- Seeing kindness as a natural capacity that allows us to receive and give love.
- Using an orange to explore interconnection, and inviting the group list all the links between themselves and the orange. The hands it passed through to get to the hospice; the sun and rain and soil contained within it. Then eating it mindfully.
- Guiding a simple loving kindness practice at the end of the class.
- Extending the practice to include all others who suffer.

Dedicating The Practice

Dedicating the practice and the group experience is openly welcomed by palliative participants, who are deeply motivated to be of use to others and frequently see themselves as a burden. It also relieves worries they have about leaving vulnerable family members behind.

Hilary, who attends the Tuesday group, has a 40 year old son with multiple sclerosis who lives in a care home and is very emotionally dependent on her. He phones her, up to three times a day. She feels that she is the only one who understands him, and worries about how he will cope when she is gone. She dedicates her practice for him.

Frequently we dedicate our practice for people on the in-patient unit. This has very tender benefit, when weeks later, a group member will be on the unit themselves.

Dedication Practice

'As we come to the end of the class we share the work and learning of the class with all who are in our hearts today. We remember all who have attended the group and send our kindness and good wishes wherever they are, here, at home, on the ward or in other hospitals'.

Reflection Session: The Loss of a Group Member

The loss of a group member can occur from one group session to the next. The nurse manager informs the mindfulness teacher before the session and then attends the session. The group are told of the loss at the beginning and the manager is there to answer any questions about the details of the death.

A ritual is designed and, if possible, our pastoral care chaplain attends. The five elements (Groves, 2005) of good ritual are:

- story
- space
- symbol
- action
- community.

In group, we create a space into which we can bring story, symbol and action. By dimming lights, lighting a candle, and using flowers, poetry or any symbol that the group chooses.

We call on familiar practices – such as mindful breathing, and always include a dedication for the person that has died. This often reflects the tradition of an Irish wake, where stories about the person are shared. We end with a prayer or a favourite poem of hers / his.

These are often very still groups. Members tentatively inquire about the details and listen carefully. It is a time when fears about the actual physical nature of death are raised and answered. There are tears and laughter and wonderings about the beyond.

We often return to Rilke's image:

> May what I do flow from me like a river,
> no forcing and no holding back,
> the way it is with children.
>
> Then in these swelling and ebbing currents,
> these deepening tides moving out, returning
> I will sing to you as no one ever has,
> streaming through widening channels
> into the open sea.
>
> R M Rilke (1996)

This poem links the work that Trish and I undertake. Though we are separated by the Irish Sea, our little communities in Blackrock and Bangor gather every week to journey mindfully, with gentle warriors, who travel before us in life. We often end by remembering that with us, when we sit are many people around the world, who support us at any moment in time.

So Many Things To Tell You

All day I sat and watched you slip away,
a schedule that was out of my command.
So many things to tell you that last day,

and hearing is the last to go they say.
It wasn't any speech that I had planned.
All day I sat and watched you slip away,

knowing you had to leave and I to stay.
Speaking words I hoped you'd understand,
so many things to tell you that last day.

All day I sat and watched you slip away,
my words a kiss I folded in your hand,
so many things to tell you that last day.

With words alone I thought I might delay
those final hours, searching for a strand.
All day I sat and watched you slip away,
so many things to tell you that last day.

Jill Teague
(North Wales, 2010)

Chapter Ten
After The Eight Week Course

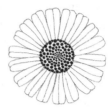

There exists in myself acres of my nature which are still undiscovered:
one has been opened by grief – what others may be known in the
future? ... The time that is left is savoured now, dwelt upon, treasured. I
have learned the strength of my own creativity: that, called upon, it
never fails to respond, and joyfully. It rushes to heal; and for that I am
grateful.

(Christopher Leach, 1981)

Introduction

We now move to the teaching issues and processes that arrive after the end
of each course. We want to support the growing community of mindfulness
participants who have attended MBCT-Ca courses and are living with cancer.
We also want to continue to develop and sustain the programme and our
teaching practice. With this in mind, there now follows the outline of a
review process that we engage in after each MBCT-Ca course. We then go on
to discuss the ways we offer follow up support to 'graduate' participants. At
the end of this chapter, there is a short section introducing examples of one
to one work with people with cancer.

Mindfulness-Based Cognitive Therapy for Cancer: Gently Turning Towards,
First Edition. Trish Bartley.
© 2012 Trish Bartley. Published 2012 by John Wiley & Sons, Ltd.

Programme and Course Review

At the end of each course, we take time to review the programme, the participants' experience, and the teaching choices we have taken. Issues that need more reflection and discussion – that are perhaps unclear, unusual or interesting – we take to supervision.

We have been making ongoing process notes week by week as the course has progressed. These are included in our review. We specifically look at themes that emerge in the way the programme unfolded – noticing trends and patterns that are particular to this group and others that link to other courses and groups.

Having looked at the programme, we then might reflect on each participant, consulting any notes written at the orientation process that recorded what s/he wanted from the course and any specific issues or challenges s/he was bringing. We look at the questionnaires (see below) that were completed before the course and at the end – collating and comparing the scores to see whether they confirm our impressions of the group as a whole.

We also consult notes made from relevant supervision sessions that might add to our reflection about the teaching choices we made – looking out for any new or deepening understandings in relation to ways of working with people with cancer.

We then bring the information together in a simple review process that in short hand looks like this: + – ?

1. + What has gone well? What positive outcomes were there? What did I (as teacher) enjoy / feel inspired by / learn?
2. – What has been challenging? What negative / disappointing outcomes were there? What was difficult / problematic / draining?
3. ? In the light of 1 and 2, what needs changing?
   - within the course programme,
   - in relation to the orientation and assessment process,
   - in relation to the context of the programme,
   - in connection to my teaching practice.

We record and put into action any decisions that come out of this process.

Course measures

We regularly use two measures that feed into the review process. Averaged out over the whole group, we feed these back to the medical team who refer patients to the courses.

WHO-Five Well-being Index (Bech et al., 1996) has five items that broadly ask about participants' experience of happiness, calm, energy, sleep, and interest over the last two weeks. The participant is invited to circle or tick one of five possibilities that go from all the time, to none of the time. The measure has the great advantage of being easy to fill in and to analyze.

Self Compassion Scale (short form) (Neff, 2003; Raes et al., in press) has 12 items, calculating an overall self compassion score, through six subscale scores relating to kindness and self-judgment; common humanity and isolation; and mindfulness and over-identification. The results from this scale offer useful information and correlate well with the wellbeing measure.

Having gathered the learning from the review, all participant papers are destroyed except for the group contact sheet, which is added to the data base for follow up session reminders–and the anonymous measures, which are filed.

Follow Up

We offer a follow up class to each group four weeks after the last session (*see Chapter 6, The Follow Up Class*). Monthly drop in sessions are open to anyone, who has completed an eight week course with us. Participants are also welcome to attend All Day sessions that run three times a year.

Through these sessions, we are building a supportive mindfulness community of practitioners living with cancer. Each one and a half hour follow up session tends to follow a similar pattern. We start with a practice (body scan, movement or sitting), and include a dialogue, (sometimes in small groups), a story and / or a poem, and a group discussion. We tend to have a theme. 'Anxiety' has been the hottest topic thus far, by a long way. We had a full house with standing room only! This speaks volumes about the experience of this population.

Sometimes we run a series of three or four sessions around one theme, such as kindness. Recent themes have included: Coming Back to the Present; Connecting to what matters to me; Living with everyday difficulties; Breathing with Kindness; Pausing to choose; Every day practices; Sharing tiny mindful practices; Turning Towards not Turning Away; Mindful Movement – and many more.

We have a small lending library of mindfulness books that are available to borrow. Thanks to a recent donation, we have a good range, which is there to inspire and motivate practice and learning. Follow up sessions offer a way of supporting emerging teachers. We invite them to co-lead sessions, gaining experience in guiding practices and facilitating dialogues in small groups. A more experienced teacher offers mentoring before and after the session to support their teaching practice development.

Working One To One

Some people cannot get to the follow up sessions. Others are keen to attend a course but may be unable to, due to distance or ill health. Sometimes, one of these people might make contact to ask for individual support. Maybe they have had a recurrence or are poorly, and want support to manage symptoms. Anxiety in relation to the future is invariably an issue. Occasionally a member of staff, concerned about a patient, may ask us to get involved.

We are guided by what each person brings. The sessions take place over the phone or in person on the oncology ward. We have drawn out three examples, to offer a taste of what they might involve.

Francis

Francis, age 59 was receiving palliative care. He had enjoyed his eight week course and seemed to have got a lot of benefit from it.

Francis maintained his practice fairly successfully at first. Then he needed more treatment to manage his symptoms and was left afterwards feeling quite poorly. He and I met at his request on three or four occasions over the following twelve months, to help him reconnect with his practice. We would talk about how he was feeling, often exploring his emotions through the resonance of physical sensations in the body – or gently turning towards the pain and discomfort of his disease symptoms, if that seemed right to him at the time. We would always do a breathing practice together, which I would guide, sometimes including some kindness phrases. On our last session, he told me that he was glad to be regularly practising on his own with the breath. 'It helps me to feel steadier somehow'. He died peacefully a few weeks later, at home.

Freddy

Freddy was too ill to attend an eight week course. He was twenty nine and had incurable cancer. I was asked by an oncology colleague if mindfulness might have anything to offer him, as he was extremely agitated and anxious about the future.

We met five or six times over the next few months. I recorded a CD for him to use at home. In the middle of this period, he became very ill and was admitted onto the ward, but after some weeks, he pulled through and we resumed our work together.

During our sessions, he would practise breathing with the agitation he felt in his body. I would guide him and practise alongside him. On his own at home, he found it hard not to become overwhelmed. By practising together, he could find the courage and presence to breathe into the intensity and be with it. It was challenging to find a practice that would offer him a strong enough anchor to come back to. He found the Body Scan difficult to tolerate and was not well enough to practise mindful movement, although walking was sometimes helpful.

When nearing the end of his life, he talked about his regret at how little he felt he had done to help others. We sat with this, sometimes exploring a felt sense of these feelings in his body. He wore a thought on a thread (see www.thoughtonathread.co.uk) and gained comfort in sending good wishes to people like him, who were ill, young and frightened. We talked about the book I was writing and I told him that I would write about our work together. He said that he hoped it might help others. This was one of our last conversations. He died on the unit a week or so later.

Hannah

Hannah, age 36 has advanced cancer. She is receiving chemotherapy and is married with two young children.

I met Hannah soon after she was diagnosed. She asked me straight away about mindfulness. We talked, and I introduced her and her husband to a simple breath practice. They seemed to get on well, so I sent her a Body Scan CD and heard some weeks later that she was practising it every day.

We set up regular sessions over the phone and Hannah quickly learnt a number of short practices. She now regularly uses Coming to the Breath, 3MBS, sitting in mountain, and turning towards her pain and discomfort, exploring the sensations and breathing into them. She also likes to bring kindness in on the breath – and is happily surprised to discover that the pain often eases when she does this. Her medical team are supportive of mindfulness, even though they do not yet have courses on their unit. This is helpful and encourages her to keep going with her practice.

Hannah now connects with a short sitting practice (15 minutes) most days and uses the Body Scan about once a week, in additional to her short practices. Her courage and commitment to practise is remarkable, for someone managing high levels of challenge and uncertainty, experiencing the side effects of treatment – and who has not attended a course or practised before. She says that mindfulness helps her a lot.

Issues in one to one work

It requires a considerable level of practice experience to be able to hold people who are managing intense distress. It is not for those of us just starting to teach. Nor it is what we, as teachers, necessarily plan to get involved with. Requests like these tend to arrive unannounced and unplanned. We respond to them as best we can. This work is usually unpaid and we may never know how many sessions there will be, or when the last one will take place. Even if prepared for this, logically, it is always sad not to have the opportunity to connect again or say goodbye.

It is surprising what we can do over the phone. Practising together always features strongly and short practices are invariably more useful than longer ones. Short practice CDs are helpful to give out or we might make a tailor made practice CD to suit the individual.

We tend to respond spontaneously to whatever is current for the person we are working with. Some planning ahead may be possible, but it seems important always to have in mind what it is we are focusing on. Usually the approach is simple, perhaps helping someone find an 'anchor' to come back to; a practice that feels robust enough to lean on when things are difficult; some kindness phrases folded into the day; a familiarity with the breath to steady and be present with. One to one work like this can be emotionally demanding, but by its nature, it often facilitates deep connection, which is always enriching.

Tonight I Heard That You Had Died

In memory of Nokwanda Gomede (1982–2006)

Images are clear.
Fitful rondavel fire smouldering
smoke wafting up towards the blackened thatch,
rounded mountains under vast spacious sky.

Nokwanda, do you know that I weep for you?
For all those who have died young, poor,
Lying on a thin little bed on red earth floor,
quietly coughing – you taught me
what it is to wish in the guts and the heart of it
that you are now enlivened by the source of all rivers,
flowing beside mountains and cool waters
peach trees and mimosa forests;
circling in the air as Veraux black African eagle,
strong and proud, watching over all that is below,
most beautiful, honoured, dignity.
Free At Last.

October, 2006

Chapter Eleven
The Third Circle – Being and the Circle of Presence

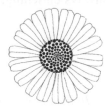

Introduction

As we approach the end of this section, we return to the three circle diagrams to consider the last one.

The third circle relates to the experience of people who are practising mindfulness to support them to *be present,* as they live with cancer – hence we call this, the Circle of Presence. The first circle drew out the psychological patterns of distress in having cancer, see chapter 4. The second traced the movements learnt through the MBCT-Ca programme which develop the practice of mindful awareness, see chapter 7. Now, we move beyond the eight week course to understand how the practice of mindfulness might be integrated into the lives of people living with cancer – and see what this might offer.

Mindfulness-Based Cognitive Therapy for Cancer: Gently Turning Towards,
First Edition. Trish Bartley.
© 2012 Trish Bartley. Published 2012 by John Wiley & Sons, Ltd.

The Circle of Presence

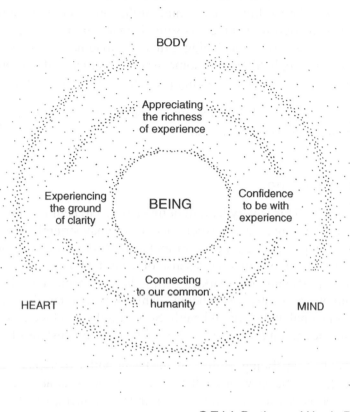

BODY

Appreciating
the richness
of experience

Experiencing
the ground
of clarity

BEING

Confidence
to be with
experience

Connecting
to our common
humanity

HEART

MIND

© Trish Bartley and Ursula Bates

Figure 11.1 Circle of Presence – Being.

The circle is more spacious and open. The markings are the lightest of the three. Called the Circle of Presence, it brings an emphasis to the practice of being present, which was first learned on the eight week course and is now being practised in everyday life. The aspects of this circle are not goals or outcomes to aim for, but they name and acknowledge the subtle shifts which course participant's experience as their practice deepens. Reduction of distress is achieved not just by lowering symptoms, but also by supporting the development of a more spacious experience of self, within which the distress is experienced, and contained.

This circle brushes up against some edges that might appear 'spiritual' in language and experience. It is hard to avoid this. Any of us who practise mindful awareness will probably encounter moments that take us beyond our usual rational understanding of ourselves and our lives. Rather than attempting to make sense of this, instead perhaps we can acknowledge the mystery, much as we wonder at the workings of the mind or the functioning of the body. It may help us to recognize that there is something about the practice of mindfulness that seems so much bigger than we imagined. This circle does not try to explain; it simply highlights some aspects of practice that support the capacity to be with difficulty, by being present and fully open to life.

We meet Jane, David and Sheila again. As before, their experiences will illustrate some aspects of the circle.

Inner ring – Being

What is 'Being'? This is very hard to define or even to begin to articulate. Wise teachers with much more experience than I, may struggle. Perhaps we might get a glimpse through the use of metaphor. Can we liken 'being' to fresh, newly baked bread that has a sense of natural wholesomeness? Or might it be like a clear stream, that sparkles with light, movement, and clarity? With this in mind, we remember 'well-being', which incorporates all aspects of physical, emotional and spiritual health. So we might conclude that 'being' involves an integration and a connection with many dimensions of experience.

We can also look at 'Being With' – as in 'being with experience', or 'being with difficulty' or 'being with kindness'. This suggests an absence of obstruction or barrier to whatever is there in that moment, whether pleasant or unpleasant. There may be no thoughts that get in the way, no conceptual ideas to analyze, or if they are there, they are simply coming and going in the space of awareness. There is a sense of being present in a direct way to what we are experiencing in this moment. Openness, spaciousness and connectedness seem to be a part of the qualities of being, which appear to be qualitively different to 'doing'. Being also suggests a direct and very present 'knowing' within experience.

It is only with the heart that one can see rightly. (de Saint-Exupery, 1943)

So, there seems to be a connection between being and wisdom or 'wise mind'. Perhaps, it is connected to the natural goodness that is there when fully present; settled and open, gentle and aware. Being appears naturally to involve a warmth and intrinsic kindness – the open wisdom of the heart. It certainly underpins and connects with the four qualities in the circle that surround it in the middle ring.

Middle ring – Four Qualities

1. Appreciating the richness of experience.
2. Experiencing the ground of clarity.
3. Confidence to be with experience.
4. Connecting to our common humanity.

Mindfulness practitioners who have attended an eight week course and are continuing to practise, describe some of these four qualities. They may not experience them for sustained periods, but even a few moments connection will have some impact, often offering insight and even inspiration. Touching into this deepens their intention and practice of mindfulness. These qualities are not conceptual ideas. They only have relevance and significance through direct experience that has a sense of immediacy and spaciousness within it.

Appreciating the richness of experience

This might be experienced outside in nature. Perhaps a vivid sense of the abundance and beauty of the world brings some moments of deep appreciation. Maybe as part of a seeing practice that involves focusing in on some detail, and then expanding out into the wider landscape. As the practice deepens, there may be a connection with some moments of experiencing beauty and richness in everything – even in those objects that we usually ignore.

Sheila was sitting in her car outside the school gates, waiting for her children to come out. She had completed a short sitting practice just before leaving home. As she sat there, the sun came out and shone directly onto her through the side window. She soaked up the warmth, and looking up, saw patterns of sun and clouds moving over the hills. She breathed it all in, feeling so grateful to be alive in this moment, surrounded by such beauty. As her children ran out from school, she felt filled with love for them. This sense of appreciation of her life and those she loved stayed with her. In those moments she knew what it was to be whole, utterly present and strangely grateful despite everything.

David had a similar experience whilst singing in his choir. He was completely focused on the music and felt them all singing together in a way they had rarely managed before. He could feel his lungs breathing deeply and experienced the resonance of the music directly in his chest. And for some moments, everything expanded for him into a sense of pleasure and inspiration. David felt uplifted and like Sheila, he felt very grateful to be well – and appreciative of his capacity to experience all of this. The moment passed, but his sense of appreciation for the richness of his life remained for some days – and he noticed that it had an effect on his daily practice.

> If you ally yourself with nature, with her sheer existence, with the small things that others overlook and that suddenly can become so huge and immeasurable: if you have this love for what is plain. ... then everything will become easier for you, more coherent, and somehow more reconciling, perhaps not in your conscious mind, but in your inner most awareness (Rilke, 1934).

Experiencing the ground of clarity

We emphasize a simple grounding practice on the programme. Participants become very familiar with the invitation to place awareness into the contact of their feet on the floor. Many of them often come back to this and through it are drawn to the mountain practice (Kabat-Zinn, 1994). With a strong sense of the embodied presence of mountain, it is as if we are seated almost immovable, with roots that go all the way down into the earth, and a feeling of tallness that rises all the way up into the sky. This stretch that pulls us down and extends us up at the same time, is strongly physical and strangely settling too. It links us with an intention to sit and sit with the dignity of a mountain, which abides forever.

Sometimes a natural sense of spaciousness opens out of this which acts as a container for whatever arises and dissolves within it. This links with choiceless awareness in the sitting practice and the third step of the breathing space. It is almost as if you are sitting on your seat on the very top of the world with a vast clear view – stretching out, above, and on all sides. Resting in this, there is a sense of calmness, openness and deep stillness – rooted to your seat and spacious like the sky above. There is a possibility of a new relationship to how we thought things to be. Previously, we might have experienced things quite solidly and personally. Now, with a vaster vision, it seems possible to find some space and air around what was intense and claustrophic. Practitioners moving towards the end of their life may gain much comfort from experiencing this quality of grounded openness and clarity, which contains and allows everything to come and go, impersonal and impermanent.

Many practitioners 'stand in mountain', especially at times of agitation or irritation. Jane found this was very helpful when her children were especially demanding. If she could get a moment to herself, she would go and stand in mountain, looking out of the window. Quite quickly, she would feel more gathered and present and, as a result, was able to respond to the children more patiently. There was more space around them and within her somehow, and this enabled her to be more kindly towards them. A friend of hers took her on a walk to the top of a mountain. She told me that they sat there for some time on what she called 'King Arthur's Seat'. She practised with her breath and described feeling really grounded and spacious at the same time. 'It was so peaceful', she said, 'I felt completely at ease with my life. Nothing was a problem and my mind felt incredibly clear – just like the blue sky above me'.

> When we stop tensing against life, we open to an awareness that is immeasurably large and suffused with love (Brach, 2003).

Confidence to be with experience

Confidence tends to build with experience of practice. The more a practitioner stays connected to her awareness practice, and turns to it when things are difficult, the more her confidence in the practice grows.

Sheila had a scare about her health. It was the first significant health challenge since finishing the course. She noticed some bleeding and immediately became very anxious. Her thoughts went straight away to the possibility that this was a sign of a recurrence. She felt her pulse start to race, experienced tightness in her chest and a lurching in her belly. However, she had a strong and regular practice of the three minute breathing space and straight away knew to come back to her body and her breath. She sat on a chair in the corner of the sitting room, where she usually did her practice, with a clear intention of breathing with the sensations in her body, as best she could.

As she felt her pulse get steadier, although the anxiety was still there in her belly, she was able to breathe into it, riding the waves of her experience, and trusting her practice to keep her safe. She remembered the phrase, 'whatever it is, let me feel it', and as she repeated this, she could feel some of the tightness and resistance opening out and easing off. Later she phoned her specialist nurse and they talked things through. She was quite surprised at herself for managing so well, and pleased that she had not moved into panic. Everytime her anxiety returned, she came back to her breath.

As a sense of confidence develops, that the practice has the capacity to contain and hold us even in intensely difficult times, the threat of being overwhelmed recedes. Each time the practitioner trusts her practice to hold her, her confidence in the practice grows, the practice itself deepens and it becomes possible to be with experience, whatever it is. Confidence here is a reliance on something that is shown to be dependable. Of course, this is not a static encounter. Some days, however committed we are, 'being with' experience may prove very difficult, but every time we practise by turning towards what is challenging us, we learn to trust ourselves and our experience a bit more.

> Just keep on, quietly and earnestly growing through all that happens to you. You cannot disrupt the process more violently than by looking outside yourself for answers that may only be found by attending to your innermost feeling (Rilke, 1934).

Connecting to our common humanity

Many MBCT-Ca participants express a sense of connection with their fellow course participants. More often than not, at some point, someone will comment, 'This is such a special group', and the others will often agree. Connecting through shared experience offers a rich learning environment.

People with life threatening illness often feel isolated and alone, even if they are well supported. As they practise kindness towards their experience, in the context of growing connectedness within the group – a sense of common humanity may naturally develop that extends out beyond the group. This changes the sense of aloneness, by offering a poignant link to others in the same or worse situation, no matter who or where they are. In itself, this is deeply healing – promoting openness, love and compassion. We feel an interconnectedness with others, which offers us an experience of being part of a larger whole. At this point, intention to practise for support one's own well-being naturally seems to open into a heart intention for the well-being of others in the group – and from there, sometimes this goes wider still to wish for the wellbeing of all.

Jane remembered feeling this a bit on the Oncology Day Unit. She had felt close to the people she had treatment with, especially the younger women like herself. She cared what happened to them. She felt similarly in her mindfulness course group – not at first – but eventually, especially after she had learned to be more kind to herself. She liked to repeat the kindness phrases for herself and others:

'May I be safe and protected'
'May you be safe and protected'
'May we all be safe and protected'

> We all face suffering. To have a body is to experience illness and pain and eventually death. To have a mind is to experience confusion, turmoil, and agitation. To have a heart is to feel hurt, loneliness, and fear. To love is to feel loss and grief (Feldman, 2005).

When Jane started the course, her own worry and fear left her feeling scrambled and very alone. When she connected with others in the group, or with the women she had treatment with, she no longer felt so alone. Her feelings for these others was comforting somehow, and seem to ease her own fear. When she could open to them in compassion, she found she could connect in kindness for herself too. She was touching into a sense of being part of a wider common humanity of people who will all eventually die, just as she will. With a gentle compassion for herself and them all, she could breath this in and send it out too.

Outer ring – Body – Mind – Heart

As with the all of this circle, the outside ring is characterized by openness. When experience arises and dissolves within a spacious container of awareness, an integrated and interconnected sense of Body, Mind and Heart can be present. They are not merged, but neither are they completely separate. There is the possibility of resonance between them. Perhaps one of the characteristics of 'being' is that body, mind and heart come together in an alignment of experience, place and time.

Summary

We have sought to capture in this last circle, a taste of how what a mindfulness practice might offer someone living with cancer.

We have come to the end of this second part of the book, which has focused on the MBCT-Ca programme. In the next and last part, we turn to issues that relate to the teaching of the programme.

Grounded in The Earth, The Body and The Heart

I came feeling that I carried the world on my shoulders,
I leave knowing that it is the earth that carries me.

I came thinking that awareness of the mind was important,
I leave knowing that awareness of the body is indispensable.

I came as a follower of my thoughts,
I leave in the service of my heart.

Peter Milligan
(South Africa, 2007)

Part Three
The Practitioner Teacher

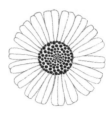

When you are free of self improvement projects, you are free of yourself.

(Reb Anderson, 1995)

Introduction

The final part of this book explores some areas relevant to those who teach mindfulness to people with cancer or planning to at some point.

First, we discuss the potential challenges to working in an oncology context and briefly touch into the training and practice we need to start teaching people with cancer. We then look at the ways that we can support our development as teachers through three evolving areas of intention, practice and reflection. In the last of these 'teaching' chapters, we investigate the learning process within MBCT-Ca, and explore the role of the group, and the teacher as facilitator of learning.

Finally, we return to the circle diagram. Bringing the three circles together in an integrated model offers us a formulation or map for Mindfulness Based

Mindfulness-Based Cognitive Therapy for Cancer: Gently Turning Towards,
First Edition. Trish Bartley.
© 2012 Trish Bartley. Published 2012 by John Wiley & Sons, Ltd.

Cognitive Therapy for Cancer. This final chapter is co-written with Ursula Bates. We track the journey from a cognitive model of cancer distress; through to the development of the practice of mindful awareness; and finally to living mindfully with cancer. Finally, we trace the connection between the circles and discuss what happens in the event of a recurrence of cancer or other life crisis

Chapter Twelve
Introducing the Teacher

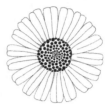

You cannot teach a man anything; you can only help him find it within himself.

(Galileo)

Introduction

In this chapter we explore the qualities that we need, and potential challenges that we face, when we teach mindfulness to people with cancer.

There are many rewards. Although cancer can be an intensely challenging experience, people with cancer are generally very motivated to learn and practice mindfulness – and paradoxically, those who are moving closer to their own mortality, can more easily get in touch with a sense of aliveness.

Mindfulness Practice and Teacher Training

Many of us arrive in the field of mindfulness-based teaching through a professional work context. Perhaps we have worked in palliative care or in oncology. Maybe, people with cancer have been amongst our clients.

Mindfulness-Based Cognitive Therapy for Cancer: Gently Turning Towards,
First Edition. Trish Bartley.
© 2012 Trish Bartley. Published 2012 by John Wiley & Sons, Ltd.

At some point, we come across mindfulness. An opportunity arises to attend a mindfulness-based approaches 'taster' session, or similar. If our interest is engaged, the next step might be to go on an eight week mindfulness-based course as a participant. Even if convinced that this is work we want to embark on, we discover that it is vital for each of us to develop a personal mindful awareness practice. This would include the core practices of Body Scan, Mindful Movement and Sitting Practice, and also involve ways of bringing mindfulness into everyday life, through short practices, such as breathing spaces; and through informal practices that fold mindfulness into our ordinary activities. We need to experience the eight week course as a participant, ideally more than once, before we start to instruct others. Everything we teach is rooted in mindful awareness, so developing a practice is the best possible way for us to prepare.

Having brought mindfulness into our lives for some time, preferably for some years, we might then start training as a teacher, I have included a list of resources at the end of the book. There are various avenues we can take. In the US, UK, Europe, and Australia, teacher training retreats are run to support health professionals to develop their practice, and acquire and deepen their teaching skills in mindfulness-based approaches. The training is a vital part of learning to teach. We then need a lot of additional time to develop our practice, teaching materials, skills and understanding.

Most of us, if we are wise, start teaching people such as friends, neighbours or colleagues, as we gain confidence and develop experience. It is best not to teach a clinical population until we have a grounded experience of the programme with people, who are likely to be less vulnerable. Once we are ready to work with clinical groups, we are encouraged only to teach those who we are already qualified to work with professionally.

However, there may be times when a mindfulness teacher experienced in working in another clinical context, might be invited to teach a group of cancer patients. Before embarking on this, it might be wise to pause and reflect on whether this is right for you, at this time. At first sight, people with cancer appear to be an attractive population to work with. Their suffering is evident and mindfulness is effective in reducing suffering. However, there are issues that we may not have considered.

Cancer in our Society

The 'Plague' of cancer

Currently, there appears to be two dominant dialogues in relation to cancer. One presents cancer as the plague of the twenty first century. Celebrity diagnoses, research news, and drug treatment decisions all feature frequently in the media. No other condition takes up nearly as much airtime or newspaper coverage. This emphasizes the sense of the illness as running out of control, which might 'attack' at any time. Yet, 40% of cancer deaths worldwide are preventable (WHO, 2007) and year on year, treatment is more effective at extending and saving lives.

The other current dialogue represents cancer as a potentially life transforming experience. Heroic individuals accomplish astonishing physical feats or raise vast sums of money whilst 'battling' with cancer. The very language of survivorship entreats people to 'fight' the disease and 'not let it get you'. Celebrities filmed at every stage of their illness contribute to the myth that if you are brave enough, and strong enough, you will 'beat' it – or die heroically in the attempt. It becomes very hard to be just an ordinary person going through cancer.

The Challenges of Working with People with Cancer

Until you are involved, it is difficult to know how this work might affect you, or how you will respond. As mindfulness teachers working in an oncology or cancer support context, we are bound to hear about aspects of the physical and psychological experience of cancer (in and out of class). This is bound to impact on us. It is part of the territory. Keeping our hearts open when others are distressed is probably our most telling quality and yet hardest challenge.

There are three broad areas to issues of working with people with cancer.

1. Working with death and dying

The first is a close involvement with death and dying – and with fears of death and dying. Even participants who have positive prognoses, and seem to be amongst the 'curative' group (see chapter 3, the Medical Implications), may experience intense anxiety about the future. Others may be coming to terms with facing their deaths much sooner than they envisaged. For some, this is a progressive development – for others, thoughts of dying, engender incipient panic and dread – waking them in the night, and impacting them by day in a very distressing way.

There will be times on the course, when as teachers, we will need to hold strong feelings within the group, perhaps triggered by thoughts of recurrence and/or dying. In assessment and orientation meetings, we will hear many stories that involve intense personal distress, trauma and challenge.

It is equally inevitable that some of our participants will die. As already mentioned, some stay in touch so that when recurrences occur, we are able to continue working with them, one to one, sometimes up to their death. Being a mindfulness-based teacher of cancer patients will sometimes involve us in attending funerals, being contacted by relatives (who may have found your phone number in an address book) to be told that a participant has died, or talking to ward staff and hearing about the last moments of someone you have been actively supporting.

How would that be for you? What would help you stay open and available? How could you support yourself in this process? And significantly, how will you manage your own thoughts around death and dying, as you hold others in their experience of this? Your own issues are bound to arise.

2. Medical challenges

The second area involves the treatments that many of our participants will have gone through – or be going through. Some of them involve some very challenging medical interventions. As mindfulness teachers we are not directly involved in these, but we will hear about them and need to have some clear understanding of what is involved, in order to support people to be with their experience, or memories of treatment. Any sense of aversion or personal discomfort around hospitals and cancer treatments (such as chemotherapy, surgery, radiotherapy, drug treatments, taking of blood, bone marrow procedures, etc.) might suggest that this context is not for you. In class, there may be issues around hair loss, stoma bags, sickness, and pain to negotiate and offer participants support with.

3. Health anxieties

Being around people with cancer for some period may trip us into health anxieties of our own. We may find ourselves becoming hyper-vigilant about some symptom or other. Even an unconscious sense of contamination may creep in. We may develop rituals, perhaps involving hand or clothes washing. One colleague disinfects all her saucepans and crockery in the kitchen sink after working on an oncology unit. Patterns like these are not unusual and highlight the impact of working in this context.

Adapting to oncology from other health settings

Working one to one with people facing medical crises, such as cancer, can be fulfilling. Holding this within a group might be a step further than we want to take at this time.

A colleague once proposed that those who are considering teaching mindfulness to cancer patients might spend a day or so on the oncology ward, where people are obviously ill, and where some are moving towards the later stages of the disease and the end of their life. It might also help to have time on a day treatment unit, where patients wearing wigs and scarves receive treatments that they know will make them sick and miserable.

Of course we are all touched by personal feelings of fear, distress or even disgust at times – and this on its own is no reason to keep away from working with people with cancer. It is probably more important to look at how we might work with these feelings when they arise – for it is inevitable that they will. Do we have or can we find personal supervision resources that can help us process whatever arises? Do we have a practice that enables us to be with feelings of distress, fear or concern?

Some of us may have worked with people who have contemplated suicide or have experienced close bereavement. We might wonder if this will offer insight into working with people facing issues of death and dying. In our experience, both suicidal ideation and bereavement are very different to receiving a cancer diagnosis. The patterns of reactivity are not the same. Having said that, depression is widespread in people with cancer and some may reach a place of hopelessness and helplessness that draws them into wanting to put an end to their suffering.

Whilst some of us working in a mental health field might have experienced mental health difficulties ourselves, many of us have a sense of our dominant vulnerabilities. Personal issues may well be triggered for us in the work we do with others, but with cancer this can happen a little differently. Although there are genetic predispositions, cancer invariably arrives unheralded and unexpected. People with otherwise perfect health can develop symptoms or attend a regular screening that results in a cancer diagnosis. Those of us working in this field are therefore not immune to the very experience that our participants are going through. We are aware of this and our work frequently reminds us of it.

Patterns of personal responses

When we first start working in this context, we may feel inspired and enthusiastic. Perhaps we have a sense that this work is special, and that we can make a significant difference. With high energy, idealized notions of what is possible begin to form. Of course, these responses may not be limited to work with people with cancer. However, at some point, anxiety about one's own personal health may creep in, perhaps accompanied by fears about being contaminated in some way, which may be experienced as quite shameful. Self doubt inevitably surfaces – often triggered by the first experience of a recent participant's death.

Two possible paths seem to emerge. Either, the teacher is able gradually to develop her capacity to balance care of herself with her work alongside others. Or a cycle of boom and bust gets established, with periods of enthusiasm and activity, followed by periods of exhaustion and despair. In other contexts, many of us may have experienced similar patterns.

Qualities of Teacher

The qualities needed in mindfulness teachers working with people with cancer may not read so very differently to those teaching with other groups and populations. Above all, we need to possess warmth and compassion, and a capacity to be embodied and grounded – in order to hold people who are working with strong feelings of fear, anxiety and uncertainty.

However, issues of personal reactivity to cancer need some reflection, as we have sought to highlight. Without taking these into account, and if we do not find ways to support ourselves as personal challenges arise, there is a risk that we will avoid them, much like our participants would like to. We may find ourselves teaching a group of people with cancer, with no mention of cancer, illness, or death ever arising in the group – because we and they collude in our joint denial. We may resist the very issues that participants are there to work with.

There is a representation of compassion that uses the image of figure holding a lotus flower – which has its roots in the dirt and mud, and yet produces a beautiful and fragrant flower. This is a helpful metaphor.

Some of us may find that we tend to get stuck in the 'mud' of the suffering of others. It seems to draw us in deep and we can find ourselves in a place where we are so empathetically involved that we ourselves become distressed and unable to function. Some of us may feel quite distant, not threatened by the distress of those we work with. We can work above it somehow, uncontaminated. In this position, it may be tempting to believe that we can make more of a significant difference. However, as mindfulness teachers, if we do not connect with those we work with, we will ultimately be as ineffective as those who are drowning in the 'mud'.

Finding a balance between these two positions is the challenge, like so much else in this work. We practise being able to 'pitch our tent' in touch with the grim reality of sickness and death on the one side – and open, on the other, to moments of beauty, meaning and connection, with those walking the razor's edge of life. Grounded, we sit with both the suffering and the possibility of wonder, without overly dwelling on or being committed to either. It is in this place that we are best able to open our hearts in compassion for ourselves and others.

Grief is an Open Door

Look in and see all
that has been.
I took love in through
your flame and fed its fire.
The crimson rowan berries
that lined our path,
sweet fallen plums
and soured apples.
The hunger for it all.

Look out and see all
that is.
The oak tree, bare now
with crow its one dark leaf
ready to fly.
And you, my beloved,
like the one yellow flower
that refuses to yield
until it is time.

Jill Teague (2010)

Chapter Thirteen
Embodying the Practice

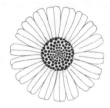

Good teaching is an act of generosity .... a craft that may grow with practice .... a maddening mystery ... Good teaching cannot be equated with technique; it comes from the integrity of the teacher, from his or her relation to subject and students, from the capricious chemistry of it all.

(Parker Palmer, 1998)

Introduction

We now move on to look at the ways that we can continue to nurture our development as teachers. Over time, we develop skills, creativity and experience in this work. This is not in order to become expert – and indeed if we do, we risk losing our capacity to stay open and fresh to learning from and with our participants – and this may be how we serve them best.

In the following pages, we bring together three processes that for us are central to our learning and development as teachers. Each of the three: Intention, Practice and Reflection; contain many evolving possibilities. They may have relevance to those of you who teach in other contexts and with other populations. We bring a particular focus to teaching mindfulness to people with cancer.

Mindfulness-Based Cognitive Therapy for Cancer: Gently Turning Towards,
First Edition. Trish Bartley.
© 2012 Trish Bartley. Published 2012 by John Wiley & Sons, Ltd.

Teaching

Sustaining the heart of learning

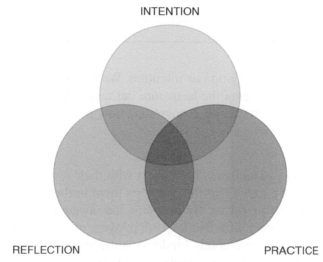

Figure 13.1 Circles of Intention, Practice and Reflection.

1. Intention

> When the basic inspiration is that of benefiting others, it creates true utopia (Shikpo, 2005).

What is intention? It has appeared in this book in a number of places. We start in the first session of the eight week programme, when we guide participants into cultivating a personal intention for their wellbeing. After that, we repeat this at the start of each session. Intention is the first of four movements that develop mindful awareness practice in the second of the circle diagrams. Now, in this chapter, we turn again to the intention of the mindfulness-based teacher, seeing this as one of the foundations that sustains the heart of her teaching.

Cultivating intention

What do we intend in relation to this work and this mindfulness teaching practice?

> Is it possible to connect with our heart intention? – asking ourselves as we sit in practice:
>
> - *What brings me to this work?*
> - *What is my heart wish in relation to my teaching?*

By doing this, we are clarifying our intention. We may choose to deliberately cultivate an intention to bring the heart into our teaching practice, both for ourselves and for those we teach, recognizing how powerful and potentially skilful this is.

We invite our course participants to connect with their own personal intentions because we know that this supports them in their practice. As teachers, the same is true for us. By dropping into awareness of what lies in the heart, we can connect with the deepening layers of our intention. This gives us an opportunity to embody kindness and compassion, supporting us both in how we are in relation to others – and how we connect in this moment to ourselves.

Intention develops as we do. It can be viewed as an opportunity to connect with a natural movement towards love, compassion, truth and awakening or aliveness. Like the sun coming out from behind the clouds, it has the potential to shed its light and warmth on all it touches. Perhaps this view of intention links with the natural goodness that we all intrinsically share.

Intention is a:

> … commitment that when 'spoken' from the heart, brings tremendous power for good. (Bartley, 2003).

Connecting to intention

As we start each class with an invitation to connect to intention, we are aligning ourselves and our participants to each other in our hearts, and joining to what supports us best.

'As we sit (at the start of this class) – inviting you to connect to your intention ... perhaps linking with what brought you here – with your deepest wish to be well ..... to cultivate your well-being ... to live in a way that develops mindfulness and kindness ...

Intention might not be formed in words. Maybe it is a sense or a feeling in your heart ... just opening to the possibility that what lies there can support you during this session and this week ...'

At any moment, as we teach, there is intention waiting to connect us into the heart. At times of concern and anxiety in or between classes, we can come to our practice and reconnect with our heart's intention. This supports us to move beyond any personal concern connected to the teaching. It connects us to a wider appreciation and trust in the process, and the heart of what we teach.

Transforming my limited skills into an intention to benefit others, I open to what is true and let *that* 'teach'.

Appreciation of having practised with intention

Intention supports the way the class is both 'held' and brought to a close. At the end of the session, we connect in appreciation of our shared intention to learn and practice together in a way that supports well-being. Later, we may widen this out to include others, such as people on the ward. This links to a growing sense of the common humanity that connects us all. It might be one of us in hospital. It probably has been at some point. Some participants have had relatives who have died on the oncology ward. Some of us may die there in the future. We practice with the intention that wellbeing and kindness may grow in us all. May it be so.

A closing practice

'As we come to the end of this class, appreciating the learning and practice of this session that we have all contributed to ... and connecting us with our shared intention to support the well-being of everyone in this group ... and if you want to, widening this out to include those on the oncology ward down the corridor and anyone resting in your heart at this time ... sending them our kindness and good wishes.

This may not suit everyone who teaches. We may choose to start slowly and build gently, staying within comfort zones – and guided by what feels right in each context and each moment. Anything else would not be genuine.

These practices of connecting with intention at the start and end of the session seem to be especially supportive when someone in the group has had a recurrence, and needs to withdraw from the course. It offers comfort and connection when a member of the group is becoming poorly. Participants feel concern for others in the group and bring them to mind during the week, wanting what is best for them. We might sometimes include those who are coming for treatment in the day unit and members of staff helping them. Many participants have been there themselves – and naturally think about others going through what they did.

As teachers our intention helps us to teach in a way that supports the wellbeing of our participants. We never know what participants will gain from their mindfulness-based course – and any attempt to guess will be misplaced. Instead we can let go and settle into our teaching practice with a heart intention to support their wellbeing in whatever it unfolds.

2. Practice

Mindfulness is a generous practice. It is always possible to start again. ... It requires a 'cup of wisdom, a bucket of kindness and an ocean of patience.'
(Feldman, 2008)

We can only teach what we practice. The process will always be the poorer when we work 'technically' or automatically. This is highlighted when insight illuminates something we have been struggling to practise for a while. There is a shift of understanding. It is as if we have never *not* known. This connects us with how to teach it in a fresh and direct way. Teaching out of our own embodied practice enables us, strangely, to get out of the way, and allow the teaching itself to come through in *its* own way.

Teaching and practice are not really different. One appears more 'inward' and one more 'outward', but both are grounded in present awareness and openness, connecting self with other. Practice is the way we align to the wise intention of the heart, to be present in the moment and aware of the habits of mind. It is like housework that needs doing and doing. Sometime, way down the line, the 'self' that strives will let go and 'love and compassion will be constant rather than vacillating and partial.'(Feldman, 2008)

Why do we practise? On the one hand, there is obvious personal benefit. We are more able to ride the weather of our lives. We may feel happier and less troubled by events. We are more present as we teach and on a good day, we have the capacity to make more skilful choices.

What if the richest potential of practice also points in another direction?

We would not be in this work without the wish to help others – but strong challenges lie in the way. Mindfulness teaching feels important. Working with people with cancer, we want to make a difference. We may be doing things that have not been done before. We may find ourselves comparing our teaching to others, who have been doing this longer or not so long. There are many ways that we strive for this or that in our teaching – wanting to be as good as it is possible to be.

> A mindfulness colleague attended a prestigious international conference. He had left behind a rather unpleasant dispute amongst his colleagues. On the flight to the conference, he relaxed into his seat, luxuriating in anticipation of reconnecting with people whom he respected, who were the 'real thing' – mindful and genuine.
>
> On arriving at the conference, a senior teacher who he knew quite well, walked straight past him, barely saying hello. As the days went by, he kept encountering examples of people behaving much like his colleagues at home. Seeking out a friend and long time mentor, he shared his deep disappointment. 'How come you believed that the world of mindfulness would be different?' His mentor responded kindly, 'It just highlights how important our practice is. None of us are safe from our egos!'

How can we return to our practice and explore things honestly? We often wish that we could remove those competitive hooks, but there they are – even as we hoped they were loosening. It is only through practice that we can hope to hear the subtler voices that come closer to the truth in our hearts. We practice both to reduce the impact of our striving and to enable us to help others. Why else would we do this work?

In 2004 at a conference in Bangor in Wales, Jon Kabat-Zinn suggested that mindfulness based teachers might make a solemn undertaking to benefit others, at the start of their teaching careers. He talked about the inspiration of the bodhisattva, a being who practises with compassion for the good of others and who has vowed to be born again and again in the world until all suffering is ended.

> *May no one's encounter with me be without benefit for them.*
>
> *Whether it gives rise to anger or faith in them, may any encounter with me,*
>
> *Be the seed for accomplishing all their wishes* (Shantideva, translated by Hookham, 1997).

Kindness and compassion practice

MBCT-Ca has a particular emphasis on kindness and compassion in the face of suffering.

When a participant has a recurrence; when a patient is dying; or when we are working with someone who is struggling with intense difficulty, there is sometimes little else we can do to support them and support ourselves in the process? Participants touch our hearts – and rightly. In working with those whose suffering resonates within us, practice may be the only way can keep our hearts open and ourselves grounded. When a participant seems resistant and defensive, after we have reflected and tried a number of approaches, what is left but to open our hearts in compassion? We come back over and over again to a practice of compassion – for ourselves and others.

Teacher as practitioner

As mindfulness-based approaches go 'mainstream', there is an inherent risk that it will become just another intervention. From the view of someone already experienced in psychological approaches, getting hold of a book like this, learning to run the processes described within it, and maybe going on a short mindfulness course might seem enough to start teaching the approach. However, when coming from a conceptual and skill based perspective, the mindfulness courses we offer may be of limited use.

As already mentioned, we are required as teachers to develop our own personal practice before we start to teach. A senior American MBSR teacher used to muse out loud that it probably takes 20 years of practice to develop into being a reasonable teacher. Some of us may need longer!

The old adage serves us well – we teach what we most need to learn. The trouble is that we learnt how to succeed in life in ways that now, coming to mindfulness, no longer *do* serve us well. Working with a group of health professionals, who were struggling to find ways of getting mindfulness 'right', a mindfulness teacher wrote them a letter.

Here is an excerpt:

This work that we are doing involves us in learning to BE with ourselves. Most of us find this very difficult. We do a lot to fill up the spaces to avoid ourselves. But our suffering is right in there. Even though we've been told that mindfulness isn't another 'fix', most of us hope that somehow it is – only different!

We can't 'do' mindfulness using the ways that have worked before....... the hard work needed now, we are discovering, is to practice with patience, gentleness and kindness. A new language for most of us! So how do we work with the heart   not just with others but with ourselves too?

Using effortless effort, knowing there's no right way – Caring a lot and yet not much at all – Practicing as if our lives depended on it – and yet just doing it every day.

Living our lives as we tasted the raisin – as if for the first time.

And seeing what happens if we blend tiny traces of kindness into the next routine activity – or add a few drops of patience to the next body scan or mindful movement – as an experiment ... We have to start with our own personal struggles. ...... then we might begin to be of some use to others, on a good day.

Even when aligned to a practice intention to benefit others, it is never possible to relieve suffering as we would like. Illness, old age and death are unavoidable. Working with cancer highlights this every day. Bringing this to our cushions, we practice to stay present and open to whatever arises in the heart, moment by moment.

Mindfulness does not reject experience. It lets experience be the teacher (Kornfield, 2008).

3. Reflection

> In the new paradigm ... the 'swamp' or mess becomes the primary ground for understanding and learning. The challenges grow; the sense of vulnerability and anxiety (as well as excitement) grows .... The result of this (is) a recognition of the need to reflect consciously and critically on my own practice. (Bell, 1998)

Reflecting seems to be a form of practice. By widening the vision of our own activity and exploring our congruence, we begin to understand a little more. Just teaching – just doing it, is not enough, it seems. We look into the 'swamp' and see things from a new perspective – both close up and wide angle.

Sometimes all we seem to see is our own experience. Like Narcissus, we may be more interested in that, than in the other images, shapes and colours. However, as we gain experience, we may notice more. We invite others' ideas – opening to hear what we may not want to hear, to see what is often not always complimentary, to touch into the doubt and fear of not being good enough. This opening to the unknown is our only way of experiencing the water we swim in – for unless we ask others, we may never know what is there.

> We need to develop the faculty of self-reflection, of humility in the face of unpredictability and uncertainty in life. We must recognize that we are most often in the dark when we are most certain and the most enlightened when we are most confused'. (Kaplan, 1996).

Process notes

Finding some way to reflect on the class just taught, we first loosely pour out written impressions onto the page. What went well? What was difficult or felt awkward?

> If we continue to work with this raw matter, it will draw us deeper and deeper into ourselves ... we will begin to see the rich garden we have inside us (Goldberg, 1986)

As we write, we may become aware of the unsatisfactory moments. These are always there to be experienced within the body – even if also involving the group. How else do we notice? Pausing to explore some more – we might ask if this was something in me, as teacher – an expectation, tiredness, or automatic moment. Or was something else going on as well? Might it be the stage the group is at? Does this often happen at this point in the course? Does it highlight a gap in the session or something relating to one of the participants?

Sometimes, just asking and reflecting on questions like these is enough. Equally, we may become aware of changes that need making. Perhaps it is evident that we rushed our preparation. The ten minutes sitting that we squeezed in before the class, we may realize, is not enough, after being frantically busy all day. As a result of this, we may choose to do something – perhaps in relation to the next class – or in connection with a participant – or perhaps in deciding to make an adjustment to the course. Equally these issues may be rich topics for supervision, or to discuss with our peers.

Peer feedback

Reflecting first on our own, perhaps through writing and also on the cushion – we may invite a colleague to sit in on our classes, and maybe teach with us. We practice turning towards their feedback as best we can. Our egos are fragile, and when criticized, most of us defend, shut down and turn away from the comments. Instead on a good day, we can hear what is said – and use it to teach more congruently.

This process, like much else in mindfulness, needs trust, courage and integrity. It is both a gift and an exchange. As we get more used to the process, it gets easier. Teachers regularly giving each other feedback can develop confidence in the other and the process – and learn a lot.

Supervision and mentoring

Working with more experienced others is important in our maturing as teachers. Supervision offers something similar to peer feedback, but with the great advantage of connecting with someone with more experience and wisdom. We approach those we respect. We identify skills, qualities and areas of experience which we would like to develop – and choose someone who in some way embodies these. It is a privilege to be asked to supervise someone – a trust.

Relationships build over time. At best it is an exchange which is mutually beneficial. We use these sessions to reflect deeply on the edges of our teaching – the inquiry that was a bit 'off' – the process that did not quite work – an aspect of personal practice – the participant who is not really connecting to the course. We expose the grey areas, where things are neither clear nor somehow wholesome.

In teaching people with cancer, we have particular needs. Our own patterns surface as we have explored earlier. If we are lucky, we find someone who can support us to keep our hearts open, help us be present with what arises and honour our learning process, in the thick of the challenges.

At times, a meditation instructor may be what we most need. Finding someone who can offer new commitment to our mindfulness practice will greatly support our teaching.

Retreat and teachings

Simplifying our lives and spending time on retreat, going deeper into ourselves, allows us to come closer to practice. When the sediment settles, we can see what is there. No longer quite so strongly attached to the 'I' and the 'mine', we connect with a more spacious mind that opens to inspiration and understanding.

Silence is a wonderful context for personal reflection. Of course when we slow down and start practising, there is no guarantee that the mind *will* be silent. Most of us discover plenty of chatter and probably a fair bit of physical pain. In trusting inner wisdom that needs no improving – just a settling into what is there – we come back to the direct immediacy of experience – and perhaps find moments of simply being.

Whilst on retreat, we may connect with a teacher, priest, or spiritual friend, whose teachings we feel drawn to. Some traditions emphasize the importance of connecting with a teacher. Most of us receive teachings from many different people in many different ways. There is also much benefit in connecting to a specific teacher or meditation instructor who can support us on our path. This may be one of the most significant connections we ever make.

Conclusion

Teaching mindfulness seems to be a corrective process. Aligning ourselves to our deepest intention, we engage with an open heart and trust what unfolds. If the conditions are right, the practice and the teaching will bear fruit and participants' learning will flourish. If the conditions are wrong, as teachers we may not practice, we may feel tired and find excuses not to teach. It is important to respect that in ourselves. This may not be our time. Those of us who pause, and come back to the work later, often return to find that the ground of our teaching is all the richer for the composting of time and practice.

It is through:

- Intention that we align ourselves to what is compassionate and wise.
- Practice that we open to awareness and compassion.
- Reflection that we come to see what is hidden to us.

Through the interconnection between them, we are able to mature as practitioners and learn as teachers.

Who would like to ring The Bells?

'But that's marvellous' she said –'isn't it?'
And wasn't it? That we should all be brought together
Strangers, yet so swiftly joined
Not presuming intimacy but
Connected and compassionate, settling

'Who would like to ring the bells?' she said
I watched my thoughts and almost cried
That in this room I could have rung those bells
And not feared failure – or success

'With a gentle curiosity' she said
Perfectly embodying the two

'Feet on the ground' she said
And thus rooted, we branched out

'Everything let go' she said
Didn't we?

Bridget (April, 2009)

Chapter Fourteen
Facilitating The Learning

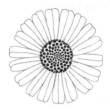

Be patient towards all that is unsolved in your heart and try to love the questions themselves like locked rooms and like books that are written in a very foreign tongue. Do not now seek the answers, which cannot be given you because you would not be able to live them. And the point is, to live everything. Live the questions now. Perhaps you will then gradually, without noticing it, live along some distant day into the answer.

(R M Rilke, 1996)

Introduction

Having considered how we can support our development as teachers, we now move on to explore aspects of the learning process itself, within the course. The group has a vital role in MBCT-Ca. We see it as central to how our participants learn. This requires us, as teachers, to develop a role as facilitator of the group process. This is not to suggest any separation from practice and the previous chapter – far from it. It is simply a way of looking at teaching from a different perspective.

The literal meaning of facilitator is 'one who makes things easy'. She helps people learn from their experience. She takes good care of *the process* of learning – attending to the voyage, rather than only navigating towards a

Mindfulness-Based Cognitive Therapy for Cancer: Gently Turning Towards,
First Edition. Trish Bartley.
© 2012 Trish Bartley. Published 2012 by John Wiley & Sons, Ltd.

fixed destination. This involves rather different skills from those of a conventional teacher. To learn from their experience, participants need to feel comfortable in the group. It is a complex process and learning outcomes are inevitably unpredictable. Skilful facilitators place their trust in the wisdom of the process, even whilst the journey is bumpy – maybe especially then.

Those of us who work predominantly with individuals, risk running mindfulness courses as an extension of our one to one work. Most exchanges seem to take place between individual participants and the teacher. Participants may still learn from others, but not as much as when the group is included as an important dimension.

MBCT-Ca has good reason to emphasize the significance of the group. People with cancer invariably feel isolated in their experience – even if surrounded by supportive family and friends. Coming on an MBCT-Ca course offers them the opportunity to connect with similar others. These connections are not so much based on their personal cancer journeys, but on a direct here and now experience of practice and dialogue, with cancer as a shared context. A sense of common humanity can develop which reduces feelings of isolation and promotes compassion. The group becomes the home of this radical shift of perspective. It is possible for a profound and even intimate community of experience to develop, which can continue to be healing and supportive long after the course has finished, even if group members never see each other again.

The Experiential Nature of Learning

I hear and I forget. I see and I believe. I do and I understand (Confucius, 1979)

Learning from the truth of experience

Mindfulness-based courses are essentially experiential in relation to learning – so how can we help people to learn from their experience?

Traditional education models are not very transferable – but there is much else to draw on. Learning to ride a bike (through persistently getting up and being encouraged to try again); cooking (often as an apprentice in the family kitchen); using a computer (through trial and error and gleaning solutions from others) are all examples.

Experiential education is all about discovering learning and applying it to life. In a poem written in the thirteenth century, called *Two Kinds of Intelligence* (Rumi, 1995), Rumi aptly describes learning that is gained from absorbing facts and concepts. He juxtaposes this with learning that comes from within the learner – and moves out into the world. He calls this 'a freshness from within the centre of the chest'. 'The wisdom we discover' or 'the faculty to discern the truth in our experience' (Shikpo, 2007) suggests that experiential learning includes a strong sense of personal value and purpose. We are therefore facilitating a process that enables people to learn from the heart and the truth of their experience.

Due to the significance and scope of this, absolute congruence is called for. Walking our talk, as teachers, requires us to practice genuine respect for everyone involved. This determines how we work with people from different backgrounds, races, abilities, religions, genders, and ages. If 'inclusion' is what we seek to facilitate, we practise this with each and every individual and group. Participation is clearly a key. (Jeffs & Smith, 1996, 2005). People learn most when they feel confident about exchanging with others in a group.

Facilitating Learning within the Group

Identifying three phases in the development of the group offers a chance to explore:

1. Forming the Circle – when individual participants join the course.
2. Holding the Circle – when participants have formed sufficient connection to feel safe within the group – enabling them to learn from and with each other.
3. Moving out Beyond the Circle – when the course finishes and participants use their practice in their everyday lives.

2. Forming The Circle

At the beginning, there is not yet a group. Separate individuals arrive, unsure of themselves, and each other. They are strangers feeling strange. All have had cancer or are closely connected to someone who has had cancer, and all of them come into the room with their own personal histories that directly influence their interactions with others.

If all goes well, they move from a collection of strangers to being a coherent group (Whitaker, 2001).

Learning to belong

How to transform this initial unease into one of eventual *belonging*? Full belonging in this context involves 'more and more to understand and feel his or her influence on the life of the group in the moment' (McCown et al, 2010).

Inevitably there are obstacles. Before the group has even met, the participant-to-be has formed her own expectations of how it will be. The relationship with teacher and other group members is largely laid down by her early relationships with parents and siblings. The group 'imago' (Berne, 1963) may well be drawn in her mind with a picture of herself (the participant) as isolated and separate; the group leader as 'above' the rest; and all other participants in an undifferentiated 'clump' away from her.

> Because the individual's first exposure to a group is in his or her family, this becomes the matrix for his or her most enduring and profound injuries or permissions. (Clarkson, 1991).

As connections are made, hopefully this changes. If conditions are conducive, eventually all projections about others in the group eventually dissolve. 'She is not a bit as I first thought', might be expressed. The teacher is experienced more fully in the present and less as a projected parent or authority figure. If the group eventually manages to reach the optimal stage of 'performing' (Tuckman, 1965), and the impact of early history and dynamics modifies – the 'clump' of undifferentiated others will have been transformed into different connections that together form a sense of belonging within the group.

Drawing the boundaries

A clear periphery needs to define where the 'circle' of the group starts and finishes. This is an explicit boundary (Mardula, 2008) which determines membership. If the boundary is fractured, damaged or unclear, it will impact on both the group and the entire course process.

This is more than just the obvious physical boundaries (affected by factors such as interruptions, or changes of venue). The safety of the group container may also be compromised by inadequate internal boundaries, affected by issues of group membership (e.g. inappropriate participants); or course information (e.g. inadequate orientation); or unclear ground rules, persistent lateness, absent group members and so forth.

This underlines the importance of the orientation and assessment process (see chapter 5, Starting Out). The one-to-one meeting that takes place with the teacher before the course begins, helps the participant gain a basic understanding of the purpose and process of the course – and begins the connection between them.

Forming connections

The group is where much of the learning takes place. Feelings of belonging can evolve and develop from the very first session, as early connections are made and barriers gently start to dismantle. The sharing of experience is facilitated by processes of inquiry and dialogue, in the whole group, in pairs and in small groups.

Any form of intimacy involves a process of 'warming up' – that enables us to be ready to engage. Working in depth with someone too early has a risk of over exposing them. If we go 'horizontally[1]' at first in the inquiry process with participants, (after the practice has finished), then gradually the group learn to deepen together. This helps to normalize experience, develops confidence in sharing, and promotes group cohesion.

For example:

Participant No.1: 'I fell asleep in the Body Scan'
Teacher: 'Did anyone else feel sleepy?' (scanning round the group). 'I see some nods from some of you – did anyone have a very different experience'?
Participant No.2: 'I felt restless and irritated'. ...

... and so on – drawing out a few words from several people, in order to allow the group to map the general experience. For individual participants, it offers an opportunity to feel secure that their experience was similar to others. This naturally helps bonds to form.

[1]Horizontal inquiry is a term developed by colleagues in North America. It is a way of inquiring that invites a very brief response from a number of members of the group about their experience of the practice, before going on to explore in more depth ('vertical' inquiry) with one or two individual participants.

Exchanging with another in a small group discussion will support participants to have the courage to share again, perhaps in the larger group. With luck, they learn that this is a safe place to contribute ideas. The teacher's role is to establish an environment, which is open, warm, affirming and accepting. This will then be mirrored within the group.

Forming Connections

Some practical ideas

- Inviting people to talk to someone they don't know / haven't spoken to yet / didn't speak to last week (*in order to expand the group imago, continue to form and renew connections, and reduce projections* [Clarkson, 1991]).
- Reminding people to share names again each time they talk (*widening connections; breaking down barriers.*
- Separating out couples or pairs who came together (*discouraging splitting, widening learning*).
- Putting solos together for support (*for example; staff with carers, non cancer patients*).
- Arranging the groups so that quieter ones are put with people who might help to draw them out (*some more shy participants may only ever speak in small groups*).
- Being aware of mobility issues or people in pain (*for example; asking others to move to them rather than have them move*).
- Noticing emerging leadership within the group – (*perhaps forming a small group around a participant who is attending for the second time, knowing she may help to facilitate the others*).
- Knowing why we are using a certain process in a certain way and choosing a small group in line with this (*e.g. early days in the group when building the community – small groups or pairs are more intimate; when half way through the course, sharing learning and renewing commitment might be best in larger groups*)

The impact of practice

Practices introduced in the sessions support participants to settle – enabling them to open and connect with others in the group.

For example, soon after the start of the first session, a short grounding practice is led. This brings attention to the body and its connection with the ground

– offering the mind a focus to help it steady and come back. This reduces anxious thinking, which is a natural reaction when in a group for the first time.

Soon after this, there is an intentions practice. This reminds participants of their reasons for coming on the course and what they hope to gain from it. It also speaks of a wider intention that whilst unnamed, connects participants to their hearts and each other.

By learning to come back, from the outset of the course – through practices such as the Body Scan and simple grounding – participants are practising stepping out of automatic reactivity and coming into direct awareness. This facilitates connection with oneself and also with others. The embodiment of the teacher supports this process, as she herself comes back over and over, as part of the way that she holds the group.

There are challenges, of course. Some groups find it harder to form than others. The process is not necessarily smooth. Practicing a Body Scan, lying down with people you barely know can almost seem like an infringement of the personal boundaries that have been so carefully set up. Even the Raisin Exercise, in its apparent oddness, can be difficult for people who may feel skeptical and unsure. However, as teachers, we can ride lightly but sure footedly with this – acknowledging what may seem odd or challenging; informing ahead of time that we will be lying on the floor for a practice; and always inviting a choice around participating. This helps us to navigate the early phase of the course and supports developing connections within the group.

2. Holding the Circle

> The teacher who is indeed wise does not bid you to enter the house of his wisdom but rather leads you to the threshold of your mind (Kahlil Gibran, 1926).

Facilitating the learning of the group involves a wide range of skills – including a well developed capacity to hold and respond to the group process. What does this involve?

The group is more than a collection of individuals. It might also be seen to be an entity in its own right. Reflecting internally at times, 'What is feeling tone of this group'? Exploring this lightly can allow a mindful response to what is happening.

Developing Awareness Of The Group

(an internal teacher reflection)

If the group were an animal, what would it be?

1. Pausing and imagining the group you are currently working with – in terms of overall characteristics (*e.g. talkative, engaged, tentative, heavy, sad, uncertain, pensive etc.*).
2. Invite the image of an animal to emerge – and allow some space for you to resonate with this animal (*e.g. lemurs – desert rats – who pop their heads up out of their little holes in the ground to look around; a flock of sparrows twittering excitedly, here one minute and gone the next; a large elephant, solid and grounded, taking his time to walk along the path*).
3. What does this animal tell you about your group? What new information do you gain? As group leader, how might you respond to this group animal? What does it need from you?

The group animal will change as the group develops. Tracking this changing 'creature', we respond differently at different points on the course.

Everything that occurs in a group has an impact on every individual within the group. As the group meditates, a collective 'field' develops that influences everyone's experiences.

It is very evident that every group is different. Apparently identical programmes are led, but every time we teach, the experience is unique. It is impossible to predict how a group will be – even week by week. Our task as teachers is to establish the group within a safe and grounded container and as 'steward', 'holding the space in which the group can work'. (McCown et al, 2010). Towards the end of the course, a lighter touch may be offered, as the group matures and is more able to take care of its own process.

Encountering the other

As the sessions progress, connections deepen. It is not about forming friendships, but of developing trust in a shared process. Participants are learning to connect with awareness, alongside others engaged on the same journey. *Encounter* is a key process that enables people to open to themselves, the other and the world.

> All real living is meeting ...... When a human being turns to another as another, as a particular and specific person to be addressed, and tries to communicate with him through language or silence, something takes place between them which is not found elsewhere in nature (Buber, 1958)

This place of encounter, which Buber called the 'between', may be the essence of shared community. In mindfulness groups, when people are present, there is an exchange that connects them in the moment of their encounter to their wholeness and wellness – and to that of the other.

Varying Small Groups

With an emphasis on nurturing participation, and a focus on increasing encounter and connection amongst group members, we can reduce monotony brought on by the same style of teaching 'delivery' or process by:

Mixing and matching within small groups:

- Pairs reflect on a theme that might benefit from a more intimate and personal exchange (*e.g. what activities shall I use to link to breathing spaces?*)
- Small groups of 3s and 4s which might benefit from a slightly more reflective base – hearing ideas from others – reinforcing own ideas / progress (*e.g. how can I remember to practice breathing spaces?*)
- Larger groups of 5 or 6 (or half the total group) when hearing from others might be helpful (*e.g. half way review: What am I learning from this course?*)

Facilitating the learning encounter

There are some guiding principles, which emphasise the significance of the group in experiential learning. (Freire, 1972).

The first of these is 'Dialogue' which emerges out of respect and conversation – rather than via a fixed curriculum. When this happens, the process of learning underpins *what* is being learnt. This requires the facilitator teacher to be working *with* and present *to* the participant – rather than working *on* her. Seeking collaboration between participants and teacher, we draw on our own shared experience of practice within a process of mutual inquiry.

From this naturally follows the 'Teacher as Learner'. A mindfulness teacher, we would suggest, is only '5 minutes' ahead of her participants. As said before, given different circumstances, it could be one of them who is 'teacher' – and she as cancer patient, and mindfulness participant. Her capacity to continue to learn is central to her qualities as teacher. Teacher and participant are therefore little different – both are practitioners – both are learners. They simply have different roles and different experience to offer.

Wise mindfulness elders tell us that the day we feel we have nothing more to learn as teachers is the day we should give up teaching.

'Experience' is a central principle in the process of mindfulness learning – as is the opportunity to articulate experience with people who may not have done this before.

Finally, 'Praxis' is necessary to link action with reflection. We learn from our experience of practice (action) and then after dialogue in the group (reflection), we apply our learning to our lives (action). Within this is a value base, which views group praxis as a means of increasing personal dignity and well being.

Turning towards

The journey into a life of awareness begins for most of us in a moment of helplessness (Tarrant, 1998).

There comes a time on the course, if conditions are right, when participants shift focus and move up closer to difficulty. This involves courage and resolve. In order to be willing to start turning towards and *being* with difficult experiences, group members need to have developed a deep trust in each other and in the safety of the process. Implicit in this is the capacity of the teacher to hold the group.

How do we do this? It is, at best, a willingness to be with what is arising in the group. Sometimes an intervention is necessary, if the safety of the group is threatened or support is needed. Often it is not about *doing* anything. The teacher is in parallel with the participants – being with what is difficult. She is not turning away, or defending, or trying to fix things. She is co-traveller on the journey, bringing her presence and attention to what is being felt in the group.

> Attention is the most basic form of love: through it we bless and are blessed (Tarrant, 1998).

Participants who feel unsure will not turn towards difficulty. It may not be safe for them. However, as some engage, so the rest are helped to find courage when they are ready. Distress may ripple around the group as this happens, affecting one then moving along to others. Since the group is a whole system in itself, this is inevitable. As teachers, we are about

> ... holding their vulnerability and finding it beautiful (Hough, 2007).

Recurrences

Inevitably, there will be times when someone in the group has news that their disease has returned or progressed. This may be shared directly in the group, or the news may come to the teacher by phone, who then shares it with the group in the next session.

These situations are very challenging. For most people with cancer, this is the very worst possible fear. Getting close to someone who has a recurrence is very upsetting – both in relation to feelings for the person involved, and also in terms of the resonance for others with cancer. 'It could be me', is an immediate thought.

Sharing the news gently, and acknowledging its challenge, the teacher leaves space to hold whatever arises in the group. The programme takes a pause, for as long as necessary, and the group are given time to express what this means to them. Giving voice to what is arising in the group and turning towards it is our practice. At some point, we bring the breath to our awareness, not to reduce the pain, but to hold it tenderly.

Kindness and self compassion

Kindness is the last of the four core movements[2] within MBCT-Ca. It is not so much an emotion or a feeling, but an intention. Kindness can really only be learnt through a resonance within the group, 'co-created ... from moment

[2]Intention, Coming Back, Turning Towards, Kindness are the four movements first outlined in chapter 7, The Second Circle - Mindful Awareness and the Circle of Practice

to moment. This gift of the group touches and helps to optimize the freedom and belonging of each of the participants.' (McCowan, 2010). We practice kindness by connecting to a sense of compassion for the distress and suffering of others. People with cancer easily judge and blame themselves. It is often through seeing this habit in others and responding with genuine compassion towards them, that participants are able to open and soften in kindness to their own emotional pain.

Enlivening the Group Process

- Different combinations of small group process – ringing the changes (see previous box for ideas).
- Standing up and moving *(e.g. mountain standing; breathing space (responding); taking a standing pause – and highlighting choice for those with mobility or pain issues).*
- Changing chairs in later classes *(bringing awareness to experiencing the group and the room from another position – new perspectives; beginners mind).* Noticing the pull to become 'homing pigeons' and stay in the same seat.
- Placing paper on the floor to make learning connections *(e.g. when reviewing the course – formal practices; short practices; informal practices; in the Sea of Reactions; when highlighting the underpinning themes of Intention; Coming back; Turning Towards; and Kindness)* Using paper on the floor within the group circle will have stronger impact than writing on a flipchart or whiteboard.
- Using a white board or flipchart to record and acknowledge contributions from participants *(e.g. as in 'Walking Down the Street' or Pleasant / Unpleasant Events exercises).*
- Inviting one of the group to ring the bells at the close of the session *(sharing the ritual, breaking down barriers between teacher and participants).*

---

3. Moving Out Beyond the Circle

Our true suffering is the shared lot of humanity. ... Our false suffering appears when we add unnecessary pains to our necessary ones (Tarrant, 1998).

By the end of the course, participants may be able to recognise moments when they add extra to their suffering. A participant, who has made strong and present connections with others in the group may speak of how she feels when others describe their difficulty or pain. This may connect her to a wider sense of suffering in others. 'My' suffering becomes 'the' suffering, which instead of being isolating can feel strangely inspiring, poignant and consoling.

This sometimes seems like a flowering – when group members widen their awareness into a more spacious and compassionate connection with others. This does not always occur for everyone, but it does seem to be a fairly frequent development for many. The resonance of this often touches others.

Group members then leave the course with a new relationship to 'the other', which may start in their group, and then expand beyond it. Many report the impact this has on relationships outside the group.

The ending of the group

Each group is unique and lives for the duration of their 8 week course. It may continue on in the hearts and minds of its members for longer, but is dissolved in a practical sense at the end of the course. Participants may anticipate the ending of the group and may feel a sense of anticipatory loss, even as early as at the half way point in the course.

Known as the adjourning or mourning stage of the group process (Tuckman, 1965), it is an opportunity to turn towards and be with what arises. Acknowledging the feelings, noticing sensations in the body, naming the thoughts that may arise, and bringing gentle attention to the breath in the body, we share our experience of the loss of the group.

This may be strongly felt amongst people with cancer, who are finely tuned to issues of loss. All endings need care. As the end of the course draws near, awareness of the sensitivity of this stage may allow the possibility of being with the experience of loss in a more compassionate and gentle way. This may be a unique opportunity for many participants with cancer to express and experience loss in safety, perhaps through ritual or through a group process using objects, such as pebbles, that they can keep.

Conclusion

There may be a concern that too much attention to group process might steer the intervention towards an overly 'therapy' / support group approach. We have not found this to be the case. By having clear boundaries and investing in the group process, there are more opportunities for group members to learn from and with each other and for the group to play a bigger role in the healing journey of mindfulness (of themselves and others). This may also reduce dependence on the teacher.

Becoming aware of all the ways that mindfulness based courses are influenced and have developed – and the lineage of teachings and teachers that contribute to this – we can reflect on what it is within the process that results in the learning. It would seem to be only partly due to the teacher and her specific skills and qualities. It is surely true that what also underpins the process is the opening of each participant to awareness of her direct personal experience with gentleness and kindness, alongside others.

LETTING GO

Letting go in order to let in
releasing in order to receive
nature's coded messages become clearer
the less we try to see
Trying hard, trying harder and harder,
trying so very hard, is not the way;
we need commitment, yes
and focus,
and hope and faith and trust
but most of all we need ease,
a discipline of ease
not trying too hard at all.
You see trying hard has a cell-mate
called giving up, admitting defeat
like black and white
like pushing and pulling
no peace there.
"Not yet," you say
"I'm not ready yet to take the step beyond."
I know, I've stepped so slow myself, still do
but love, sweet sister, like death
comes in a moments heartbeat
then goes;
there are no ways to hold,
except by letting go
and letting it be a part of you
and you of it.

Stewart Mercer (2002)

Chapter Fifteen

The Three Circle Model: A Formulation of MBCT for Cancer (MBCT-Ca)

Trish Bartley and Ursula Bates

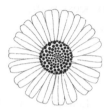

Introduction

Our work is strongly informed by clinical work with seriously ill patients. The three circle model that we use guides us in our struggle to maintain personal equanimity, and supports our patients to find stability in the face of very difficult internal and external experiences.

Cognitive Behavioural Therapy (CBT) has been well developed and researched as a therapeutic intervention for cancer patients. It is recommended for the treatment of cancer distress in a number of national guidance (including UK NICE guidance and US NCCN guidelines). MBSR has been shown to hold much promise as an intervention in cancer care (Shennan et al., 2010). MBCT-Ca, drawing as it does on CBT, MBSR and MBCT for Depression, is well placed to demonstrate ways of targeting the two underlying mechanisms of rumination and avoidance that greatly contribute to the incidence and maintenance of anxiety and depression in people with cancer.

MBCT-Ca is targeted and adapted to the needs of a clinical population of cancer patients. The programme described in this book is delivered in a

Mindfulness-Based Cognitive Therapy for Cancer: Gently Turning Towards,
First Edition. Trish Bartley.
© 2012 Trish Bartley. Published 2012 by John Wiley & Sons, Ltd.

hospital oncology setting, although it could be offered in a community setting to people with cancer. Drawing on the considerable evidence of the psychological impact of cancer (see chapter 2, Cancer – The Psychological Implications), and a cognitive model of cancer distress drawn from Moorey and Greer (2002), the Three Circle Model that we have developed serves as a formulation for MBCT-Ca.

Up to now, we have examined the three circles one at a time. We bring them together here to form a model that we suggest outlines some of the ways that mindfulness practice impacts on people with cancer.

The first circle, The Circle of Suffering, describes patterns of difficulties commonly experienced by participants coming onto eight week MBCT-Ca programmes. One of these, which we are calling the cognitive model of cancer distress, demonstrates the way that cancer patients easily become trapped in vicious cycles of anxious pre-occupation. This serves to maintain their distress.

The second circle, The Circle of Practice, illustrates the 'movements' or gestures that participants learn on the course, which when brought together, develop mindful awareness practice. We are proposing that the Four Movements in MBCT-Ca (Intention; Coming Back; Turning Towards; and Kindness) are central to enabling cancer patients to learn to relate differently to their patterns of distress. Kindness and compassion have a central role in this intervention.

The third circle, The Circle of Presence, takes us up to and beyond the eight week programme, to people who have completed the course and are now integrating mindfulness into everyday life, as they live with cancer. We suggest that mindfulness practice is a way for these practitioners to connect with qualities that have the potential to profoundly enrich their lives and expand their capacity to be with difficulty.

The Three Circle Model

An inherent drawback to a diagram such as this is the attempt to conceptualize what is essentially experiential, subtle, developmental, individual and complex. However, some notion of progression from left to right, from cancer diagnosis, through the programme, to living mindfully with cancer – whilst never as linear as in the model, may offer something to our understanding of the MBCT-Ca intervention.

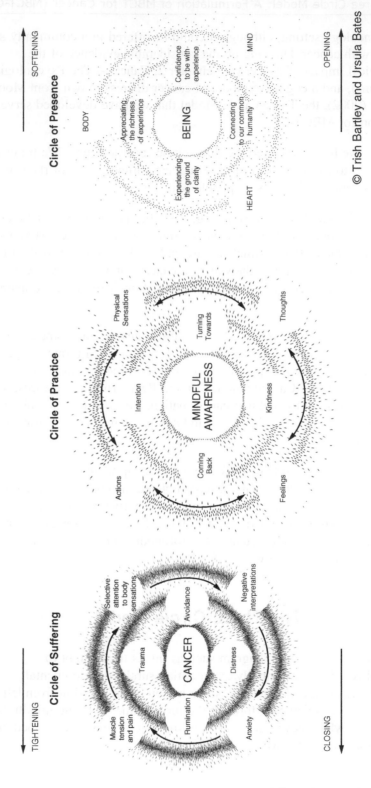

Figure 15.1 The Three Circle Model.

The Three Circle Model: A Formulation of MBT for Cancer (MBCT-Ca)

© Trish Bartley and Ursula Bates

Circle of Suffering

TIGHTENING

CLOSING

Selective attention to body sensations

Negative interpretations

Avoidance

Trauma

CANCER

Distress

Muscle tension and pain

Rumination

Anxiety

Circle of Practice

Physical Sensations

Turning Towards

Thoughts

Intention

MINDFUL AWARENESS

Kindness

Actions

Coming Back

Feelings

Circle of Presence

SOFTENING

OPENING

BODY

MIND

Confidence to be with experience

Appreciating the richness of experience

BEING

Connecting to our common humanity

Experiencing the ground of clarity

HEART

Relating across the Circles

Looking at the model, we can appreciate that there is a relationship between the circles as they progress across the page – remembering that this is only a map, and all development is unique and dynamic. Some participants' stories illustrate how this unfolds.

The Inner Rings

The obstructed, problematic and often claustrophobic experience of CANCER – is brought to the practice of MINDFUL AWARENESS – which may develop into allowing the practitioner to have moments of glimpsing an open spacious experience of BEING fully present with whatever is there.

> You know that the flower bends when the wind wants it to, and you must become like that – that is, filled with deep trust. (Rilke, 1949)

The Middle Rings

Trauma – Intention – Appreciating the richness of experience

TRAUMA is triggered by an event or a series of events. It results in an inability to integrate thoughts and feelings with what has happened, and variously involves panic, shock, and intense aversion. Trauma is inevitably isolating and is invariably accompanied by intrusive memories that rekindle and re-stimulate strong emotions. The reaction of trauma when moving across to the Circle of Practice is offered the resolve, commitment and steadying inspiration of INTENTION – to practise in ways that support personal wellbeing, to stay with the course until the end, and to bring a kind heart to judgement and self blame. As practice deepens in the Circle of Presence, and the practitioner settles into herself, she sometimes opens quite naturally into APPRECIATING THE RICHNESS OF her EXPERIENCE.

> Suffering from a life threatening disease also helped me to have a different attitude and perspective. It has given me a new intensity to life, for I realize that there is much that I used to take for granted – the love and devotion of my wife Leah, the laughter and playfulness of my grandchildren, the glory of a

splendid sunset, the dedication of colleagues, the beauty of a dew coloured rose. I responded to the disease not morbidly, but with a greater appreciation of that which I might not see and experience again (Tutu, 1999).

Sheila kept seeing the look on her mother's face when she received her cancer diagnosis. By the end of her treatment, Sheila had become highly agitated. She was conscientious on the MBCT-Ca course, although she chose not to close her eyes during any of practices, for fear of remembering that expression of her mother's again. Over the weeks, her mindfulness practice developed and became an established part of her life. Her intention to practise and her commitment in doing this helped her feel a lot steadier. She also found it easier to get off to sleep. Some months after the end of the course, Sheila was continuing to practise most days for five or ten minutes. Her anxiety was still around at times, but she found she could usually breathe with it. She often felt great appreciation for being alive, and much love for her family. She enjoyed noticing the changing countryside and the mountains around her. This offered a new dimension to her life.

Rumination – Coming back – Experiencing the ground of clarity

When the mind starts to move into RUMINATION, the mood inevitably spirals downward, fuelled by judgement and self blame. The practice of pausing and COMING BACK to the direct experience of the breath in the body offers opportunity to step out of rumination, and step into the anchor of being present to what is happening now. Later as practice develops, the practitioner finds that at times she moves into what we call 'EXPERIENCING THE GROUND OF CLARITY', even if just for a moment. This is often accompanied by a strong physical sense of the body, grounded and stable – and a spacious clear awareness within the mind. This enables the practitioner to experience what is arising and dissolving, coming and going, 'held' in the space of awareness. Then, there may be a glimpse of knowing fear as just fear, or sadness as just a collection of sensations. In those moments, there is possibility of connecting with the very impermanent nature of experience. Grounded, spacious, and present with the immediacy of experience itself.

> Whenever our minds are completely open … our bodies and minds can sit still, in the heart of all suffering beings. That is all we have to do. Everything else will take care of itself … if I can let this body settle into itself, then it is empty and open … We have to experience and accept our share of suffering every day, and then it can drop away, leaving us ready to live. (Anderson, 2005)

David was quite depressed when he started his MBCT-Ca course. He blamed himself both for getting cancer and for feeling low. Although sceptical about the programme, he committed himself to the home practice. As the course progressed, he became intrigued by the workings of his mind. By the end, he came to value his mindfulness practice. Whenever he felt judging thoughts returning, or his mood dipping, he would stand in his garden in mountain posture, taking a breathing space. He liked to remember the phrases: 'weight going down, rooted – height going up, tall – standing with the dignity and presence of a mountain'. Sometimes, he had a tangible sense of feeling 'grounded', whilst at the same time very spacious and clear. Then, it was as if he had stepped out of the spiral of rumination, and into a clear sense of his experience simply coming and going, like the sounds around him or the breeze on his skin.

Avoidance – Turning Towards – Confidence in being with experience

AVOIDANCE is very common in all forms of suffering. It is an instinctive reaction in even the simplest of organisms, to turn away and pull back from what is painful or unwanted. Yet this directly maintains and even strengthens difficulty. TURNING TOWARDS what is not wanted with curiosity and interest, although counter intuitive, is how we can be with difficulty, though this requires considerable courage and practice. Eventually, even with tough challenges, we may find that we can be with what arises, breathing into it, giving it some air, holding it in wider awareness. When the practice has been tested and has been found to be dependable, then we can trust it. Over time, we develop CONFIDENCE in our mindfulness practice IN BEING WITH EXPERIENCE.

> It might be possible to deal with problems that seem to be insoluble without translating them into something you can already understand. Taking such a course would mean accepting and even embracing being in the dark ... When something precious is damaged, almost everyone tries at first to mend it. However, if you rely on the inconceivable, you cannot know what will happen ... (it) might give you your life and even unexpected joy (Tarrant, 2004).

When Jenny returned to work after treatment, she found she was often distressed and anxious. Anxiety tended to be a bit of a pattern in her family, evident in her father. Jenny tried to push her difficulties at work to the back of her mind, for her job was important to her – but things got worse. On the MBCT-Ca course, she learnt about the value of turning towards difficulty, cultivating curiosity about how the anxiety felt in her body. This helped her manage things at work and she felt a lot more settled by the end of the course and more able to cope with the everyday stresses of her job. She invested in her practice, and came to follow up sessions, whenever she felt the need. On returning home, after one of these sessions, she got a call from her mother. Her father was very ill in hospital and unlikely to survive the night. Jenny drove the two hour journey to Manchester and on arriving, found she was able to sit with her father and be really present to him, holding his hand and talking quietly to him. She was able to draw directly on her practice – in supporting her mother, comforting her father as he died, remaining centred and calm, and also compassionate, loving and grateful. She described a sense of peacefulness within the experience – and a confidence that all was ultimately well, despite the sadness of losing her father.

Distress – Kindness – Connecting to our common humanity

DISTRESS is a widespread reaction in those diagnosed with cancer, and those closely connected to them. As people with cancer come onto the course, they learn to practise KINDNESS towards their experience and themselves. This is a powerful practice and affects many of us profoundly – enabling us to open and soften to ourselves. Extending and developing this alongside others in the group, and taking it out into everyday life, we find we are more easily able to connect in compassion for them and their difficulties. We can feel for them too. CONNECTING TO OUR COMMON HUMANITY – *my* suffering becomes *the* suffering – no longer so personal and isolating, but ultimately something we all share and experience.

> The wisdom and compassion you most deeply yearn for will not be found outside of your body, mind, heart, or story but within them. Understanding their nature deeply, you come to understand the nature of all bodies, minds, and hearts. Learning to heal the sorrow and anguish within yourself, you learn the lessons of healing all sorrow and anguish. Learning to meet every moment of suffering and pain in your life with compassion and wisdom, you find the vastness of genuine compassion that embraces all suffering (Feldman, 2005).

Jo has an eighteen year old son, who has a rare and aggressive brain cancer. Frequent operations and medical crises have meant that he now needs 24 hour care. Jo came onto an MBCT-Ca course, as one of two carers in the group. In the orientation meeting, she spoke of feelings of intense pain 'deep down inside'. Her way of coping was to push the pain away, and keep very busy. Through her practice, she found an 'anchor' in her feet. (She had some difficulty being with the breath, as she associated it with her son's difficulty in breathing). Little by little, she learnt to come back to her feet on the ground, and this helped her feel steadier.

When given a thread (www.thoughtonathread.co.uk) to wear in week 4 on the course, and was told of others wearing the thread, some of whom are caring for their young who have Aids, she was heard to say quietly, 'I feel less alone'. After that, her two key practices involved coming back to her feet on the floor, and touching the bead on the thread and connecting in compassion with others like her. By knowing their suffering, she was more able to open in kindness to her own and allow her pain to be there.

The Outer Rings

A VICIOUS CIRCLE in ANXIOUS RUMINATION (Moorey and Greer, 2002) – our cognitive model of cancer distress – is mapped out into differentiated, and interconnecting layers of experience – PHYSICAL SENSATIONS, FEELINGS AND EMOTIONS, THOUGHTS, and Actions. When these move across to relate to the Circle of Presence, the different layers open and soften into more of an alignment between BODY, HEART and MIND.

Recurrence

Return to suffering

At times of crises, when a recurrence occurs or a period of difficulty arises, the practitioner with cancer may well move back to the first circle of suffering. However, there will be differences to the experience she had before she participated on the programme. She may be better able to recognize her personal reactivity for what it is. Her experience may still be very uncomfortable – perhaps even more intense than before – but there may be some possibility that she is aware of what is happening. This may be enough to move her to reconnect with her practice of mindful awareness – and reconnect with practices, long or short, that she may not have done for some time (such as Body Scan or Breathing Spaces). In taking this step, she is moving back into the circle of practice. Other helpful actions may follow – such as going back to her action plan, deciding to attend a follow up session or making contact with a fellow participant or teacher.

This will change the experience. Even when the difficulty is very intense, as long as there is still a link with the practice, with some remembering to come back to the breath and the body, then it may be possible to pause, notice and acknowledge what is happening, and thereby create a possibility of being with the intensity in a different and kinder way. Most of us revisit our suffering repeatedly, sometimes with intensity, sometimes with our own personal brand of dissatisfaction. Being with this *is* the practice of mindfulness.

For people with cancer, uncertainty is a given. Follow up appointments, aches and pains and traumatic memories all have the potential to bring difficulty to life. People with advanced disease have ongoing experience of loss, fear and anger. Those moving towards the end of their lives have much to be with. A daily practice does not make the practitioner immune from difficulty. However it makes being caught in difficulty and overwhelm less likely – and coming back more possible.

Compassion and Kindness

Many people with cancer experience 'existential' distress. It is as if the universe has turned against them. They wonder about the world, their future, and sense of self. For some, this involves a deep loss of trust in the world and can lead to immobilizing tightness that can twist and turn against the self. All too common questions arise such as 'Why me?' 'What did I do wrong?'

We end this chapter with what seems to us to be most important – both in relation to the practice and the teaching of this intervention – and also in relation to relieving the distress of people with cancer.

Through the course and the practices, the practitioner with cancer cultivates and connects with an intention to support her own wellbeing. She learns to come back, to be present, to step out of automatic reacting and return to her body and to awareness of the movements of her mind. Slowly, she learns to turn towards what is difficult, by exploring her physical experience of difficulty within the body with interest. Throughout, she learns to practise with kindness and tender compassion for herself.

The four movements in our model might appear to suggest that kindness comes last. This is not so – kindness is integral to them all and to the very heart of this programme. From the beginning intention for wellbeing has kindness at its heart. 'Coming back' and 'turning towards' need kindness as pivotal to these movements of mind. Kindness is like the colour on the palette – the warmth in the sun – the smile of the child. It is at the centre of our being – yet often buried out of sight. Through the practise of kindness, we remember how to love again.

The longing for love and the movement of love is underneath all of our activities. The happiness we discover in life is ... this capacity to love, to have a loving, free, and wise relationship with all of life. Such love ... arises out of a sense of our own well-being and connection with everything ... Out of love, our path can lead us to learn to use our gifts to heal and serve, to create peace around us, to honor the sacred in life, to bless whatever we encounter, and to wish all beings well (Kornfield, 1994).

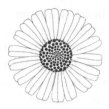

Personal Story

Geraint

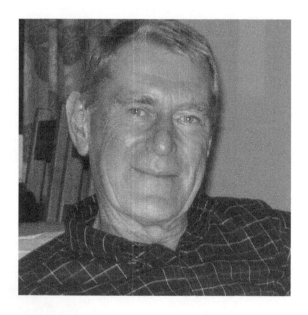

Mindfulness-Based Cognitive Therapy for Cancer: Gently Turning Towards,
First Edition. Trish Bartley.
© 2012 Trish Bartley. Published 2012 by John Wiley & Sons, Ltd.

Introduction

Geraint was in his early 60's when diagnosed with incurable oesophageal cancer in 2008, just before his retirement. He had a successful career as a vet, in private practice, and as a University academic and set up a practice in partnership with his wife Bridget, who is also a vet. Geraint was a keen sailor and hill walker. His two daughters have both received treatment for cancer. Geraint died on 3rd July 2010[1].

Diagnosis

'I suspected something for quite a few months before I was properly diagnosed. I had some symptoms and was pretty certain it was cancer. When I was told about it, it didn't really hit home for a few hours. The surgeon said that he had found a lump at the bottom of my oesophagus. He said we'd have to wait for the biopsies. My first reaction was basically 'oh damn – all the things I wanted to do'. We didn't know for the first few weeks whether they could remove it by surgery.

Then they did an ultrasound scan and discovered there was spread. I was told that surgery wasn't appropriate and I started on chemotherapy. Basically they gave me a year average, with the emphasis on that being average. One possible outcome might be that the tumour would disappear, but they said that this was very unlikely. So essentially within two weeks of diagnosis, I was told I had a year or so left.

It was shocking because I was retiring. In fact I started chemo on the first day of my retirement. All the things I'd mentally prepared myself to do, I couldn't do them. I couldn't go sailing. I couldn't finish the boat I'd been working on. I couldn't go hill walking again. I'd ill-prepared myself for a life of inactivity. I was going to be an active, striding up mountains, brown-legged septuagenarian. I was going to live to a ripe old age. Both my father and mother lived until 87. My grandfather died at 94. So I had high hopes of longevity.

Being a cancer patient

Once you've had cancer – you are a patient. It is almost a definition of you. This involves a giving away of independence. You become someone who travels back and forwards to institutions. Your life is defined by the disease.

[1] Interview recorded 9 September 2009.

The word cancer has some pretty bad connotations. There is still stigma. People don't recoil from you as they might have done 50 or so years ago – but there is still that sort of 'oh gosh you've got cancer'. It is almost like it might be catching. People's reactions are interesting.

I'm feeling quite weak these days. There are things I can't do now and probably will never be able to do again. It is a sort of sepia tint on your photograph. Your whole world is coloured by cancer.

Eventually, the whole thing begins to settle in your soul somehow. You accept the fact that you've got cancer – and that it is incurable. It begins to influence everything you do and everything you think about. This took several months to happen.

When a cancer diagnosis first happens, it is all very special and rather dramatic. Then time passes and you become just another patient. It is a bit like being possessed – it is always there. You wake up in the morning and think 'Gosh isn't it a lovely day – and then – 'Oh, I've got cancer'. Whether that is the same for cancer sufferers who have a realistic chance of cure, or long term remission, I don't know.

Chemotherapy

Once I moved onto chemo, I felt a bit more secure. Somebody was doing something. There was a certain rhythm of three-weekly cycles and three-weekly bouts of feeling like death. Even so, there seemed to be a purpose to it and this made me feel supported. The people I met were very nice. They seem to choose the chemo nurses for their kindness and their smiles. This was hugely important.

Mindfulness

Then when chemo stopped I felt quite vulnerable – like a lot of people do apparently. It was around about that time that J (specialist oncology counsellor) suggested that a mindfulness course might be helpful.

You look for all sorts of handholds to grab hold of. I asked whether Bridget would be able to join in. I thought if we did it together, we would have a joint reference point.

The 8 week course

Essentially I had no idea what I was letting myself in for. It came as a bit of a shock on that first day in February 2009, when we were given that raisin. I was sceptical – but then I was intrigued. It seemed such a trivial thing to do, but it obviously had quite enormous resonance, once you grasped the fact that eating the raisin is a metaphor for all sorts of things. After that, I began to look at it all with more interest.

The way in which the course developed was good. There was a lot of discipline involved and that was difficult for someone like me, who has always been an anti-disciplinarian. Bridget was a help and I suspect that if she had not been there, I wouldn't have done half so many practices. But we did a lot together. There were many weeks that we practised every day. It became almost an obligation to myself. If I didn't do it, I felt a bit of a gap as if something was missing.

Effects of the practice

Probably about half way along, I began to find that the practice had become a little supportive prop. It helped in the bad times, when we were fraught or scratchy with each other. Doing a practice seemed like a bit of a lifeline. It would be as if you were saying, 'Stop now. Let's start again'.

Recurrence and losing the practice

I was pretty sure even before I went to Turkey that I was having a recurrence but I was damned if I was going to miss out. Based on what they told me and on what I thought was happening, it was likely that it was going to be the last holiday and it will be.

We were doing our practices very regularly until I started radiotherapy in July (two month earlier) for about a month. Because it made me so nauseous – appallingly nauseous – they put me on all sorts of drugs. Some were ones which make you forget things. That put paid to my practice. I feel like I've lost 6 weeks of my life.

We have now just started again to try to practice. It is fascinating how difficult it is to get back to where we were. By the time I'd done choiceless awareness for a while, I could just conjure it up out of nothing. Thanks to radiotherapy, I seem to have lost the knack somehow and just can't practice like that anymore. I couldn't wait for choiceless awareness. Something expanded in my mind and there was this great big balloon of emptiness. It was actually quite fascinating. It stopped somewhere beyond my head but it was pleasurable. I don't think I was in control of it and I'd be quite disappointed when something interrupted it. It was an interesting phenomenon that I never imagined I could do.

The Future

I don't know what mindfulness will offer me from now on. I hope I can restart and keep up the discipline of the practice. I hope it may do the same as before – flatten out the excesses of emotion. Depending on what they find on the next scan, I may go in for another session of chemotherapy. Whether that will allow me to carry on with meditation, or whether I will be feeling too yucky to do it – I'm not sure. In some ways I miss it.

One of the things about the practice is to let whatever thoughts come into your mind, be there. I'm worried about opening my mind and finding all these thoughts will flood in. I'm hoping that mindfulness practice will be another thing that I can just hold onto – a bit of ritual in life – that will calm me down and keep me from the excesses of these thoughts.

Looking Beyond

Basically death is an absence of me. I've no religious feeling about it all. But I'm not an atheist. I don't think I have any worries about dying. It is the leaving behind. It is the absence of everything. I don't think death frightens me but it is huge regret for everything that is left behind.

You certainly exist in memories, don't you? You leave ripples in the pond – it would be nice if you did exist a bit … It is interesting how you can forget about these things. You can push them away for a bit, and then suddenly if you are made to face them, a whole new world opens up – of possibilities. Yes, we don't know, do we? It might be the biggest mystery of them all. It might be the biggest adventure or voyage that you have ever had – yes – let's hope so'.

Buffalo

Still they come, my thoughts
Trampling like a herd of buffalo
Through the green prairie of my mind
Leaving their black footprints in the smooth pasture

But I am Mountain Man
They do not scare me now
And I watch them moving by
With no more than passing interest

Geraint (April, 2009)

Epilogue

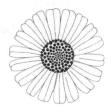

Maybe at root our minds are not so separate.

(Rigdzin Shikpo, 1992)

As I reflect on this ending, those of you planning to start teaching mindfulness to people with cancer may be focused on your beginnings. Every ending is a beginning. Those of you new to mindfulness may be considering starting your own mindfulness journey. As teachers, the ending of each group heralds the beginning of recruiting the next. Some beginnings may be more memorable than others. Most of us who teach probably remember our first mindfulness groups – wondering now, how they got anything from the experience!

Fortunately our skill and experience as teachers grows with time, given the right conditions. A plant needs light, nourishment, water and warmth. What do we need to develop and grow as teachers or practitioners? Opening to uncertainty seems to be an essential ingredient.

> The process of learning and deepening that is connected to our practice encourages us to realise how much we do not know (Feldman, 2008).

So as I pause at the end of this book, to reflect on the development of this programme, I become aware of all the many networks and interconnections

---

that have fed into it. An interesting mix of personal and professional comes into view. And when tracing the connections, it becomes apparent that the haphazard way they came together would be impossible to plan or organize.

The context

We start in Alaw, the oncology unit in Ysbyty Gwynedd Hospital. Dr. Huw Parry and Sister Beryl Roberts attended an eight week course at Bangor University in 1999, connected to the first MBCT for Depression trial. I was receiving my first chemotherapy treatment in the Unit. Due to their enthusiasm, a course for Alaw staff was organized the following year, taught by Becca Crane, (herself teaching on the first MBCT trial at that time) and supported by me. This directly laid the foundations for the development of MBCT-Ca courses for patients on the Unit.

Since then, Professor Nick Stuart, a senior oncologist in the Alaw Unit and contributing author of a chapter in this book, has picked up the role of championing mindfulness. Without his support, the courses would never have thrived. When asked recently why he has supported them so consistently – he unhesitatingly replied that he believes in mindfulness. 'The evidence base for MBCT-Ca is still to come, but I think it works', he said.

From Alaw, we move to all the people who have attended courses, who have directly added to the knowledge and experience gained over these eleven years. They have been generous in agreeing to allow their learning to be shared, through videos, writing, interviews, feedback, questionnaires, poems and many other ways. Whenever asked, they always affirm that they are willing to do anything that might help others. This is a noble practice.

Mindfulness developments

The development of MBCT for Depression through the work of John Teasdale, Mark Williams and Zindel Segal has of course been a major inspiration and guiding influence to MBCT-Ca. This has played out at a number of levels. Firstly the courses themselves are drawn directly from and adapted out of the original MBCT for Depression programme. The material that we use in our workbooks, and some key processes, approaches and practices, such as the Breathing Spaces, come from MBCT and 'The Green Book' (Segal et al., 2002).

At another level, two of the three founders of MBCT have given significant support to the Alaw courses. In the early days, Mark Williams offered encouragement and guidance, as the courses were getting off the ground. Without this, I doubt they would have started. His advice was clear and wise, 'Stick to the MBCT for Depression programme (removing the direct depression material), until you are clear that you know what are doing and what needs changing, and why and how'. His advice was sound and I followed it. It was some years before I made any major adaptations to the programme.

John Teasdale has been a very significant influence and support to me personally and the Alaw courses directly. From the early days on the 1999 Bardsey retreat, I was intrigued by the mix of John's brilliant and sharp mind and deeply compassionate heart. Finding the courage to ask if he would supervise me in 2003, I now look back on the years of our connection, in which John has been a true guide through rocky times and balmy. He has become a dear friend and wise counsel, for whom I have the greatest respect. The foundation of MBCT-Ca is the stronger for his wisdom and kindness.

The final layer of the MBCT influence comes out of the connections to the original trial, which involved Bangor, Cambridge and Toronto. I was lucky enough to have just moved to North Wales, near Bangor, and was invited on the Bardsey retreat, met the international MBCT 'cast', and was included in the mindfulness teacher developing process that followed.

The MBCT story and its close interconnection with MBSR has a direct bearing on all of this. Jon Kabat-Zinn has been incredibly generous in the way he has supported and taught us all. I count him as one of my closest teachers, and continue to be profoundly inspired by his heart commitment to this work.

The Centre for Mindfulness Research and Practice (CMRP)

At the same time that courses were starting for Alaw cancer patients, a group of us were coming together to form what was to become the Centre for Mindfulness, Research and Practice (CMRP). Mark Williams, as our founding director, tasked us to develop a centre which would train mindfulness teachers. Centre for Mindfulness teachers from the US helped us a great deal, especially Jon Kabat-Zinn, Ferris Urbanowski, Melissa Blacker, Pam Erdman, Saki Santorelli and Elana Rosenbaum.

The business of learning, practising, teaching and eventually training together has enriched both the development of CMRP and also our individual and shared development as mindfulness teachers. Working with students on the masters programme, supervisees and teachers in training has extended this further. The Alaw courses have directly benefitted from this process.

On another level, the Bangor teaching colleagues have offered their own clear contributions. Through co-leading courses and offering feedback, and finding time to reflect and discuss issues, my peers have offered their ongoing encouragement and inspiration, which has supported the way that these oncology mindfulness courses have matured. Cindy Cooper, Jody Mardula, Mariel Jones and Becca Crane have been especially significant within this process.

Psycho-oncology and mindfulness – an Irish/Welsh collaboration

A fruitful and significant collaboration began with Ursula Bates in 2007. At the time, she was working as a psycho-oncologist in a Dublin hospital. She later moved to work at Blackrock hospice, as head of psychological and bereavement services. After being invited by her to lead a practice day in Dublin for cancer patients and professionals, we started sharing ideas about mindfulness-based approaches with people with cancer. At the time, neither of us was in touch with anyone else working in the field. We shared a genuine concern at the levels of sadness, anxiety and anger that people with cancer were holding. Whilst we had great respect for the commitment and skill of our medical colleagues, and the progress being made in the treatment of cancer – we both felt that the medical system radically underestimates the subjective distress of a cancer diagnosis and treatment.

From 2007, we started taking it in turns to catch the Dublin to Holyhead ferry to spend weekends together to develop our ideas. When it was my turn to go to Ireland, Ursula would walk me round Dublin, showing me her favourite haunts, while we thrashed out ideas around psychological and mindfulness issues for people with cancer. We were searching for common ground, each coming from our different perspectives and backgrounds. Our discussions were very stimulating and by the end of the weekend, I would return to the peace of my mountain, tired but happy, with pages of notes to write up in preparation for this book, which was beginning to take shape.

It was on one of these weekends in 2008, that the genesis of our three circle MBCT-Ca model took form. We saw straight away that this had the potential for clarifying much of what we had been discussing. Although it has evolved over time, the finished model is easily recognizable from the sketches we drew on Ursula's kitchen table.

She has offered much in developing my theoretical understanding of the psychological challenges for people with cancer. She has lent her support to my work in a number of ways. Not only has she written her own chapter on mindfulness and palliative care, but she has been directly instrumental in two other chapters, her shared one with Stirling Moorey, and within the last chapter where the three circle model comes together. Our connection has facilitated many of the ideas and developments described here. It is in reality 'our' book. I have written most of it, but Ursula's influence has been very significant.

Dharma colleagues

In 1998/99, I spent some months in a monastery in Nepal. On moving to Wales on my return, I began looking for a teacher. I looked first in London. However, soon after buying a mountain house on Pen Llŷn overlooking the Irish Sea and Cardigan Bay, I was told about teachers who had a centre only five miles away. In due course, I met Rigdzin Shikpo and have been fortunate in being connected to him and his teaching since then. This has offered me much inspiration and I am immensely grateful to him. Others have also been significant – notably Andrew Patching, who has been my meditation instructor for many years.

Overview

This book was delayed when I received treatment for cancer in 2010. At the time, it was a great disappointment not to be able to get it finished and depart for South Africa. I now see that in many ways, my illness has supported this work – both in offering me a clear teaching about ways of being with treatment and difficulty – but also in giving me the gift of time and practice to develop the writing a bit further.

Looking back on all of this, I am inspired and moved by all the contributions that the course participants themselves have made. I always hoped that their voice would be significant, but their personal stories, poems, anecdotes and experiences form the heart of this book. Their journeys are the thread that holds the text together. We open to inspiration from many sources, especially from those we teach.

Out of the network of our interconnectedness, may kindness, awareness and awakening grow.

I Believe In All That Has Never Yet Been Spoken

I believe in all that has never yet been spoken.
I want to free what waits within me
so that what no one has dared to wish for
may for once spring clear
without my contriving.

If this is arrogant, forgive me,
but this is what I need to say.

May what I do flow from me like a river,
no forcing and no holding back,
the way it is with children.

Then in these swelling and ebbing currents,
these deepening tides moving out, returning,
I will sing you as no one ever has,
streaming through widening channels
into the open sea.

R M Rilke (1996)

Resources and Links

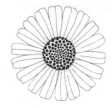

Resources

Centre for Mindfulness Research and Practice (CMRP)
School of Psychology, Bangor University, Dean Street Building,
Bangor, UK. LL57 1UT
+44 (0)1248 382939

www.bangor.ac.uk/mindfulness – *CMRP offers mindfulness-based teacher training through a range of Continuing Professional Development courses (including eight week distance learning courses) and through part-time Masters and post-graduate programmes in mindfulness-based approaches / teaching.*

Centre for Mindfulness in Medicine, Health Care and Society, (CFM)
55 Lake Avenue North , Worcester, Massachusetts, 01655, US.
+ 1 508-856-2656

www.umassmed.edu/cfm - *CFM has pioneered the integration of mindfulness meditation and other mindfulness-based approaches in mainstream medicine and healthcare through patient care, research, academic medical and professional education.*

Mindfulness-Based Cognitive Therapy for Cancer: Gently Turning Towards,
First Edition. Trish Bartley.
© 2012 Trish Bartley. Published 2012 by John Wiley & Sons, Ltd.

Web Links

www.mbct.co.uk *website provides information about Mindfulness-Based Cognitive Therapy.*

www.bemindful.co.uk *is a UK campaign, by the Mental Health Foundation, raising awareness about the benefits of mindfulness*

www.mbct.com *Mindfulness Based Cognitive Therapy (North America) – offers information on books, founders, research and workshops.*

www.oxfordmindfulness.org *was founded to promote the well-being of people in their world of work, home and family life.*

www.gaiahouse.co.uk *Gaia House in Devon, UK offers insight meditation retreats.*

http://health.groups.yahoo.com/group/MBSR-MBCT_ANZ/ *Australia and New Zealand network provides information on mindfulness practitioners plus information about local training courses, retreat and research articles.*

Materials

www.trishbartley.co.uk – including practice CDs for MBCT-Ca course participants.

mindfulnesscds@trishbartley.co.uk to order:

- CD 1 Body Scan (30) and Sitting Practice (30);
- CD 2 Mindful Movement (30) Mindful Walking (20);
- CD 3 Short Practices including Sitting Practice (15) The Physical Barometer (5), 3 minute Breathing Space; Extended Breathing Space (Responding) (10); and Bells (20)

www.stressreductiontapes.com – Tapes and CDs recorded by Jon Kabat-Zinn

www.bangor.ac.uk/mindfulness – Practice CDs recorded by CMRP teachers

www.octc.co.uk – Practice CDs recorded by Mark Williams

www.thoughtonathread.co.uk – for information on obtaining simple black cotton bracelets with red beads on – used in week 4 of MBCT-Ca as aide-memoires to 'come back' to the present moment.

Bibliography

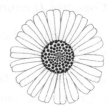

Allen, D. (2002). *Myth and religion in mircea eliade*. New York: Routledge.

Anderson, R. (1995). *Warm smiles from cold mountains: Dharma talks on zen meditation*. Berkeley: Rodmell Press.

Andrykowski, M.A., & Kangas, M. (2010). Posttraumatic stress disorder associated with cancer diagnosis and treatment. In J.C. Holland, W.S. Breitbart, P.B. Jacobsen, M.S. Ledernerg, M.J. Loscalzo, & R. McCorkle (Eds.), *Psycho-oncology* (2nd ed, pp. 348–357). New York: Oxford University Press.

Andrykowski, M.A., Brady, M.J., & Hunt, J.W. (1993). Positive psychosocial adjustment in potential bone marrow transplant recipients: Cancer as a psychological transition. *Psycho-oncology*, 2, 261–276.

Arrow, H., Henry, K.B., Poole, M.S., Wheelan, S.A., & Moreland, R.L. (2005). Traces, trajectories, and timing: The temporal perspective on groups. In M.S. Poole, & A.B. Hollingshead (Eds.), *Theories of small groups: Interdisciplinary perspectives*. Thousand Oaks, California: Sage.

Bachelaed, G. (1994). *The poetics of space*. Boston, Massachusetts: Beacon Press.

Baer, R.A. (Ed). (2006). *Mindfulness-based treatment approaches: Clinician's guide to evidence base and applications*. Burlington, Massachusetts: Elsevier.

Bartley, T. (2003). *Holding up the sky: Love power and learning in the development of a community*. London: Community Links.

Bech, P., Gudex, C., & Staehr Johansen, K. (1996). *The WHO (Ten) well-being index: Validation in diabetes*. Psychother Psychosom, 65, 183–190.

Bell, S. (1998). Self-reflection and vulnerability in action research: Bringing forth new worlds in our learning. *Systemic Practiceand Action Research*, 11(2), 179–191.

Berne, E. (1963). *The structure and dynamics of organizations and groups*. New York: Grove Press.

Bion, W. (1961). *Experiences in groups*. London: Tavistock.

Boorstein, S. (1995). *It's easier than you think: The buddhist way to happiness*. New York: HarperCollins.

Brach, T. (2003). *Radical acceptance: Embracing your life with the heart of the Buddha*. New York: Bantam Books.

Breitbart, W., Bruera, E., Chochinov, H., & Lynch, M. (1995). Neuropsychiatric syndromes and psychological symptoms in patients with advanced cancer. *Journal of Pain and Symptom Management, 10*, 131–141.

Brennan, J. (2001). Adjustment to cancer – coping or personal transformation? *Psycho-Oncology, 10*, 1–18.

Buber, M. (1958). *I and Thou* (Translation: R. Gregory Smith) (2nd ed). Edinburgh: T. & T. Clark.

Buber, M. (1973) *Meetings*. (Translated by M. Friedman). La Salle, Illinois: Open Court Publishing.

Burgess, C., Cornelius, V., Love, S., Graham, J., Richards, M., Ramirez, A. (2005). Depression and anxiety in women with early breast cancer: Five year observational cohort study. *British Medical Journal, 330*, 702–707.

Carlson, L.E. (2010). Meditation and yoga. In J.C. Holland, W.S. Breitbart, P.B. Jacobsen, M.S. Lederberg, M.J. Loscalzo, & R. McCorkle (Eds.), *Psycho-oncology* (2nd ed.). Oxford: Oxford University Press.

Carlson, L.E., & Speca, M. (2010). *Mindfulness-based cancer recovery: A step by step MBSR approach to help you cope with treatment & reclaim your life*. Oakland: New Harbinger Publications.

Carlson, L.E., Speca, M., Patel, K.D., & Faris, P. (2007). One year pre-post intervention follow up of psychological, immune, endocrine and blood pressure outcomes of mindfulness-based stress reduction (MBSR) in breast and prostate cancer out patients. *Brain, Behaviour and Immunity, 21*, 1038–1049.

Carlson, L.E., Ursuliak, Z., Goodey, E., Angen, M, & Speca, M. (2001). The effects of a mindfulness meditation-based stress reduction program on mood and symptoms of stress in cancer outpatients: Six month follow up. *Supportive Care in Cancer, 9*, 112–123.

Chah, A., (2004) *A still forest pool*. Adyar, India: Quest Books.

Chödrön, P. (1997). *When things fall apart: Heart advice for difficult times*. Boston & London: Shambhala Publications.

Clarkson, P. (1991). Group imago and the stages of group development. *Transactional Analysis Journal, 21*(1), 36–50.

Confucius. (1979). *The Analects* (Translated by A. Waley) London: Penguin Classics.

Cordova, M.J., Cunningham, L.L., Carlson, C.R., & Andrykowski, M.A. (2001). Post-traumatic growth following breast cancer: A controlled comparison study. *Health Psychology, 20*(3), 176–185.

Coyne, J.C., Lepore, S.J., & Palmer, S.C. (2006). Efficacy of psychosocial interventions in cancer care: Evidence is weaker than it first looks. *Annals of Behavioral Medicine, 32*, 104–110.

Crane, R. (2009). *Mindfulness-based cognitive therapy: Distinctive features*. London and New York: Routledge.

Crane, R.S., Kuyken, W., Hastings, R.P., Rothwell, N., & Williams, J.M.G. (2010). Training teachers to deliver mindfulness-based interventions: Learning from the UK experience. *Mindfulness, 1*, 74–86.

Derogatis, L.R., Morrow, G.R., & Fetting, J. (1983). The prevalence of psychiatric disorders among cancer patients. *Journal of American Medical Association, 249*, 751–757.

Didonna, F. (Ed.). (2009). *Clinical handbook of mindfulness*. New York: Springer Science and Business Media.

Edgar, L., Rosberger, Z., & Nowlis, D. (1992). Coping with cancer during the first year after diagnosis: assessment and intervention. *Cancer, 69*, 817–828.

Feldman, C. (2005). *Compassion: Listening to the cries of the world*. Berkeley, California: Rodmell Press.

Feldman, C. (2008). From a talk at a mindfulness-based teachers retreat at Gregynog Hall, Powys, Wales organised by the Centre for Mindfulness Research and Practice, Bangor University, UK.

Feldman, C. (2001). *The Buddhist Path to Simplicity: Spiritual Practice for Everyday Life*. London: Thorsons.

Ferlay, J., Shin, H.R., Bray, F., et al. (2010). Estiminates of worldwide burden of cancer in 2008: Globocan 2008. *International Journal of Cancer, 127*(12), 2893.

Foley, E., Baillie, A., Huxter, M., Price, M., & Sinclair, E. (2010). Mindfulness-based cognitive therapy for individuals whose lives have been affected by Cancer: A randomised controlled trial. *Journal of Consulting and Clinical Psychology, 78*(1), 72–79.

Frankl, V.E. (1959). *Man's search for meaning: An introduction to logotherapy*. New York: Simon & Schuster.

Freire, P. (1972). *Pedagogy of the oppressed*, Harmondsworth: Penguin.

Friedrich, R. (Ed). (1961). *The Frontiers of Medicine*. New York: Liveright Publishing Corp.

Galileo, G. (1564–1642) http://www.quotationspage.com/quotes/Galileo_Galilei/

Garland, C. (1998). *Understanding trauma: A psychoanalytical approach*. London: Duckworth.

Gibran, K. (1926). *The Prophet*. London: Heinemann.

Goldberg, N. (1986). *Writing down the bones: Freeing the writer within*. Boston: Shambhala Publications.

Goldstein, J. (2002). *ONE dharma: The emerging western buddhism*. San Francisco: HarperCollins.

Greer, S. (1985). Cancer: Psychiatric Aspects. In Granville Grossman, K. (Ed.). *Recent advances in clinical psychiatry*. Edinburgh: Churchill-Livingstone.

Greer, S., Moorey, S., Baruch, J.D., Watson, M., Robertson, B.M., Mason, A., et al. (1992). Adjuvant psychological therapy for patients with cancer: a prospective randomized. *British Medical Journal, 304*, 675–680.

Groves, R. (2005). *The american book of dying*. Berkeley, California: Celestial Arts.

Hayes, S.C., Strosahl, K., & Wilson, K.G. (1999). *Acceptance and commitment therapy*. New York: Guilford Press.

Helgeson, V.S., Reynolds, K.A., & Tonlich, P.L. (2006). A meta-analytic review of benefit finding and growth. *Journal of Consulting and Clinical Psychology, 74*, 797–816.

Hoffman, C. (Personal communication). MBSR doctoral research study.

Hookham, M. (1985). *On freeing the heart: A series of transcribed talks*. Oxford: Longchen Foundation.

Hookham, S. (1999). *Discovering the heart of buddhism*. Coursebook Four: Sensitivity and Mandala. Shrimala Trust (www.ahs.org.uk).

Hough, A. (2007). (Personal communication) In mindfulness based teacher training process. KwaZulu Natal, South Africa.

Ingram, L.C. (2005). (Unpublished) *A qualitative evaluation of mindfulness-based cognitive therapy for oncology outpatients*, MSc dissertation. Bath, UK: University of Bath.

Jeffs, T., & Smith, M.K. (1996). *Informal education. Conversation, democracy and learning*, Ticknall: Education Now.

Jeffs, T., & Smith, M.K. (2005). *Informal education. Conversation, democracy and learning*, Ticknall: Education Now.

Johnson, D.W., & Johnson, F.P. (2003). *Joining together. Group theory and group skills*. Boston: Allyn and Bacon.

Journal of Clinical Oncology, 20(14), 3137–3148.

Kaasa, S., Malt, U., Hagen, S., Wist, E., Moum, T., & Kvikstad, A. (1992). Psychological distress in cancer patients with advanced disease. *Radiotherapy and Oncology, 27*(3), 193–197.

Kabat-Zinn, J. (1990). *Full catastrophe living: Using the wisdom if your body and mind to face stress, pain and illness*. New York: Delta.

Kabat-Zinn, J. (1994). *Wherever you go, there you are: Mindfulness meditation in everyday life*. New York: Hyperion.

Kabat-Zinn, J. (2000). Indra's net at work: The mainstreaming of Dharma practice in society. In G. Watson, S. Batchelor, & G. Claxton (Eds.), *The psychology of awakening: Buddhism, science, and our day-to-day lives*. York Beach, Maine: Samuel Weiscr.

Kaplan, A. (1996). *The development practitioner's handbook*. London: Pluto Press.

Kelly, B., Raphael B., Smithers M., Swanson C., Reid C., McLeod R., et al. (1995). Psychological responses to malignant melanoma. An investigation of traumatic stress reactions to life-threatening illness. *General Hospital Psychiatry, 17*, 126–136.

Kenny, M.A., & Williams, J.M.G. (2007). Treatment-resistant depressed patients show a good response to Mindfulness-based cognitive therapy. *Behaviour Research & Therapy, 45*, 617–625.

Khyentse, D., & Sangye, P. (2006). *The hundred verses of advice: Tibetan buddhist teachings on what matters most*. Boston & London: Shambhala.

Kingston, T., Collier, C., Hevey, D., et al. (Submitted). Mindfulness-based cognitive therapy for psycho-oncology patients: A randomised control trial.

Kissane, D.W., Grabsch, B., Love, A., Clarke, D.M., Bloch, S., & Smith, G.C. (2004). Psychiatric disorder in women with early stage and advanced breast cancer: A comparative analysis. *Australian and New Zealand Journal of Psychiatry, 38*, 320–326.

Kolb, D.A. (1984). *Experiential learning experience as a source of learning and development*. New Jersey: Prentice Hall.

Kornblith, A.B., & Ligibel, J.A. (2003). Psychosocial and sexual adaptation of women with breast cancer. *Seminars in Oncology, 30,* 799–813.

Kornfield, J. (1993). *A path with heart.* New York: Bantam Books.

Kornfield, J. (1994). *Buddha's little instruction book.* London: Rider.

Kornfield, J. (2008). *The wise heart: Buddhist psychology for the west.* New York: Random House.

Kramer, G. (2007). *Insight dialogue: The interpersonal path to freedom.* Boston & London: Shambhala.

Kuyken, W., Byford, S., Taylor, R.S., Watkins, E.R., Holden, E.R., White, K., et al. (2008). Mindfulness-based cognitive therapy to prevent relapse in recurrent depression, *Journal of Consulting and Clinical Psychology, 76,* 966–978.

Kuyken, W., Watkins, E., Holden, E.., White, K., Taylor, et al. (2010). How does mindfulness-based cognitive therapy work? *Behaviour Research and Therapy, 48*(11), 1105–1112.

Lawrence-Lightfoot, S. (2000). *Respect: An exploration.* Cambridge, Massachusetts: Perseus Books.

Leach, C. (1981). *Letters to a younger son.* London: J.M. Dent & Sons, Ltd.

Ledesma, D., & Kumano, H. (2009). Mindfulness-based stress reduction and cancer: a meta-analysis. *Psycho-Oncology, 18,* 571–579.

Lee, L-Y. (1986). *Rose.* New York: BOA Editions.

Lepore, S.J., & Coyne, J.C. (2006). Psychological interventions for distress in cancer patients: a review of reviews. *Annals of Behavioural Medicine, 32*(2), 85–92.

Levine, S. (1987). *Healing into Life and Death.* Bath: Gateway Books.

Lewin, K. (1951). *Field theory in social science.* New York: Harper Collins.

Lewis, G. (2002). *Sunbathing in the rain: A cheerful book about depression.* London: Flamingo.

Linehan, M.M. (1993a). *Cognitive-behavioural treatment of borderline personality disorder.* New York: Guilford Press.

Linehan, M.M. (1993b). *Skills training manual for treating borderline personality disorder.* New York: Guilford Press.

Ma, S.H., & Teasdale, J.D. (2004). Mindfulness-based cognitive therapy for depression. Replication and exploration or differential relapse prevention effects. *Journal of Consulting and Clinical Psychology, 72,* 31–40.

Mackenzie, M.J., Carlson, L.E., & Speca, M. (2005). Mindfulness-based stress reduction (MBSR) in oncology: Rationale and review. *Evidence-based Integrative Medicine, 2,* 139–145.

Macmillan. (2006). *Worried sick – the emotional impact of cancer.* Macmillan Cancer Support.

Mardula, J. (2008). *The external and internal group boundaries* Centre for Mindfulness Research and Practice, Bangor University.

Massie, M.J. (2004). Prevalence of depression in patients with cancer. *Journal of the National Cancer Institute Monographs, 32,* 57–71.

Massie, M.J., & Holland, J.C. (1992). The cancer patient with pain: psychiatric complications and their management. *Journal of Pain and Symptom Management, 7,* 99–109.

Mc Bee, L. (2008). *Mindfulness-based elder care*. New York: Springer.

McCown, D., Reibel, D., & Micozzi, M.S. (2010). *Teaching mindfulness: A practical guide for clinicians and educators*. New York: Springer Science and Business Media.

Moorey, S. (2007). Breast cancer and body image. In M. Nasser, K. Baistow, J. Treasure (Eds.), *The female body in mind: The interface between the female body and mental health*. New York: Routledge.

Moorey, S. (2010). The six cycles maintenance model: Growing a 'vicious flower' for depression. *Behavioural and Cognitive Psychotherapy, 38*(2), 173–184.

Moorey, S., & Greer, S. (2002). *Cognitive behaviour therapy for people with cancer*. Oxford: Oxford University Press.

Moorey, S. (2010). Cognitive Therapy. In J.C. Holland, W.S. Breitbart, P.B. Jacobsen, et al. (Eds.). *Handbook of Psycho-oncology* (pp. 402–407). Oxford: Oxford University Press.

Moorey, S., Greer, S., Bliss, J., & Law, M. (1998). A comparison of adjuvant psychosocial therapy and supporting counseling in patients with cancer. *Psycho-Oncology, 7*, 218–228.

Moorey, S., Greer, S., Watson, C., Gorman, L., Rowden, R., Tunmore, R., Greer, L., et al. (1994). Adjunctive psychological therapy for patients with cancer: Outcome at one year. *Psycho-Oncology, 3*, 39–46.

Moyers, B.D., & Grubin, D. (Directors). (1993). *Healing and the Mind*. (DVD). New York, New York: David Grubin Productions.

Mundy, P., Delgado, C., Block, J., Venezia, M., Hogan, A., & Seibert J. (2003). A manual for the abridged early social communication scales (ESCS). Retrieved from: http://www.ucdmc.ucdavis.edu/mindinstitute/ourteam/faculty_staff/ESCS.pdf.

National Cancer Institute. (2009). *Depression*. Retrieved from: http://www.cancer.gov/cancertopics/pdq/supportivecare/depression/Patient/page2.

National Institute for Health and Clinical Excellence (NICE) (October 2009). *Depression: The treatment and management of depression in adults (partial update of clinical guideline 23) Clinical guideline 90*. (1.9.1.8 & 1.9.1.10).

Neff, K. (2003). *Self-Compassion: An alternative conceptualization of a Health Attitude towards Oneself. Self and Identity* (pp. 285–101). Psychology Press.

Nelson, P. (1994). *There's a hole in my sidewalk: the romance of self discovery*. Hillsboro: Beyond Words Publishing.

Newell, S.A., Sanson-Fisher, R.W., & Savolainen, N.J. (2002). Systematic review of psychological therapies for cancer patients: Overview and recommendations for future research. *Journal of the National Cancer Institute, 94*(8), 558–584.

Nhat Hanh, T. (1988). *The sun my heart*. Berkeley, California: Parallax Press.

Noyes, R., Holt, C.S., & Massie, M.J. (1998). Anxiety disorders. In J.C. Holland (Ed.), *Psycho-oncology* (pp. 548–559). New York: Oxford University Press.

Nye, N.S. (1994). *Words under the words: Selected poems* (A far corner book). The Eighth Mountain Press.

Oliver, M. (1992). *New and selected poems*. Boston: Beacon Press

Ott, M.J., Norris, R.L., & Bauer-Wu, S.M. (2006). Mindfulness meditation for oncology patients: A discussion and critical review. *Integrative Cancer Therapies, 5*(2), 98–106.

Palmer, Parker. J. (1998). *The courage to teach. Exploring the inner landscape of a teacher's life*, San Francisco: Jossey-Bass.

Palmer, S.C., Kagee, A., Coyne, J.C., & DeMichele, A. (2004). Experience of trauma, distress, and posttraumatic stress disorder among breast cancer patients. *Psychosomatic Medicine, 66*, 258–264.

Passik, S.D., Dugan, W., McDonald, M.V., Rosenfeld, B., Theobald, D.E., & Edgerton, S. (1998). Oncologists' recognition of depression in their patients with cancer. *Journal of Clinical Oncology, 16*, 1594–1600.

Pitcaethly, C., Maguire, P. (2003). The Psychological impact of cancer on patients' partners and other key relatives: a review. *European Journal of Cancer, 39*(11), 1517–1524.

Potter, D. (1994). *Without Walls*. Channel 4 television (UK).

Pugh, S. (1990). *Sometimes* from *selected poems*. Bridgend: Seren Books.

Raes, F., Pommier, E., Neff, K.D., & Van Gucht, D. (in press). Construction and factorial validation of a short form of the Self-Compassion Scale. *Clinical Psychology & Psychotherapy*.

Remen, R.N. (1996). *Kitchen table wisdom*. New York: Riverhead Books.

Remen, R.N. (2000). *My grandfather's blessings: stories of strength, refuge and belonging*. New York: Riverhead Books.

Ricard, M. (2003). *Happines: A guide to developing life's most important Skill*. New York: Little, Brown and Co.

Ries, L.A.G., Eisner, M.P., Kosary, C.L., Hankey, B.F., Miller, B.A., Clegg L., et al. (Eds) (2004). *SEER Cancer Statistics Review, 1975–2001*. National Cancer Institute. Bethesda MD. Retrieved from: http://seer.cancer.gov/csr/1975_2000/.

Rilke, R.M. (1934). *Letters to a young poet*. Trans. by Herter Norton, M.D. New York: W.W. Norton.

Rilke, R.M. (1949). *The notebooks of Malte Laurids Brigge* (Trans. by M.D. Herter Norton). New York: W.W. Norton.

Rilke, R.M. (1996). *Rike's book of hours: Love poems to God* (Trans by Barrows, A. & Macy, J.). New York: Riverhead.

Rinpoche, S. (1992). *The Tibetan Book of Living and Dying*. London: Rider.

Roemer, L., & Orsillo, S.M. (2002). Expanding our conceptualization of and treatment for generalized anxiety disorder: Integrating mindfulness/acceptance-based approaches with existing cognitive-behavioural models. *Clinical Psychology: Science and Practice, 9*, 54–68.

Rosenberg, L., & Guy, D. (1998). *Breath by breath: The liberating practice of insight meditation*. Boston: Shambhala.

Rosenfeld, B., Breitbart, W., Krivo, S., & Chochinov, H. M. (2000). Suicide, assisted suicide, and euthanasia in the terminally ill. In H. M. Chochinov, & W. Breitbart (Eds.), *Handbook of psychiatry in palliative medicine* (pp. 51–62). New York: Oxford University Press.

Rumi, J.B. (1995). *The essential Rumi* (Translated by Barks, C., & Moyne, J.). London and New York: Penguin Books.

Sage, N., Sowden, M., Chorlton, E., & Edeleanu, A. (2008). *CBT for chronic illness and palliative care: A workbook and toolkit*. Oxford: Wiley Blackwell.

Saint-Exupery de, A. (2009). *The little prince* (Translated by Katherine Woods). London: Egmont.

Salzberg, S. (1995). *Loving kindness: The revolutionary art of happiness*. Boston: Shambhala.

Santorelli, S. (1999). *Heal thyself: Lessons on mindfulness in medicine*. New York: Bell Tower.

Santorelli, S. (2010) http://mindful.org/mindfulness-practice/meditation-in-action/practice-befriending-self.

Saunders, C. (1965). Watch with me. *Nursing Times, 61*(48), 1615–1617.

Savard, J., Simard, S., Giguère, I., Ivers, H., Morin, C.M., Maunsell, E., Gagnon, P., Robert, J., & Marceau, D. (2006). Randomized clinical trial on cognitive therapy for depression in women with metastatic breast cancer: psychological and immunological effects. *Palliative and Supportive Cure, 4*, 219–237.

Schneiderman, N., Antoni, M.H., Saab, P.G., & Ironson, G. (2001). Health psychology: Psychosocial and bio-behavioral aspects of chronic disease management. *Annual Review of Psychology, 52*, 555–580.

Searles, H.F. (1955). The informal value of the supervisor's emotional experiences. *Psychiatry, 18*, 135–146.

Segal, Z.V., Williams, J.M.G., & Teasdale, J.D. (2002). *Mindfulness-based cognitive therapy for depression: A new approach to preventing relapse*. New York: Guilford Press.

Sen, J. (1996). *Healing Foods Cookbook: of the Bristol Cancer Help Centre*. London: Thorsons.

Shantideva. (1997). *The Bodhicharyavatara* (Translated by Hookham, S.) Oxford: Longchen Foundation.

Shapiro, S., Carlson, L., Astin, J., & Freedman, B. (2006). Mechanisms of Mindfulness. *Journal of Clinical Psychology, 62*(3), 373–386.

Shapiro, S.L., & Carlson, L.E. (2009). *The art and science of mindfulness: Integrating mindfulness into psychology and the helping professions*. Washington: American Psychological Association.

Shennan, C., Payne, S., & Fenlon, D. (2010). What is the evidence for the use of mindfulness-based interventions in cancer care? A review. *Psycho-Oncology* DOI: 10.1002/pon.1819.

Shikpo, R. (1992), *Openness, Clarity and Sensitivity*. Oxford: Longchen Foundation.

Shikpo, R. (2003) Public teaching Oxford, UK.

Shikpo, R. (2005) The highest maha ati teachings: Chögyam Trungpa in Great Britain. In F. Midal, *Recalling Chögyam Trungpa*. Boston: Shambhala Publications.

Shikpo, R. (2007). *Never turn away: The buddhist path beyond hope and fear*. Boston: Wisdom Publications.

Shikpo, R. (2007). Public teaching Oxford Town Hall, UK.

Shunryo, S. (1973). *Zen mind, beginner's mind*. New York and Tokyo: Weatherhill.

Singh, N.N. (2010). Mindfulness: A Finger Pointing to the Moon. *Mindfulness, 1*, 1–3.

Smith, J.E., Richardson, J., Hoffman, C., & Pilkington, K. (2005). Mindfulness-Based Stress Reduction ass supportive therapy in cancer care: systematic review. *Journal of Advanced Nursing, 52*(3), 315–327.

Söllner, W., DeVries, A., Steixner, E., Lukas, P., Sprinzl, G., et al. (2001). How successful are oncologists in identifying patient distress, perceived social support, and need for psychosocial counselling? *Br J Cancer, 84*(2), 179–185.

Soulsby, J.G., Morrison, V., Bartley, T., Stuart, N.S.A, Parry, D.H., & Williams, J.M.G. (2006). (Unpublished). *Evaluation of mindfulness-based cognitive therapy for oncology and haematology outpatients.* Unpublished Report to Funders : The North Wales Research Committee.

Speca, M., Carlson, L.E., Goodey, E., & Angen, M. (2000). A randomised, wait-list controlled clinical trial: The effect of a mindfulness meditation-based stress reduction program on mood and symptoms of stress in cancer outpatients. *Psychosomatic Medicine, 62,* 613–622.

Speca, M., Carlson, L.E., Goodey, E., & Angen, M. (2006). Mindfulness-Based Stress Reduction (MBSR) as an Intervention for Cancer Patients. In Baer, R.A. (Ed.), *Mindfulness-based treatment approaches: Clinician's guide to evidence base and applications.* Burlington, Massachusetts: Elsevier.

Stark, D., Kiely, M., Smith, A, Velikova, G., House, A., & Selby, P. (2002). Anxiety Disorders in Cancer Patients: Their Nature, Associations, and Relation to Quality of Life.

Talbot, A. (1990). The importance of Parallel Process in Debriefing Crisis Counsellors. *Journal of Traumatic Stress, 3,* 265–277.

Tarrant, J. (2004). *Bring me the rhinoceros: And other zen koans that will save your life.* Boston and London: Shambhala.

Tarrant, J. (1998) *The light inside the dark: Zen, soul, and the spiritual life.* New York: HarperCollins.

Teasdale, J.D. (2006). Mindfulness-Based Cognitive Therapy for depression. In D.K. Nauriyal, M.S. Drummond & Y.B Lal (Eds.). *Buddhist thought and applied psychological research: Transcending the boundaries.* London: Routledge Curzon.

Teasdale, J.D. (2008). from a talk at a mindfulness-based teachers retreat at Gregynog Hall, Powys, Wales organised by the Centre for Mindfulness Research and Practice, Bangor University, UK.

Teasdale, J.D., Segal, Z.V., Williams, J.M.G., Ridgeway, V.A., Soulsby, J.M., & Lau, M.A. (2000). Prevention of relapse/recurrence in major depression by mindfulness-based cognitive therapy, *Journal of Consulting and Clinical Psychology, 68,* 615–623.

Thomas, R.S. (1993). *Collected Poems 1945–1990.* London: Orion Books.

Trungpa, C. (1981). *Journey with goal: The tantric wisdom of the Buddha.* Boston & London: Shambhala.

Trungpa, C. (1984). *Shambhala: The sacred path of the warrior.* Boston & London: Shambhala.

Trungpa, C. (1991). *The heart of the Buddha.* Boston & London: Shambhala.

Trungpa, C. (1995). *The path is the goal: A basic handbook of buddhist meditation.* Boston & London: Shambhala.

Trungpa, C. (2004). *Shambhala warrior slogans: 53 principles for living life with fearlessness and gentleness*. Boston & London: Shambhala.

Tuckman, B.W. (1965). Developmental sequence in small groups. *Psychological Bulletin, 63*, 384–399.

Tutu, D. (2000). *No future without forgiveness: A personal overview of South Africa's truth and reconciliation commission*. London: Rider.

Walshe, T. (1998). *Favourite poems we learnt at school*. Cork: The Mercier Press.

Watson, M., Law, M., dos Santos, M., Greer, S., Baruch, J., & Bliss, J. (1994). The mini-MAC: Further development of the mental adjustment to cancer scale. *Journal of Psychosocial Oncology, 1* (3), 33–46.

Weisman, A.D., Worden, J.W. (1976). The existential plight in cancer: significance of the first 100 days. *International Journal of Psychiatry in Medicine, 7*, 1–15.

Whitaker, D.S. (2001). *Using groups to help people*. Philadelphia: Taylor & Francis Inc.

Wilde, O. (2001). (Originally published in 1893). *An Ideal Husband*. Dover Publications Inc.

Willcox, B.J., Willcox, D.C, & Suzuki, M. (2001). *The Okinawa programme*. New York: Three Rivers Press.

Williams, J.M.G., Duggan, D., Crane, C., & Fennell, M.J.V. (2006). Mindfulness-based cognitive therapy for prevention of recurrence of suicidal behaviour. *Journal of Clinical Psychology, 62*, 201–210.

Williams, J.M.G., Teasdale, J.D., Segal, Z.V., & Kabat-Zinn, J. (2007). *The mindful way through depression: Freeing yourself from chronic unhappiness*. New York: Guilford Press.

Williams, M. & Penman, D., (2011) *Mindfulness: a practical guide to finding peace in a frantic world*. London: Piatkus.

Wilson, K.G., Chochinov, H.M., Skirko, M, Allard, P., Chary, S., Gagnon, P.R., et al. (2007). Depression and anxiety disorders in palliative cancer care. *Journal of Pain Symptom Management, 33*(2), 118–129.

World Health Organization. (2005). *WHO cancer control programme*.

World Health Organization. (2007). *The World Health Organization's fight against cancer: Strategies that prevent, cure and care*.

World Health Organization. (2001). *Occupational health: A manual for primary health care workers*. Cairo: Regional Office for the Eastern Mediterranean, World Health Organization.

Wurtzen, H., Elsass, P., Sumbundu, A., Flyger, H., & Johansen, C. (2008). Mindfulness-based stress reduction (MBSR): preliminary results of an RCT of MBSR intervention amongst Danish women diagnosed with breast cancer. *Psycho-Oncology, 17*, S276–277.

Yalom, I.D. (1995). *The theory and practice of group psychotherapy*. New York: Basic Books.

Yalom, I.D., & Graves, C. (1977). Group therapy with the terminally ill. *Am J Psychiatry, 13*(4), 396–400.

Zabora, J., BrintzenhofeSzoc, K., Curbow, B., Hooker, C., & Piantadosi, S. (2001). The prevalence of psychological distress by cancer site. *Psycho-Oncology, 10*, 19–28.

Sources and Permissions

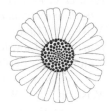

'A Vicious Cycle of Anxious Preoccupation' – a cognitive model developed by
  Stirling Moorey and Stephen Greer in *Cognitive Behaviour Therapy for People
  with Cancer* (Oxford University Press 2002) copyright © Moorey & Greer.
  Reproduced with permission, pp. 20, 26, 131, 148, 361.
'From Blossoms' and 'The Gift' by Li-Young Lee from *Rose* (BOA editions 1986)
  copyright © Li-Young Lee . Reproduced with permission, p. 22.
'Ich Glaube an Alles noch nie Gesagte' by Rainer Maria Rilke translated by Anita
  Barrows and Joanna Macy from *Rilke's Book of Hours: Love Poems to God*
  (Riverhead Books, an imprint of Penguin Group (USA) Inc., 1996) copyright ©
  Anita Barrows and Joanna Macy. Reproduced with permission, pp. 74, 82, 88,
  157, 158, 167, 168, 176, 202, 216, 223, 228, 299, 310, 314, 316, 340, 357, 375.
'The Other' by R.S.Thomas from *Collected Poems 1945-1990* by R.S.Thomas (Orion
  Books 1993) copyright © R.S.Thomas . Reproduced with permission, p. 19.

Previously unpublished poems:

'Grounded in the Earth, the Body, and the Heart' by kind permission of Peter
  Milligan, p. 317.
'The Raku Bowl', 'So Many Things to Tell You' and 'Grief is an Open Door' by
  kind permission of Jill Teague, p. 32.
'The Rush Hour' by kind permission of Pauline Kenyon, p. 90.
'The Thickening Stillness' and 'Letting Go' by kind permission of Stewart Mercer,
  pp. 268, 353.

Participants' poems reproduced with their kind permission:

'Buffalo' by Geraint, p. 369.
'Friends' by Liddy, p. 242.
'Got up Mindfully this Morning' by Ruth, p. 71.
'I just want to Live' by Helen, p. 42.
'Mooring in the here and now' by Ann, p. 110.
'My Late Night Visitor' by Liz, p. 214.
'My Journey' by Beryl, p. 52.
'What If' by Jane, p. 282.
'Who would have thought?' by Katie, p. 129.
'Who would like to ring the bells?' by Bridget, p. 339.

Other poems by the author

Subject Index

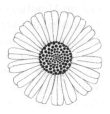

Printed and bound by CPI Group (UK) Ltd, Croydon, CR0 4YY

27/10/2024

14580296-0004